Seeking out SDGs in Dialysis Medicine—Selected Articles from the JSDT Conference, Yokohama 2022

Seeking out SDGs in Dialysis Medicine—Selected Articles from the JSDT Conference, Yokohama 2022

Editors

Ken Tsuchiya
Norio Hanafusa

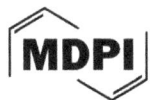

Basel • Beijing • Wuhan • Barcelona • Belgrade • Novi Sad • Cluj • Manchester

Editors

Ken Tsuchiya
Tokyo Women's Medical University
Tokyo
Japan

Norio Hanafusa
Tokyo Women's Medical University
Tokyo
Japan

Editorial Office
MDPI
St. Alban-Anlage 66
4052 Basel, Switzerland

This is a reprint of articles from the Special Issue published online in the open access journal *Kidney and Dialysis* (ISSN) (available at: https://www.mdpi.com/journal/kidneydial/special_issues/2022_JSDT_Conference).

For citation purposes, cite each article independently as indicated on the article page online and as indicated below:

Lastname, A.A.; Lastname, B.B. Article Title. *Journal Name* **Year**, *Volume Number*, Page Range.

ISBN 978-3-7258-1315-5 (Hbk)
ISBN 978-3-7258-1316-2 (PDF)
doi.org/10.3390/books978-3-7258-1316-2

© 2024 by the authors. Articles in this book are Open Access and distributed under the Creative Commons Attribution (CC BY) license. The book as a whole is distributed by MDPI under the terms and conditions of the Creative Commons Attribution-NonCommercial-NoDerivs (CC BY-NC-ND) license.

Contents

Ken Tsuchiya
Seeking out SDGs in Dialysis Medicine—Selected Articles from the JSDT Conference, Yokohama 2022
Reprinted from: *Kidney Dial.* 2022, 2, 296–297, doi:10.3390/kidneydial2020028 1

Joel D. Kopple and Maryam Ekramzadeh
Renal Nutrition—Where It Has Been and Where It Is Going
Reprinted from: *Kidney Dial.* 2022, 2, 512–533, doi:10.3390/kidneydial2040046 3

Raymond Vanholder
Green Nephrology
Reprinted from: *Kidney Dial.* 2022, 2, 454–458, doi:10.3390/kidneydial2030041 25

Shu Wakino
Trace Elements and Their Management in Dialysis Patients—Pathophysiology and Clinical Manifestations
Reprinted from: *Kidney Dial.* 2023, 3, 274–296, doi:10.3390/kidneydial3030025 30

Kosaku Nitta, Norio Hanafusa, Kenichi Akiyama, Yuki Kawaguchi and Ken Tsuchiya
Chronic Kidney Disease—Mineral and Bone Disorder (CKD-MBD), from Bench to Bedside
Reprinted from: *Kidney Dial.* 2023, 3, 46–55, doi:10.3390/kidneydial3010004 53

Katsuhito Mori, Masafumi Kurajoh, Masaaki Inaba and Masanori Emoto
Multifaceted Nutritional Disorders in Elderly Patients Undergoing Dialysis
Reprinted from: *Kidney Dial.* 2022, 3, 1–23, doi:10.3390/kidneydial3010001 63

Ryota Matsuzawa and Daisuke Kakita
Renal Rehabilitation—Its Theory and Clinical Application to Patients Undergoing Daily Dialysis Therapy
Reprinted from: *Kidney Dial.* 2022, 2, 565–575, doi:10.3390/kidneydial2040051 86

Masanori Abe, Tomomi Matsuoka, Shunsuke Kawamoto, Kota Miyasato and Hiroki Kobayashi
Toward Revision of the 'Best Practice for Diabetic Patients on Hemodialysis 2012'
Reprinted from: *Kidney Dial.* 2022, 2, 495–511, doi:10.3390/kidneydial2040045 97

Kenji Nakata and Nobuhiko Joki
Non-Ischemic Myocardial Fibrosis in End-Stage Kidney Disease Patients: A New Perspective
Reprinted from: *Kidney Dial.* 2023, 3, 311–321, doi:10.3390/kidneydial3030027 114

Yukie Kitajima
How Can We Improve the Appetite of Older Patients on Dialysis in Japan?
Reprinted from: *Kidney Dial.* 2024, 4, 105–115, doi:10.3390/kidneydial4020008 125

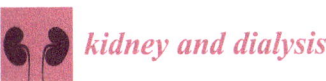 kidney and dialysis

Editorial

Seeking out SDGs in Dialysis Medicine—Selected Articles from the JSDT Conference, Yokohama 2022

Ken Tsuchiya

Department of Blood Purification, Tokyo Women's Medical University, Tokyo 162-8666, Japan; tsuchiya@twmu.ac.jp

Citation: Tsuchiya, K. Seeking out SDGs in Dialysis Medicine—Selected Articles from the JSDT Conference, Yokohama 2022. *Kidney Dial.* 2022, 2, 296–297. https://doi.org/10.3390/kidneydial2020028

Received: 31 May 2022
Accepted: 1 June 2022
Published: 2 June 2022

Publisher's Note: MDPI stays neutral with regard to jurisdictional claims in published maps and institutional affiliations.

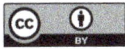

Copyright: © 2022 by the author. Licensee MDPI, Basel, Switzerland. This article is an open access article distributed under the terms and conditions of the Creative Commons Attribution (CC BY) license (https:// creativecommons.org/licenses/by/ 4.0/).

The 67th Annual Meeting of the Japanese Society for Dialysis Therapy (JSDT) was held in Yokohama City from 1 to 3 July, 2022 [1] and took as its theme 'Seeking Sustainable Development Goals for Dialysis Medicine.' The JSDT was founded in 1968 as the Dialysis Research Association and comprises some 18,000 members [2].

The Annual Meetings of the JSDT have always focused on dialysis medicine per se, but their scope is now expanding to encompass modality selection for renal replacement therapy. Since last year, cases of patients who have 'withdrawn' from dialysis have become a social issue, and the publication of a formal guide for palliative care in renal failure patients, which is essential for patients who have withdrawn from dialysis therapy, was published in 2021. The objectives of the dialysis medicine should include not only the quality of dialysis therapy but also the selection of dialysis modality, renal failure complications, the aging of the patient population, healthcare economics, thanatology, multidisciplinary team medicine, and community healthcare.

Rapid changes in society, healthcare economics and dialysis medicine present us with new challenges and opportunities, hence the relevance of the concept of the Sustainable Development Goals to our specific field.

The Sustainable Development Goals (SDGs) are a fundamental part of the 2030 Agenda for Sustainable Development. Adopted by all United Nations Member States in 2015, the 2030 Agenda for Sustainable Development provides a 'shared blueprint for peace and prosperity for people and the planet, now and into the future' [3]. The SDGs, 17 in number, are recognized by all UN Member States and apply to everyone, for the benefit of everyone.

Working together as a medical discipline to better serve our patients' needs will involve maintaining some of our tried and tested approaches, while at the same time embracing new concepts, technologies, and methodologies. The object of our own 'SDGs' must be to articulate the totality of this need and present it in a framework that is simple, accessible, memorable, and actionable.

What should we agree are our key goals? How should these be defined and measured? How should they be worded to be concise, clear and unequivocal? How many goals should we have, how many subordinate goals should each contain, and what is the timeline for achieving them? These are the key questions that the 67th Annual Meeting of JSDT in Yokohama City sought to address.

This Special Issue presents a selection of the papers presented at the conference. They discuss cardiovascular complication, renal anemia, CKD–MBD, diabetes and nutrition, frailty and sarcopenia, rehabilitation, and environmental issues. It is our hope that the papers collected in this Special Issue will take us a significant step closer to finding the answers. The Guest Editors would like to express their gratitude to all the authors who have contributed to this Special Issue.

Conflicts of Interest: The author declares no conflict of interest.

References

1. The 67th Annual Meeting of the Japanese Society for Dialysis Therapy. Available online: http://www.congre.co.jp/jsdt2022/eng/index.html (accessed on 17 May 2022).
2. The Japanese Society for Dialysis Therapy. Available online: https://www.jsdt.or.jp/english/ (accessed on 17 May 2022).
3. THE 17 GOALS. Available online: https://sdgs.un.org/goals (accessed on 17 May 2022).

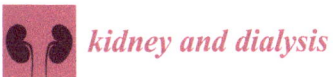

Editorial

Renal Nutrition—Where It Has Been and Where It Is Going [†]

Joel D. Kopple [1,2,3,*] **and Maryam Ekramzadeh** [1]

[1] Division of Nephrology and Hypertension, The Lundquist Institute, Harbor-UCLA Medical Center, Torrance, CA 90502, USA
[2] David Geffen School of Medicine, University of California, Los Angeles, CA 90095, USA
[3] Fielding School of Public Health, University of California, Los Angeles, CA 90095, USA
* Correspondence: jkopple@lundquist.org; Tel.: +1-310-968-5668
[†] Presented, in part, at the 67th Annual Meeting of the Japanese Society of Dialysis Therapy, Yokohama, Japan, 1–3 July 2022.

Abstract: This paper is a synopsis of an invited lecture entitled, The Future of Renal Nutrition, that was presented at the Japanese Society of Dialysis Therapy, July 2022. The purpose of this presentation is to suggest some of the advances in the field of renal nutrition that the authors think are likely to occur during the next several years. There will be continued development of methods for precisely diagnosing and classifying protein-energy wasting and developing methods to treat this disorder. Why weight loss commonly occurs when the GFR decreases to about 30–35 mL/min/1.73 m^2 and why substantial weight loss (>5%/year) is associated with increased mortality will be investigated. Clinical consequences of the interactions between gut microbiota, nutrient intake and other environmental influences will continue to be examined. The clinical value of diets high in fruits and vegetables or other plants for chronic kidney disease (CKD) patients will continue to be studied. Our knowledge of how different diets and medicines affect intestinal absorption, metabolism and excretion of nutrients will expand. Precision medicine will be extended to precision nutrition. There will be more focus on the effects of nutritional disorders and dietary treatment on the emotional status and quality of life of people with kidney disease and their families. Nutritional centers that provide centralized nutritional assessment and dietary counselling for CKD patients may develop in more urban centers. More clinical trials will be conducted to test whether nutritional management improves clinical outcomes in people with kidney disease. It is hoped that the foregoing comments will encourage more research on these topics.

Keywords: diet; nutrition; kidney disease; gut microbiota; precision medicine; protein-energy wasting; weight loss

1. Introduction

My task in this presentation is to predict future development in the field of renal nutrition. This is, at best, a hazardous exercise, as it is impossible to guess what new discoveries and novel ways of thinking may alter the direction of this field, which might be occurring even as this paper is being written. Intellectual history is rife with examples of how predictions regarding the future course of science and medicine have been erroneous, not uncommonly egregiously so. Nonetheless, since this is our assignment, we will, with humility and with the recognition that, at the least, some of our speculations are certain to be wrong, try to describe some of the future directions of this field. This paper will briefly describe the recent history of renal nutrition. We will then speculate as to what developments may occur in the near future. This paper will end by describing some of the more distant developments that possibly may occur in this discipline. Our hope is that these speculations may emphasize some of the areas in renal nutrition of great need of advancement and possibly stimulate some of the younger scientists and leaders in this field to solve some of the challenges that lie before us.

2. The History of Renal Nutrition Since the 19th Century Encompasses Several Periods

Since the 19th century, two different views have been advanced regarding the potential benefits of dietary treatment for people with chronic kidney disease (CKD) [1]. 1. Protection of the health and function of the diseased kidney. 2. Preservation or improvement of the overall health of the patient. For over 100 years, the thinking of workers in this field has often fluctuated widely between these two potential goals. Particular attention was initially focused on reduction in the quantity of protein and modification of the type of protein in the diet. From at least the last part of the 19th century until about the "teens" of the 20th century, dietary protein restriction was recommended to protect the kidney, primarily from what was considered to be overwork. It was thought that in people with kidney disease, a higher protein intake, by increasing the generation of urea which is excreted by the kidney, will increase the work of the diseased kidney and may thereby further injure the kidney. It is now understood, of course, that renal urea excretion requires little or no energy expenditure by the kidney [1].

From about the "teens" of the 1900s until the very late 1940s, low protein diets (LPDs) were still recommended to protect the diseased kidney from more rapid progression of kidney failure. However, unlike in rodents, some studies did not show that LPDs slowed progression in humans. In the 1950s, LPDs (about 40 g protein/day) and control of mineral intake (primarily sodium and potassium) were primarily recommended to maintain metabolically and clinically healthier patients with CKD [1].

In the 1960s, with the advent of chronic dialysis therapy and renal transplantation, the focus of renal nutrition changed to maintaining a healthy metabolic and nutritional status in advanced CKD patients with the use of protein, sodium and potassium restriction and provision of adequate calories. Recommended protein restriction by different renal nutrition workers was sometimes about 40 g per day and sometimes about 20 g per day (viz., the Giovannetti-Giordano Diet) [2–6]. It was contended that such diets could reduce symptoms and maintain advanced CKD patients in much healthier and asymptomatic states. Thus, if CKD patients eventually needed dialysis or transplantation, they would be physically better prepared for these treatments.

In the late 1960s and early 1970s, it became apparent that the 20 g protein/day diet provided inadequate amounts of protein [7,8]. Three alternatives to dietary protein restriction were developed, each of which was shown to be nutritionally adequate:

i. A low protein diet (LPD) providing about 0.55–0.60 g protein/kg/day diet (~40 g protein/day) [7,8].
ii. A very low protein diet (VLPD) providing about 20 g protein/day diet supplemented with about 16–20 g/day of essential amino acids (EAA). It was referred to as a EAA supplemented VLPD (SVLPD) [9–11].
iii. A VLPD providing about 20 g protein/day diet supplemented with about 16–20 g/day of a mixture of ketoacid and hydroxyacid analogues (KAs) of some EAA plus other EAA; this was called a KA supplemented VLPD (SVLPD) [12,13].

Shortly thereafter, Walser observed that KA SVLPDs seemed to slow the rate of progression of kidney failure [13]. Walser's observations precipitated a firestorm of clinical trials. Some, but not all, studies reported slowing of progressive CKD with the ketoacid SVLPD. These studies led, in turn, to the United States NIH-funded large scale MDRD Study [14]. The results of the MDRD Study were ambiguous, in part because of several inadvertent flaws that were incorporated into the design of the study [14,15]. Since the MDRD study, other clinical trials examined whether LPDs or SVLPDs can retard progression of CKD. Several of these trials showed effectiveness of SVLPDs in slowing progression [16–19]. A confounding factor is that certain medicines given to CKD patients may mimic some of the physiologic effects of LPDs on glomerular hemodynamics (e.g., angiotensin converting enzyme inhibition or blockade, or the use of sodium-glucose cotransporter-2 (SGLT2) inhibitors), thus making it more difficult to assess the independent effects of LPDs or SVLPDs on progression of CKD.

There were other advances concerning the nutritional management of renal disease that developed concurrently with the clinical trials of LPDs and SVLPDs for nondialyzed

CKD patients. These advances included greater understanding and more effective treatments of the nutritional, physiological and metabolic processes concerning:

i. Patients with acute kidney injury (AKI)
ii. Maintenance hemodialysis (MHD) patients
iii. Chronic peritoneal dialysis (CPD) patients
iv. Kidney transplant recipients
v. Children with CKD
vi. Macrominerals, especially sodium, potassium and phosphorus, in kidney disease
vii. Vitamins and trace elements, especially iron, in kidney disease
viii. Furthermore, developed during this time was the description of the syndrome of protein-energy wasting (PEW) in CKD [20]
ix. Identification of the relationships between PEW, inflammation and adverse clinical outcomes.

Precision Nutrition

Precision nutrition is based upon precision medicine and is an approach to nutritional assessment, care and research that is designed for individual patients or subgroups of patients, instead of a one-treatment-fits-all model [21]. Precision nutrition attempts to involve the complex set of factors that comprise an individual, including the person's genotype, phenotype, psychodynamics, psychosocial and economic status and past and anticipated future life experiences, among other items. Precision nutrition can be considered a general goal of renal nutrition research and also of the nutritional management of people with or at increased risk for developing kidney disease [22].

3. The Future of Renal Nutrition—The Immediate Future

3.1. Role of New Medicines That Modify Nutrient Biochemistry or Physiology

What may lie ahead in the immediate future regarding renal nutrition? Perhaps the following: Medicines that modify the intestinal absorption, urinary excretion or metabolism of nutrients will continue to be developed. The development of such pharmaceuticals has already been underway for over one century. These medicines include diuretics, intestinal binders of phosphate and potassium, HMG Coenzyme A inhibitors (statins), medicines that simulate (or replicate) the action of LPDs on glomerular hemodynamics (e.g., ACE inhibition or blockade, SGLT2 inhibitors), and purified vitamins or analogs of such vitamins as pyridoxine HCl, folate, cholecalciferol, and calcitriol (1,25-dihydroxycholecalciferol), which may have slightly different and more clinically desirable characteristics.

3.2. Reexamination of the Classification and Diagnostic Criteria for Protein-Energy Wasting (PEW) in Kidney Disease

The rationale for this reexamination is that PEW is a powerful risk factor for mortality [23–25]. As we have learned more about PEW syndrome, the classification of PEW and the current diagnostic criteria for PEW have turned out to be somewhat inadequate. There appears to be a need for more highly developed criteria. This process for more precise classification and diagnostic criteria is being conducted right now. It is led by Professor Denis Fouque and Dr. Laetitia Koppe from Lyon, France.

3.3. Examination of Why CKD Patients Often Lose Weight When the GFR Decreases to about 25–32 mL/min/1.73 m^2, and Why a Large Weight Loss Is Associated with Increased Mortality?

The majority of CKD patients appear to lose edema-free weight as they approach end-stage kidney disease (ESKD) [26]. These latter patients not uncommonly have at least some mild signs or symptoms of uremia and may have anorexia from uremic toxicity. Accumulation of uremic toxins may contribute to this weight loss. Figure 1 indicates the results of a cross-sectional evaluation of the relationship between true GFR and body mass in 1760 CKD patients undergoing screening for the MDRD Study [26]. The solid lines indicate men, and the broken lines indicate women. When the GFR, determined by ^{125}I-iothalamate clearances, reaches about 30–35 mL/min/1.73 m², body weight, expressed either directly or as a percentage of the standardized weight of normal people of the same sex, age range, height and frame size as the patients, often begins to decrease or starts to decrease at a more rapid rate. The same findings are observed when body weight is expressed as a percentage of previous body weight or body mass index. Dietary protein intake began to decline, particularly in men but also in women, around a GFR of 30–35 mL/min/1.73 m². This decline was also observed for dietary energy intake at about this GFR level in men and at a somewhat lower GFR level in women [26]. Also many pediatric and adult CKD patients lose weight when their GFR decreases to about 30–35 mL/min/1.73 m² (Figures 2 and 3) [27,28].

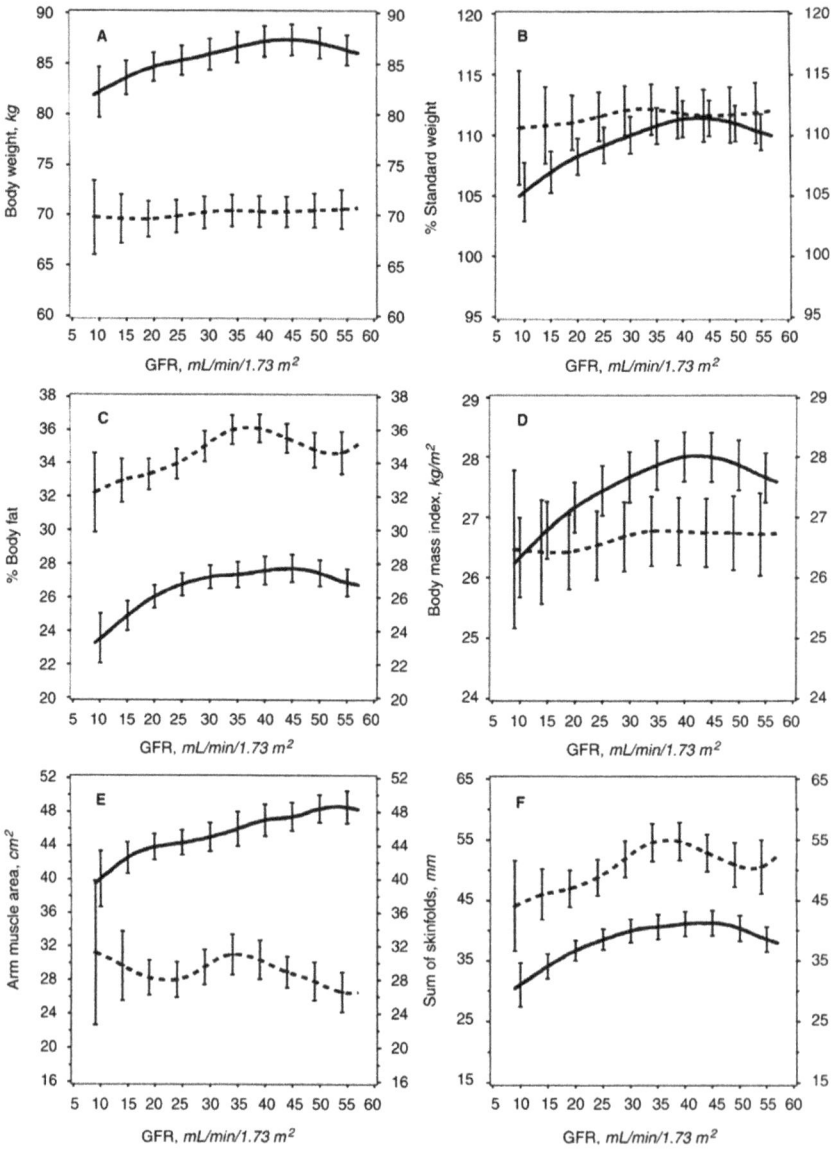

Figure 1. Mean levels of some anthropometric measures of nutritional status as a function of GFR.

The estimated mean levels with 95% confidence limits of anthropometric measures of nutritional status are shown as a function of GFR (males, solid line; females, dashed line) controlling for age, race and use of protein and energy restricted diets. (**A**) Males, $N = 1077$ ($p = 0.009$); females, $N = 702$ ($p = 0.61$). (**B**) Males, $N = 1077$ ($p < 0.001$); females, $N = 702$ ($p = 0.62$). (**C**) Males, $N = 649$ ($p < 0.001$); females, $N = 414$ ($p = 0.057$). (**D**) Males, $N = 1069$ ($p = 0.002$); females, $N = 701$ ($p = 0.67$). (**E**) Males, $N = 695$ ($p < 0.001$); females, $N = 435$ ($p = 0.26$). (**F**) Males, $N = 648$ ($p < 0.001$); females, $N = 410$ ($p = 0.11$). Reprinted from Kidney International, Vol. 57, J. D. Kopple et.al., Relationship between nutritional status and the glomerular filtration rate: results from the MDRD study, Pages 1688–1703, Copyright (2000), with permission from International Society of Nephrology [26].

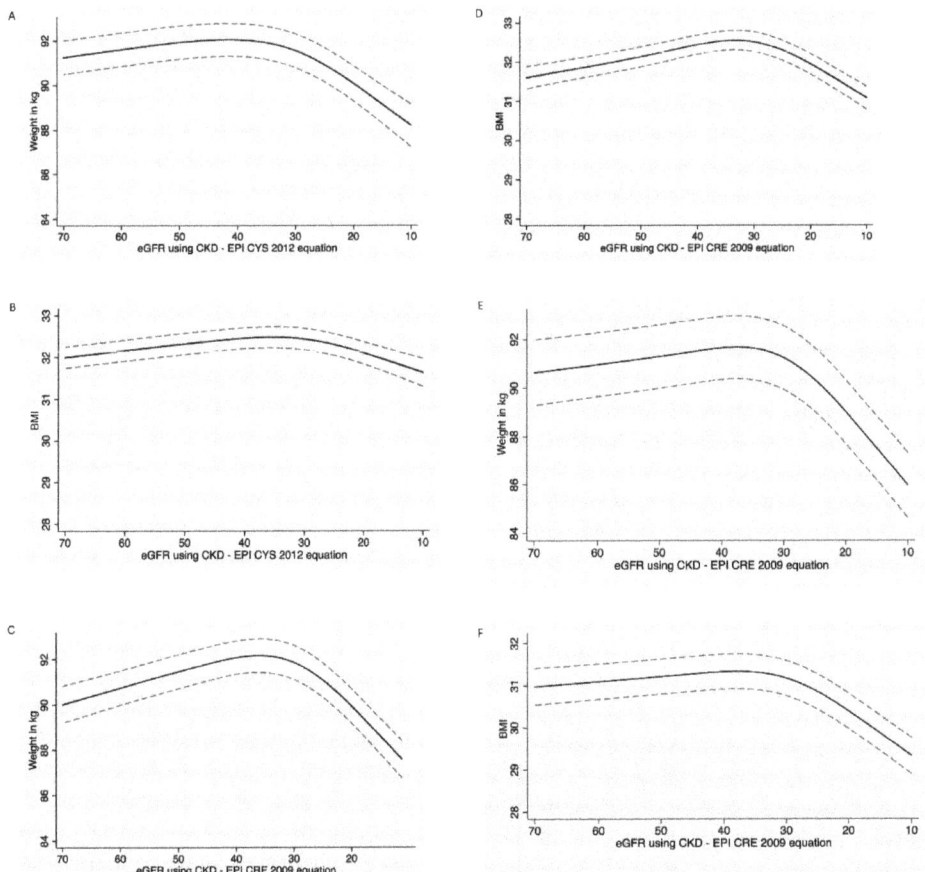

Figure 2. Repeated measures of weight and body mass index with advancing CKD. (**A**) Longitudinal repeated measures of weight with repeated measures of eGFR by cystatin C in CRIC. (**B**) Longitudinal repeated measures of BMI with repeated measures of eGFR by cystatin C in CRIC. (**C**) Longitudinal repeated measures of weight with repeated measures of eGFR by creatinine in CRIC. (**D**) Longitudinal repeated measures of BMI with repeated measures of eGFR by creatinine in CRIC. (**E**) Longitudinal repeated measures of weight with repeated measures of eGFR by creatinine in AASK. (**F**) Longitudinal repeated measures of BMI with repeated measures of eGFR by creatinine in AASK. Reprinted from Am J Kidney Dis., Vol. 71, Ku, E. et.al., Longitudinal Weight Change During CKD Progression and Its Association With Subsequent Mortality, Pages 657–665, Copyright (2018), with permission from the National Kidney Foundation, Inc., New York, NY, USA [27].

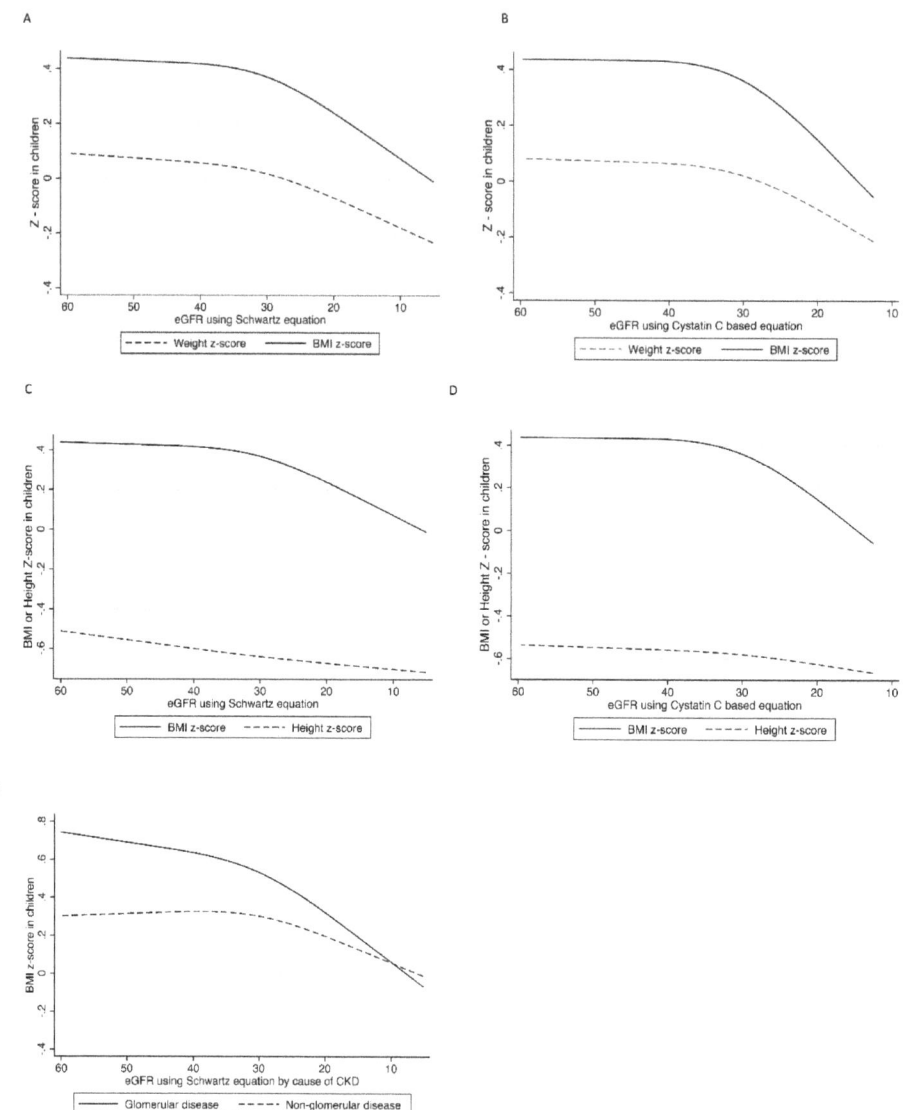

Figure 3. Association between longitudinal repeated measures of body mass index, weight, and height z score with repeated measures of kidney function over time in the Chronic Kidney Disease in Children study in the overall cohort, and by cause of CKD (glomerular versus non-glomerular disease). (**A**) Repeated measures of BMI and weight z scores with repeated measures of eGFR by serum creatinine. (**B**) Repeated measures of BMI and weight z scores with repeated measures of eGFR by cystatin C. (**C**) Repeated measures of BMI and height z scores with repeated measures of eGFR by serum creatinine. (**D**) Repeated measures of BMI and height z scores with repeated measures of eGFR by cystatin C. (**E**) Repeated measures of BMI with repeated measures of eGFR by serum creatinine by glomerular versus non-glomerular causes of CKD. Reprinted from Am J Kidney Dis., Vol. 71, Ku, E. et.al., Associations Between Weight Loss, Kidney Function Decline, and Risk of ESRD in the Chronic Kidney Disease in Children (CKiD) Cohort Study, Pages 648–656, Copyright (2018), with permission from the National Kidney Foundation, Inc., New York, NY, USA [28].

Similar results were obtained when the relationship between changes in estimated GFR and changes in weight and BMI were examined in almost 4000 people with CKD who participated in the CRIC study (Panels A–D) or in 1067 people with CKD in the AASK study (Panels E–F) (Figure 2) [27]. The data obtained from both groups of patients are longitudinal; the GFR and body weight in most of these patients were measured more than once. Again, when the GFR fell to about 30–35 mL/min/1.73 m^2 in both the CRIC study and the AASK study there was a decline in body weight [27]. Similar results were obtained when 854 children under 16 years who had an eGFR between 30–90 mL/min/1.73 m^2 and who were followed in the CKiD study in children [28] (Figure 3). At about the same eGFR level, their BMI began to decrease [28].

These data are not limited to the American experience. In the KNOW-CKD Study from South Korea, over 1800 patients with CKD stages 1–5 were evaluated [29]. None were undergoing dialysis. In this cross-sectional study, as the eGFR fell and the CKD stages increased starting with stage 3, the percentage of patients with serum albumin levels less than 3.8 g/dL began to increase. The percentage with low serum albumin levels jumped in the patients with stage 4 (eGFR 15–29 mL/min/1.73 m^2) and stage 5 CKD (eGFR <15 mL/min/1.73 m^2). Similarly, the number of patients diagnosed with PEW was rather low in South Korean patients with CKD stages 1 and 2, increased modestly in those with stages 3A and 3B, and then increased rather abruptly in stage 4 CKD patients, and rose even higher in stage 5 CKD. In stage 5 CKD, one out of four patients was diagnosed with PEW [29].

We have observed that adult CKD patients with eGFR of about 30–35 mL/min/1.73 m^2 and greater weight loss (>5% per year) had a 54% increase in mortality rate [27]. Children with an eGFR of about 30–35 mL/min/1.73 m^2 and greater weight loss (a decline in the z-score of BMI of > 0.2 kg/m^2 per year) had a 3.28 times greater increase in the rate of development of ESKD. In addition, weight loss that occurs in advanced CKD patients shortly after they commence chronic dialysis therapy is also associated with increased mortality [30].

3.4. Why Do CKD Patients Often Lose Weight When GFR Falls to about 30–35 mL/min/1.73 m^2?

CKD patients who lose weight when their GFR decreases to about 30–35 mL/min/1.73 m^2 may look normal unless they are suffering from the consequences of a systemic disease. The cause of their weight loss is unknown. Reduced energy intake is a likely cause of the weight loss, but the mechanism responsible for a reduction in energy intake in these patients is not clear. The potentially toxic metabolites that are normally excreted in urine and often accumulate in advanced CKD as the GFR, and hence urinary toxin excretion, decreases would not be expected to be sufficiently high in the body to cause anorexia in people with an eGFR of about 30–35 mL/min/1.73 m^2. This raises the question of whether the weight loss is due to anorexia caused by increased or reduced levels of one or more circulating hormones. Serum levels of many hormones may be increased at this level of reduced GFR [31,32] The paper by Kuro-O and Moe regarding bone mineral metabolism in kidney disease may be particularly illustrative in this regard [33,34].

Theoretically, anorexia and weight loss could be due to elaboration of proinflammatory cytokines in the kidney or elsewhere in the body. However, these patients seem to feel well and generally do not appear or act as if they are systemically inflamed. Another possibility is alterations in the gut microbiome that might alter energy metabolism or cause anorexia (see below).

The kidney is an endocrine organ that elaborates erythropoietin, renin and 1,25-dihydroxycholecalciferol. Is it possible that the kidney also normally elaborates an orexigenic (appetite stimulating) hormone, and perhaps when diseased or damaged, there is a reduction in the synthesis or release of this hormone by the kidney. Alternatively, could the kidney start to produce appetite suppressing hormones at this time? Although there is no evidence for these possibilities, they have never been systematically explored. The hypothesis is consistent with the weight loss occurring in CKD patients with beginning stage

4 CKD, which is a point at which the renal parenchyma can be expected to be extensively damaged. Research will be necessary to answer this question.

3.5. Why Is Large Weight Loss Associated with Increased Mortality in These CKD Patients?

In the CRIC study, CKD patients who had a GFR <35 mL/min/1.73 m^2 and who lost greater than 5% of their body weight per year, the risk of death was increased by 54% in comparison to people with no weight change. In the AASK study, CKD patients who had a GFR <35 mL/min/1.73 m^2 and who had an annualized percent weight loss greater than 5% also displayed a 56% increase in their adjusted mortality [27]. Interestingly, those people who gained weight also had increased mortality. The cause for this latter finding is particularly obscure; this weight gain might reflect accumulation of edema fluid in these patients [27].

In the CKiD study, using two different models of adjusted odds ratios, children with CKD and an eGFR <35 mL/min/1.73 m^2 who had a decline in their BMI z-score >0.2 per year had a 3.28 times greater risk of developing ESRD in comparison to children who had a stable BMI (0–0.1 z-score per year) [28]. Children who displayed a more moderate degree of weight loss or who gained body weight also showed a trend toward increased risk of ESRD in comparison to children with little or no weight change, although this trend was not statistically significant [28].

3.6. The Human Microbiome

What is the microbiome in humans? The adult human body is composed of about 30–40 trillion cells. Vastly greater amounts of microbial organisms, about one hundred trillion microbial cells, live in or on the human body [35]. Most of these microbes live in the gut, but they are also found in or on the mouth, vagina, auditory canals, skin, etc. [35]. In humans, there are ≥100 times more different genes in the gut microbiome than in the entire human genome [36,37]. Most of these microbes cannot be cultured and are identified by their DNA or RNA. However, they elaborate enzymes which may be bioactive in humans. The gut microbiota have the three domains of life: Archaea, Eubacteria, and Eukaryotes [36], and normally are rather similar in different people. However, diet, antibiotics, other medicines (such as metformin), hormones, aging, and many illnesses including CKD and acute kidney injury (AKI), can alter the gut microbiome [38]. Animal studies suggest that altered gut microbiome activity may injure the kidney and also promote conversion of a person with AKI to CKD [39]. No information is available as to whether other, non-gut, microbiomes may injure the kidney or affect the health of CKD patients. Whether nutritional intervention can modify the relation between the gut microbiome, and the risk of developing CKD or the progression of AKI and CKD and thereby protect the human kidney needs to be investigated [38,40,41].

Differences have been observed in the microbiota and the gut wall when normal people ingest a diet poor in quality versus a healthy diet. A healthy diet, predominantly composed of fruits, vegetables, fibers, plant-derived proteins, monounsaturated fatty acids (MUFAs) and n-3 polyunsaturated fatty acids (n3-PUFAs), has been associated with high microbial diversity, resistance to colonization of gut with pathogenic bacteria, immune homeostasis, a healthy mucus layer adherent to the gut wall, and a healthy gut barrier [41]. In contrast, a less healthy diet that contains more animal-derived protein (meat, including processed meat), saturated fats, refined grains, sugar, salt, alcohol and corn-derived fructose has been associated observationally with reduced microbial diversity, increased likelihood of colonization by other pathogenic microbes, inflammation, erosion of the protective mucus layer, and increased intestinal permeability [41].

3.7. The Gut Microbiome in CKD

In people with advanced CKD, several factors involving the diseased kidney and the gut predispose to increased concentrations of potentially toxic compounds:

i. Microbiota in the gut become altered (dysbiosis). The gut microbes may synthesize increased amounts or different types of compounds [42]
ii. These newly formed metabolites may be absorbed from the gut into the circulation [42–44].
iii. Blood levels of some compounds may increase due, in part, to reduced renal excretion and probably to increased synthesis [42,44].

There is degradation of the protective mucous layer adjacent to the gut wall and altered intestinal permeability. These changes may facilitate passage of intestinal bacterial matter and chemicals into the blood stream. Among the most studied of the altered chemicals produced in the CKD gut are trimethylamine and trimethylamine-N-oxide (TMAO) derived from carnitine and choline, p-cresyl sulfate and P-cresyl-glucuronide from tyrosine, and indoxyl sulfate, and indole-3-aldehyde produced from tryptophan. The gut microbiota participate in the synthesis of these compounds, and the liver usually also contributes to their formation. All of these metabolites are normally excreted by the kidney. In the presence of impaired GFR, they accumulate. Animal studies indicate that many of these gut-derived uremic toxins may induce chronic inflammation and cause nephrotoxicity in CKD [42–44].

3.8. Plant-Based Diets for CKD Patients

Diets that are high in plant-based sources of protein can generate less acid in the body, reduce the acid burden and/or decrease intestinal phosphate absorption. A more appropriate name may be *High Fruit and Vegetable Diet (HFVD)*. As conceived by Donald Wesson, MD, who has published extensively on the acid-base ramifications of this diet, the HFVD is high in fruits and vegetables but is not very low in protein. By Dr. Wesson's design, the total protein content of this diet is about 0.8–0.9 g/kg/day, including the protein provided by the fruit and vegetables (Wesson, personal communication). One reason we prefer to not just call this a plant dominant (PLAYDO) diet is that grains, which include such foods as bread, rolls, bagels, cakes and donuts, are also plants, and they may provide an acid load and therefore do not contribute to the alkalizing properties of this diet.

Table 1 from Wesson [45] shows the calculated potential renal acid load of selected relevant foods, per 100 g of an edible portion, and whole diets. Meat and seafood generate about 13.6 mmoles of acid. Dairy products also engender an acid load. In contrast, an equivalent amount of vegetables provide an alkali (negative acid) load (−24.9 mmoles acid), and fruits provide a smaller amount of alkali (−1.81 mmoles). Oils are virtually neutral with regard to acid or base production (+0.01 mmoles). As indicated in the table, grain-based foods produce a modest acid load (+6.3 mmoles) [45]. Table 1 also indicates the average intake of these acid generating foods in a rather typical United States diet, expressed in terms of acid production per each serving of a meal. As can be seen there is a generation of about 27 mmoles of acid per meal per day from a typical diet, and grains contribute about 6.4 mmoles to this acid load. A typical Mediterranean diet, which is particularly high in vegetables and fruits, low in meat/seafood, and contains a lot of grains, is essentially neutral in acid production. The DASH diet, which is high in vegetables, fruits, and low-fat dairy products, generates more acid due to the high meat or seafood content in the diet. A vegan diet provides a smaller acid load, which could be even lower if the content of grain-based foods is reduced (Table 1) [45].

Table 1. Calculated potential renal acid load of selected relevant diets. Used with permission of the American Society of Nephrology, from The continuum of acid stress, Wesson, D.E., 16, 2021 of copyright [45].

Food	USDA Recommended	Average Intake in the United States	Study Participants	Study Participants Given F + V	Mediterranean Diet	DASH Diet	Vegan Diet
Meat/seafood	13.61	22.55	27.45	25.21	6.03	22.83	0
Vegetables	−24.91	−12.46	−5.75	−13.96	−22.63	−20.19	−6.52
Fruit	−1.81	−0.91	6.23	−18.68	−10.04	−5.91	−13.72
Grains	6.34	6.43	10.64	9.57	18.26	8.15	27.6
Dairy	10.16	11.21	23.31	23.31	7.99	5.77	0
Oils	0.01	0.01	0.01	0.01	0.01	0.01	0
Total	3.4	26.83	61.89	25.46	−0.39	10.63	7.36

All values are shown in millimoles per day. USDA, United States Department of Agriculture; F + V, fruits and vegetables; DASH, dietary approaches to stop hypertension.

3.9. The Problem of Adherence to High Fruit and Vegetable Diets (HFVDs)

In the experience of one author (JDK), roughly 15% of CKD patients will adhere to a LPD (0.60 g protein/kg/d). Dr Wesson estimates that around one-third of his CKD patients will adhere to an HFVD for an extended period of time; i.e., for at least one year (personal communication). However, these latter patients tend to have low incomes, and the fruit and vegetable portion of their diet is given to them at no cost, even for as long as one year or more. It is not known what degree of long-term adherence to a HFVD can be expected if patients must personally pay for their fruits and vegetables and also ingest a LPD; for example a total daily protein intake closer to 0.60 g protein/kg/day rather than the 0.8–0.9 g protein/kg/day that CKD patients were apparently eating with the HFVD. For individuals who may have difficult adhering to the HFVD, the alkalizing benefits of this diet can be attained, without focusing so intensely on fruit and vegetable intake, by providing alkali, such as sodium bicarbonate or a sodium citrate/citric acid solution, or an alkali binding resin (veverimer). Another issue is the degree to which a HFVD or a high plant food diet will suppress intestinal absorption of phosphate. In this regard, the role for grain- and nut-based foods for CKD patients' needs to be investigated. Let us examine these questions.

3.10. What Type of Plant-Based Diets May Lower Dietary Phosphorus Uptake?

Grain-Based Foods

There has been much interest in phytates recently because they bind avidly to phosphate and reduce intestinal phosphate absorption. Table 2 shows the phytate content of various plant foods. Nuts and grain-based foods contain rather large amounts of phytate, in contrast to coconut, corn, strawberries, and polished rice that have rather small amounts [46–49]. On the other hand, grains provide an acid load (Table 1) [45]. So it would seem that the plant foods that may reduce intestinal phosphate absorption by binding phosphate with phytate may not be as effective at providing an alkaline load. Some potential benefits and limitations of plant-based diets are summarized in Table 3.

Table 2. Phytate content of different plant foods (derived from [46–49]).

Food	Phytate (In Milligrams per 100 g of Dry Weight)
Brazil nuts	1719
Cocoa powder	1684–1796
Brown rice	1250
Oat flakes	1174
Almond	1138–1400

Table 2. *Cont.*

Food	Phytate (In Milligrams per 100 g of Dry Weight)
Walnut	982
Peanut roasted	952
Peanuts ungerminated	821
Lentils	779
Peanuts germinated	610
Hazel nuts	648–1000
Wild rice flour	634–752.5
Yam meal	637
Refried beans	622
Corn tortillas	448
Coconut	357
Corn	367
Entire coconut meat	270
White flour	258
White flour tortillas	123
Polished rice	11.5–66
Strawberries	12

Table 3. Potential Benefits of High Plant Diets for People with CKD.

Potential Benefit	Potential Limitations
1. Reduces intestinal phosphorus absorption.	The reduction in intestinal phosphate absorption by plant foods is rather modest. Such medicines as phosphate binders or tenapanor also reduce phosphate absorption. LPDs are usually lower in phosphorus and therefore cause less intestinal phosphorus absorption.
2. Diets high in vegetables and fruits can alkalize blood, urine and, potentially, the kidneys.	Sodium bicarbonate, solutions of sodium citrate and citric acid, and the resin veverimer also can alkalinize, neutralize acid or bind protons.
3. High dietary fiber may enhance GI motility and reduce risk of hyperkalemia in advanced CKD.	Constipation usually is not a problem in CKD patients and often can be prevented with fiber supplements or other changes in the diet.
4. Animal studies indicate high plant diets may improve the microbiome and reduce renal inflammation and oxidative stress.	There are no randomized prospective clinical trials (RCTs) in humans with CKD that demonstrate these beneficial outcomes.
5. Animal studies show high plant diets produce less trimethylamine oxide, p-cresyl phosphate, p-cresyl sulfate and indoxyl acetic acid.	There are no RCTs that demonstrate beneficial clinical outcomes in humans with CKD from any such changes in production.

3.11. Effect of the Source of Dietary Phosphorus on Urinary Phosphorus Excretion

There have been several publications regarding the different degrees of intestinal phosphate absorption of organically bound phosphate in plant vs. animal foods and of inorganic phosphate salts [50–52]. We are of the opinion that the role of phytate in reducing phosphorus absorption and of the inorganic form of phosphate in enhancing phosphate absorption may be somewhat overstated (A. Shah et al.; unpublished observations). In most studies, the magnitude of intestinal phosphate absorption was estimated from the changes in urinary phosphate excretion. To assess more precisely the effects of these different forms of phosphorus on intestinal phosphate absorption, it would be helpful to measure net phosphorus absorption more directly in these studies; for example, by measuring dietary phosphorus intake minus fecal phosphorus excretion. These studies have yet to be done in CKD patients.

3.12. Can Medicines Substitute for Foods to Reduce Acidosis-Induced Progression of CKD or to Prevent or Treat Hyperphosphatemia?

Randomized clinical trials (RCTs) demonstrate that alkaline salts or solutions, such as sodium bicarbonate, sodium citrate and solutions of sodium citrate and citric acid, prevent or treat acidosis and slow the progression of CKD [53–58]. Other alkaline preparations, such as calcium citrate [59], potassium citrate and citric acid [60], potassium bicarbonate [61] and calcium bicarbonate [62], in rodent models of renal injury progression also slow the progression of chronic renal injury. Of course, many of these latter alkaline preparations may be contraindicated in CKD patients, because the associated cations may be toxic.

There appear to be at least two mechanisms responsible for the slowing of progression of kidney disease with alkalinization. Acidification is associated with increased synthesis and excretion of ammonium ion in the kidney which appears to stimulate complement deposition in the kidney with consequent development of interstitial fibrosis [63,64]. Acidification of the kidney also promotes the synthesis and release of endothelin 1 in the kidney which also stimulates interstitial fibrosis in the kidney [58,65,66].

With regard to the use of phosphate lowering medicines rather than diet to prevent or correct hyperphosphatemia, there are innumerable studies that show the effectiveness of these medicines at preventing or correcting hyperphosphatemia [67–70]. Although dietary phosphorus restriction is generally a necessary component of treatment to prevent or correct hyperphosphatemia in both far advanced CKD and chronic dialysis patients, the use of phosphate binders is almost always necessary as well. It is not known whether inclusion in the diet of large amounts of plants rich in phytate will enable some patients to completely avoid use of phosphate binders.

3.13. Summary of Discussion on the Use of High Plant Diets to Control Acidosis and Hyperphosphatemia in Advanced CKD and Chronic Dialysis Patients

1. A HFVD, as defined by Wesson and colleagues, is documented to reduce or prevent acidosis in CKD patients [71,72]. Since the PLAYDO diet may contain lower amounts of fruits and vegetables than the HFVD described by Wesson et al. [72] and may contain substantial animal-based protein, it is not clear how effective the PLAYDO diets are collectively at reducing the acid load and therefore, decreasing net body protein catabolism and slowing progression of CKD. It should be emphasized that grain-based foods are also plant foods, but still provide some acid (Table 1) [45].
2. Any diet, vegan or omnivorous, that provides 0.60 g protein/kg/day is likely to be deficient in calcium and certain essential micronutrients and may require supplements to prevent calcium and micronutrient deficiencies. Such LPDs that are composed entirely or almost entirely of plant foods may also be deficient in some essential amino acids, especially methionine and lysine [73]. It is therefore important that the primarily plant-based LPDs prescribed for CKD patients should be designed with the assistance of an experienced renal dietitian.
3. According to the tastes and preferences of the CKD patient, the potential benefits of plant dominant diets on alkalinization, decreased constipation, reduced intestinal phosphate absorption can be replicated with omnivorous LPDs that are augmented with alkali supplements, supplemental fiber, and intestinal phosphate binders.
4. To our knowledge, with the exception of the HFVD described by Wesson et al., there are no RCTs that demonstrate beneficial clinical outcomes (e.g., reduced rate of loss of GFR, less adverse cardiovascular events, decreased mortality) with PLADO diets as compared to similar LPDs that contain less plant protein but that have the same protein content and contain the medicines or supplements necessary to control blood pH, serum phosphate, bone-mineral disease, and fecal flow.

5. The difficulty with the term, PLAYDO Diet, is the amount of plant foods present in the diet is not well-specified. There is a similar concern with the HFVD. Perhaps it would be helpful if the amount of plant food or plant food protein in these diets was defined more precisely.

3.14. Renal Nutrition in the More Distant Future?

The following predictions can be considered highly speculative and could easily be disproven by future developments.

There will be increased development and use of medicines to facilitate the body's handling of nutrients. The following are examples of these types of medicines that are already in use:

1. Surveys of chronic dialysis patients indicate that food and fluid restriction are not uncommonly onerous [74–76]. In this regard, there are intestinal binders for potassium [77–79] and phosphorus [67–70]. An inhibitor of the Na/H exchanger iso-form 3 (NHE3) in the small intestine may suppress intestinal phosphate absorption [80]. Inhibitors of sodium absorption are under development [81–84]. Veverimer may bind hydrogen ion in the gut [85]. Diuretics, especially loop diuretics, may enhance the renal excretion of sodium, chloride and potassium, even in chronic dialysis patients who are not anuric.
2. Sodium-glucose co-transporter-2 (SGLT2) inhibitors stimulate tubular glomerular feedback to reduce intraglomerular hypertension and protect the kidney [86–88]. Glucagon-like peptide-1 (GLP-1) receptor agonists may improve serum glucose control [89–91]. Selective mineral corticoid antagonists may decrease blood pressure, improve glomerular hemodynamics and reduce renal fibrosis [92–94]. Hypoxia-inducible factor-proline hydroxylase inhibitors (HIF PHIs) enhance intestinal iron absorption and may improve anemia of CKD [95,96]. Calcimimetic medicines (cinecalcet, etalcalcetide) are used to treat hyperparathyroidism [97,98]. Oral, enteral or parenteral nutritional supplements are given to improve nutritional intake and prevent malnutrition in CKD patients. Dialysis treatments may also become more nutritionally relevant. For example, dialysate solutions may provide additional nutrients [99,100].
3. There will be more sophisticated methods for assessment of the patient's nutritional status of micronutrients. For example, more effective methods may be developed for:
    - Simple measurements of serum or blood cell concentrations that can accurately indicate the body burden of an individual micronutrient.
    - Measurements may be developed to indicate the functionality, as well as the blood and individual tissue concentrations, of a micronutrient and also the presence of inhibitors or other modifiers of the physiology, metabolism or actions of micronutrients. As examples, in the uremic state, retained endogenous metabolites, increased hormone levels, medicines or metabolites of medicines might inhibit or enhance actions of micronutrients [101–103].
    - Altered Vitamin Function or Metabolism in CKD/ESKD.

Examples of altered vitamin function in CKD and ESKD include:

- Erythrocyte transketolase (ETK) activity which requires the presence of the vitamin, thiamine pyrophosphate. However, low ETK activity has been found in patients who have normal blood thiamine levels [104].
- There is an increased daily need for pyridoxine hydrochloride (vitamin B6) in advanced CKD and chronic dialysis patients that exceeds the Recommended Dietary Allowance of vitamin B6 for normal adults [105].
- Membrane tetrahydrofolate (THF) transport is reported to be inhibited in advanced CKD [106].
- There is decreased vitamin B12 uptake by blood monocytes in advanced CKD patients [107].

- There is a reduced synthesis of 1,25(OH)$_2$D$_3$ by the diseased kidney [108]. In rats with CKD, impaired intestinal absorption of a number of vitamins, including riboflavin [109], folate [110] and vitamin D [111], have been described.
- Many medicines or other compounds, such as hydralazine, isoniazid and methotrexate, may inhibit or impair the actions of vitamin B6 [101,102] or folate [112].

These considerations have a number of implications should stimulate further research:

- How do these alterations affect dietary needs for the respective vitamins or, for that matter, trace elements?
- How can we assess the daily vitamin and trace element needs and the state of vitamin and trace element nutriture of CKD and chronic dialysis patients? By function tests? By blood levels?
- How can we know whether CKD or chronic dialysis patients are receiving adequate amounts of every essential micronutrient?

4. There will be more definitive investigations of the role of the microbiota, and particularly the gut microbiome, as contributing causes of AKI or CKD, of the clinical manifestations of these disease states, and of the general health of AKI and CKD patients. The potential role of nutrition and nutrients for modifying the microbiome and its pathogenetic or health-enhancing effects in AKI and CKD patients will continue to be investigated.

3.15. Is Nutritional Care Clinically Valuable?

We are of the opinion that a major reason why nutritional care is not as widely practiced for CKD patients is that many nephrologists are unconvinced that the benefits of nutritional prescription to the patient outweigh its negative effects. Even the use of LPDs and VLPDs to slow progression of renal failure in nondialyzed CKD patients can be considered controversial [14,15,113–115]. Previous reports suggest that nutritional support reduces the mortality risk in chronic dialysis patients with PEW [116]. However, these reports are almost all retrospective analyses of studies that were not randomized prospective controlled clinical trials (RPCTs). Although some of these studies were very well analyzed, it is hoped that in the future, there will be more RPCTs that test whether various types of nutritional management for CKD, chronic dialysis and AKI patients or renal transplant recipients are beneficial. It is likely that such trials will also inform the medical community of more effective ways to deliver nutritional care to people with kidney disease.

3.16. The SONG (Standard Outcomes in Nephrology) Initiative May Become Operative in Renal Nutrition

This initiative (viz., SONG) "aims to establish a set of core outcomes and outcome measures across the spectrum of kidney disease for trials and other forms of research. The outcomes will be developed based upon the shared priorities of patients, caregivers, clinicians, researchers, policy makers, and other relevant stakeholders. This will help to ensure that research is reporting outcomes that are meaningful and relevant to patients with kidney disease, their family, and their clinicians to support decisions about treatment" [117].

3.17. What May Be the Effects of SONG on Renal Nutrition?

The effects that SONG may have on renal nutrition are uncertain. It is clear that most CKD and chronic dialysis patients do not like to eat their prescribed diets [74–76]. We suspect that in the future there will be a greater focus on improving the comfort and enjoyment that CKD and chronic dialysis patients derive from their dietary intake. Will the combination of medicines (e.g., inhibitors of intestinal absorption of certain mineral or compounds, drugs that increase renal excretion) and chemically modified yet tasteful foods (e.g., low in various minerals and protein and higher in calorie content) enable CKD and chronic dialysis patients to eat more enjoyably? There may be increased publication of renal nutrition research on social media, and this may stimulate more interest and greater sophistication concerning renal nutrition among patients and their families.

3.18. Major Challenges to the Nutritional Treatment in CKD

Finally, there will continue to be logistical challenges to instituting nutritional therapy for advanced CKD and chronic dialysis patients. A major challenge to dietary therapy for CKD and chronic dialysis patients is the fact that many nephrologists are not very knowledgeable concerning the potential benefits of nutritional management and lack enthusiasm for prescribing renal nutrition for their patients. The time needed for a physician to introduce to CKD patients the concept of dietary therapy with its major ramifications, including explaining the importance of good adherence to the prescribed diet, can provide a disincentive for the physician to prescribe nutritional therapy. Furthermore, effective renal nutritional management requires the involvement of knowledgeable dietitians, and there is a paucity of dietitians who are experienced and sophisticated in renal nutrition therapy, especially for CKD patients who are not undergoing chronic dialysis. Moreover, many dietitians have only limited time that they can allocate to an individual patient. Many CKD patients have malaise, and they and their families or significant others may lack the motivation to acquire, prepare and eat specialized diets. The dietary prescription is restrictive of the types, variety and amounts of foods that many patients desire. Healthier foods and food supplements often cost more. Unfortunately, the less expensive foods tend to be the less healthy foods.

Figures 4 and 5 are from a study published by Angela Wang and coworkers in 2022 [118]. These figures summarize data obtained from a survey from representatives from 155 countries that responded to a series of questionnaires. This survey showed that the availability for CKD patients of renal dietitian support, or even the access of CKD patients to dietitians who do not have special expertise in renal nutrition, is actually quite low in the great majority of countries and particularly in low-income countries. The availability of dietetic counseling even by a person with some training in dietetics or nutrition and who is not necessarily a dietitian or nutritionist was only identified in 14% of low income countries. Among lower-middle income countries, this number rises to 31%. People surveyed described availability of dietetic counselling for CKD patients in 71% of upper-middle income countries and 84% of high-income countries (Figure 5). In contrast, in low-income countries for the great majority of CKD patients, consultations with a dietitian is either usually not available or never available. Some low-income countries, which may be rather populous, do not have a single university program to train students to become dietitians.

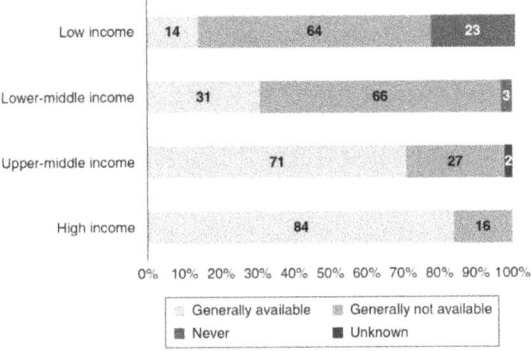

Figure 4. Global availability and capacity of kidney nutrition care. Dietitians/renal dietitians practice settings in outpatient and inpatient settings and nutrition care availability for nondialyzed CKD patients versus those undergoing maintenance dialysis for different World Bank income groups. Used with permission of the American Society of Nephrology, from Assessing Global Kidney Nutrition Care, Wang, A.Y. et.al., 17, 2022 of copyright [118].

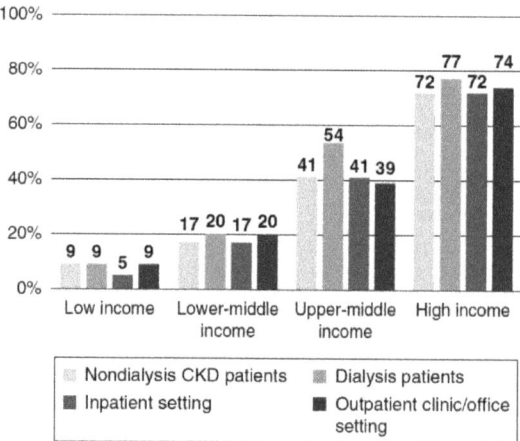

Figure 5. Global availability and capacity of kidney nutrition care. Dietitians/renal dietitians practice settings in outpatient and inpatient settings and nutrition care availability for nondialyzed CKD patients versus those undergoing maintenance dialysis for different World Bank income groups. Used with permission of the American Society of Nephrology, from Assessing Global Kidney Nutrition Care, Wang, A.Y. et.al., 17, 2022 of copyright [118].

The availability of dietitians or renal dietitians for nutritional care of non-dialyzed CKD and chronic dialysis patients varies enormously according to the patients' income status. The availability of renal dietitians for CKD and chronic dialysis patients is less than 10% for low-income patients, about 17–20% for lower-middle income patients, about 39–54% for upper-middle income patients, and about 72–77% for high income patients (Figure 5). Approximately one quarter of kidney disease patients have no access to a renal dietitian or any dietitian for their nutritional care in low income countries (Figure 4) [118]. It is the authors' experience that even in high income countries, or among CKD patients with high income, it is often difficult to access a knowledgeable dietitian who is experienced in the nutritional management of CKD patients who are not undergoing chronic dialysis.

3.19. A Different Institutional System for Nutritionally Managing People with Kidney Disease

Recently, a novel and potentially effective institution was developed in Mexico for managing the nutritional needs of non-hospitalized CKD and chronic dialysis patients and kidney transplant recipients: the Fresenius Kabi Nutritional Care Centers (CEANs). Most patients have CKD and are not receiving dialysis, but some are chronic dialysis patients or kidney transplant recipients. Patients are referred to the CEAN for nutritional care by any nephrologist in the metropolitan area. When the patient comes to this center, a renal dietitian conducts a nutritional, social and pharmaceutical history, performs anthropometry, bioelectric impedance (BIA) studies, assesses handgrip strength and reviews the patient's biochemical data. A nutritional diagnosis is then made, and a plan for personalized nutritional care is formulated. A consultation letter is sent to the referring nephrologist, usually within several workdays. The patient is counselled on his/her prescribed diet by the renal dietitian. Nutritional counseling with the patient is performed monthly until dietary adherence becomes acceptable. Patients are then seen every 3, 4 or 6 months depending upon the level of their dietary adherence and their clinical condition. Dietary adherence is assessed by both 24-h dietary records and sometimes by urine collection and measurement of protein nitrogen appearance.

Currently there are eight such CEAN centers located in different urban areas in Mexico. Attending the CEAN clinic is at no cost to the patient. If this model is to be applied widely, a method for funding these clinics would have to be devised. Possibly, funds from government or insurance companies might be allocated to support the renal nutrition centers, since these former agencies often pay for renal dietitian support in the hospital or dialysis center, and presumably the need for these latter dietitians might diminish when the renal nutrition centers become operative. These centers may also delay the need for chronic dialysis therapy with its attendant costs, thereby further defraying the overall costs to the government or other third party payers for these centers.

These renal nutrition centers may remove some of the key barriers to nephrologists offering nutritional therapy. As with a dialysis unit, much of the orientation and rationale for treatment could be provided to patients by dietitians or other non-physician workers in the renal nutrition centers. This would save nephrologists the very substantial amount of work and time that they might normally spend explaining to the patients their need for dietary therapy. We suspect that this might remove one of the major disincentives that physicians may have to starting patients on dietary therapy.

3.20. Summary: Future of Renal Nutrition May Include

- Development of new medicines to help control absorption in the intestinal tract and facilitate removal of unwanted nutrients and their metabolites.
- The refinement of the classification and the criteria for diagnosis of PEW.
- Examine why people commonly lose weight when GFR decreases to 30–35 mL/min/1.73 m^2 and why this weight loss is associated with increased mortality, or in children with CKD, an increased risk of developing ESRD.
- Continue the investigation of the gut microbiome, particularly with regard to how it influences human physiology and metabolism in CKD and ESRD and how it can be modified to make it more health enhancing.
- Continue to investigate the most effective uses of high fruit and vegetable diets and other plant-based diets vs. medicinal intake.
- Continued to explore the interactions and potential treatments of nutrient-medicine-hormonal interactions; for example, with regard to bone-mineral disorders.
- Develop and refine better methods for identifying altered vitamin and trace element metabolism, nutritional needs and deficiencies in kidney disease and kidney failure.
- Continue to develop more patient and family friendly nutritional therapy. The needs and feelings of the patients will become more central with regard to planning and implementing nutritional therapy.
- Explore the possible development of widely disseminated renal nutritional care centers, particularly in urban areas.

Author Contributions: Conceptualization and design of the editorial, J.D.K.; original draft preparation, M.E.; writing—review and editing, J.D.K.; supervision, J.D.K. All authors have read and agreed to the published version of the manuscript.

Funding: This research received no external funding.

Conflicts of Interest: The authors declare no conflict of interest.

References

1. Kopple, J.D.B.; Jerrilynn, D. History of Dietary Protein Treatment for Non-dialyzed Chronic Kidney Disease Patients. In *Nutrition in Kidney Disease*, 3rd ed.; Burrowes, J., Kovesdy, C.P., Byham-Gray, L.D., Eds.; Humana Press: Totowa, NJ, USA, 2022.
2. Giovannetti, S.; Maggiore, Q. A low-nitrogen diet with proteins of high biological value for severe chronic uræmia. *Lancet* **1964**, *283*, 1000–1003. [CrossRef]
3. Monasterio, G.; Giovannetti, S.; Maggiore, Q. The place of the low protein diet in the treatment of chronic uraemia. *Panminerva Medica* **1965**, *7*, 479–484. [PubMed]
4. Giovannetti, S. Dietary Treatment of Chronic Renal Failure: Why Is It Not Used More Frequently? *Nephron* **1985**, *40*, 1–12. [CrossRef] [PubMed]
5. Giordano, C.; Pluvio, M.; Di Guida, G.; Savoia, S.; Di Serfino, A. Modulated nitrogen intake for patients on low-protein diets. *Am. J. Clin. Nutr.* **1980**, *33*, 1638–1641. [CrossRef]
6. Giordano, C. The Role of Diet in Renal Disease. *Hosp. Pract.* **1977**, *12*, 113–119. [CrossRef]

7. Kopple, J.D.; Shinaberger, J.H.; Coburn, J.W.; Sorensen, M.K.; Rubini, M.E. Evaluating modified protein diets for uremia. *J. Am. Diet. Assoc.* **1969**, *54*, 481–485. [CrossRef]
8. Kopple, J.D.; Coburn, J.W. Metabolic studies of low protein diets in uremia. *Medicine* **1973**, *52*, 583–595. [CrossRef]
9. Alvestrand, A.; Furst, P.; Bergstrom, J. Plasma and muscle free amino acids in uremia: Influence of nutrition with amino acids. *Clin. Nephrol.* **1982**, *18*, 297–305.
10. Bergström, J.; Ahlberg, M.; Alvestrand, A.; Fürst, P. Amino Acid Therapy for Patients with Chronic Renal Failure. *Transfus. Med. Hemotherapy* **1987**, *14*, 8–11. [CrossRef]
11. Fürst, P. Amino acid metabolism in uremia. *J. Am. Coll. Nutr.* **1989**, *8*, 310–323. [CrossRef]
12. Walser, M. Keto Acid Therapy in Chronic Renal Failure. *Nephron Exp. Nephrol.* **1978**, *21*, 57–74. [CrossRef] [PubMed]
13. Mitch, W.E.; Walser, M.; Steinman, T.I.; Hill, S.; Zeger, S.; Tungsanga, K. The Effect of a Keto Acid–Amino Acid Supplement to a Restricted Diet on the Progression of Chronic Renal Failure. *N. Engl. J. Med.* **1984**, *311*, 623–629. [CrossRef] [PubMed]
14. Klahr, S.; Levey, A.S.; Beck, G.J.; Caggiula, A.W.; Hunsicker, L.; Kusek, J.W.; Striker, G. The Effects of Dietary Protein Restriction and Blood-Pressure Control on the Progression of Chronic Renal Disease. *N. Engl. J. Med.* **1994**, *330*, 877–884. [CrossRef] [PubMed]
15. Menon, V.; Kopple, J.D.; Wang, X.; Beck, G.J.; Collins, A.J.; Kusek, J.W.; Greene, T.; Levey, A.S.; Sarnak, M.J. Effect of a Very Low-Protein Diet on Outcomes: Long-term Follow-up of the Modification of Diet in Renal Disease (MDRD) Study. *Am. J. Kidney Dis.* **2009**, *53*, 208–217. [CrossRef] [PubMed]
16. Mircescu, G.; Gârneață, L.; Stancu, S.H.; Căpușă, C. Effects of a Supplemented Hypoproteic Diet in Chronic Kidney Disease. *J. Ren. Nutr.* **2007**, *17*, 179–188. [CrossRef] [PubMed]
17. Aparicio, M.; Bellizzi, V.; Chauveau, P.; Cupisti, A.; Ecder, T.; Fouque, D.; Garneata, L.; Lin, S.; Mitch, W.E.; Teplan, V.; et al. Protein-Restricted Diets Plus Keto/Amino Acids—A Valid Therapeutic Approach for Chronic Kidney Disease Patients. *J. Ren. Nutr.* **2012**, *22*, S1–S21. [CrossRef]
18. Garneata, L.; Stancu, A.; Dragomir, D.; Stefan, G.; Mircescu, G. Ketoanalogue-Supplemented Vegetarian Very Low–Protein Diet and CKD Progression. *J. Am. Soc. Nephrol.* **2016**, *27*, 2164–2176. [CrossRef]
19. Fouque, D.; Chen, J.; Chen, W.; Garneata, L.; Hwang, S.J.; Kalantar-Zadeh, K.; Kopple, J.D.; Mitch, W.E.; Piccoli, G.; Teplan, V.; et al. Adherence to ketoacids/essential amino acids-supplemented low protein diets and new indications for patients with chronic kidney disease. *BMC Nephrol.* **2016**, *17*, 63. [CrossRef]
20. Fouque, D.; Kalantar-Zadeh, K.; Kopple, J.; Cano, N.; Chauveau, P.; Cuppari, L.; Franch, H.; Guarnieri, G.; Ikizler, T.A.; Kaysen, G.; et al. A proposed nomenclature and diagnostic criteria for protein–energy wasting in acute and chronic kidney disease. *Kidney Int.* **2008**, *73*, 391–398. [CrossRef]
21. Stover, P.J.; King, J.C. More Nutrition Precision, Better Decisions for the Health of Our Nation. *J. Nutr.* **2020**, *150*, 3058–3060. [CrossRef]
22. Kalantar-Zadeh, K.; Moore, L.W. Precision Nutrition and Personalized Diet Plan for Kidney Health and Kidney Disease Management. *J. Ren. Nutr.* **2020**, *30*, 365–367. [CrossRef] [PubMed]
23. Carrero, J.J.; Stenvinkel, P.; Cuppari, L.; Ikizler, T.A.; Kalantar-Zadeh, K.; Kaysen, G.; Mitch, W.E.; Price, S.R.; Wanner, C.; Wang, A.Y.; et al. Etiology of the Protein-Energy Wasting Syndrome in Chronic Kidney Disease: A Consensus Statement from the International Society of Renal Nutrition and Metabolism (ISRNM). *J. Ren. Nutr.* **2013**, *23*, 77–90. [CrossRef] [PubMed]
24. Beddhu, S.; Chen, X.; Wei, G.; Raj, D.; Raphael, K.L.; Boucher, R.; Chonchol, M.B.; Murtaugh, M.A.; Greene, T. Associations of Protein–Energy Wasting Syndrome Criteria with Body Composition and Mortality in the General and Moderate Chronic Kidney Disease Populations in the United States. *Kidney Int. Rep.* **2017**, *2*, 390–399. [CrossRef] [PubMed]
25. Moreau-Gaudry, X.; Jean, G.; Genet, L.; Lataillade, D.; Legrand, E.; Kuentz, F.; Fouque, D. A Simple Protein–Energy Wasting Score Predicts Survival in Maintenance Hemodialysis Patients. *J. Ren. Nutr.* **2014**, *24*, 395–400. [CrossRef]
26. Kopple, J.D.; Greene, T.; Chumlea, W.C.; Hollinger, D.; Maroni, B.J.; Merrill, D.; Scherch, L.K.; Schulman, G.; Wang, S.-R.; Zimmer, G.S. Relationship between nutritional status and the glomerular filtration rate: Results from the MDRD Study. *Kidney Int.* **2000**, *57*, 1688–1703. [CrossRef]
27. Ku, E.; Kopple, J.D.; Johansen, K.L.; McCulloch, C.E.; Go, A.S.; Xie, D.; Lin, F.; Hamm, L.L.; He, J.; Kusek, J.W.; et al. Longitudinal Weight Change During CKD Progression and Its Association with Subsequent Mortality. *Am. J. Kidney Dis.* **2018**, *71*, 657–665. [CrossRef]
28. Ku, E.; Kopple, J.D.; McCulloch, C.E.; Warady, B.A.; Furth, S.L.; Mak, R.H.; Grimes, B.A.; Mitsnefes, M. Associations Between Weight Loss, Kidney Function Decline, and Risk of ESRD in the Chronic Kidney Disease in Children (CKiD) Cohort Study. *Am. J. Kidney Dis.* **2018**, *71*, 648–656. [CrossRef]
29. Hyun, Y.Y.; Lee, K.-B.; Han, S.H.; Kim, Y.H.; Kim, Y.-S.; Lee, S.W.; Oh, Y.K.; Chae, D.W.; Ahn, C. Nutritional Status in Adults with Predialysis Chronic Kidney Disease: KNOW-CKD Study. *J. Korean Med. Sci.* **2017**, *32*, 257–263. [CrossRef]
30. Chang, T.I.; Ngo, V.; Streja, E.; Chou, J.A.; Tortorici, A.R.; Kim, T.H.; Soohoo, M.; Gillen, D.; Rhee, C.M.; Kovesdy, C.P.; et al. Association of body weight changes with mortality in incident hemodialysis patients. *Nephrol. Dial. Transplant.* **2017**, *32*, 1549–1558. [CrossRef]
31. Mehta, R.; Cai, X.; Lee, J.; Xie, D.; Wang, X.; Scialla, J.; Anderson, A.H.; Taliercio, J.; Dobre, M.; Chen, J.; et al. Serial Fibroblast Growth Factor 23 Measurements and Risk of Requirement for Kidney Replacement Therapy: The CRIC (Chronic Renal Insufficiency Cohort) Study. *Am. J. Kidney Dis.* **2020**, *75*, 908–918. [CrossRef]

32. Isakova, T.; Cai, X.; Lee, J.; Mehta, R.; Zhang, X.; Yang, W.; Nessel, L.; Anderson, A.H.; Lo, J.; Porter, A.; et al. Longitudinal Evolution of Markers of Mineral Metabolism in Patients With CKD: The Chronic Renal Insufficiency Cohort (CRIC) Study. *Am. J. Kidney Dis.* **2020**, *75*, 235–244. [CrossRef] [PubMed]
33. Hu, M.C.; Shiizaki, K.; Kuro-O, M.; Moe, O.W. Fibroblast Growth Factor 23 and Klotho: Physiology and Pathophysiology of an Endocrine Network of Mineral Metabolism. *Annu. Rev. Physiol.* **2013**, *75*, 503–533. [CrossRef] [PubMed]
34. Kuro-O, M.; Moe, O.W. FGF23-αKlotho as a paradigm for a kidney-bone network. *Bone* **2017**, *100*, 4–18. [CrossRef] [PubMed]
35. Sender, R.; Fuchs, S.; Milo, R. Revised Estimates for the Number of Human and Bacteria Cells in the Body. *PLoS Biol.* **2016**, *14*, e1002533. [CrossRef]
36. Qin, J.; Li, R.; Raes, J.; Arumugam, M.; Burgdorf, K.S.; Manichanh, C.; Nielsen, T.; Pons, N.; Levenez, F.; Yamada, T.; et al. A human gut microbial gene catalogue established by metagenomic sequencing. *Nature* **2010**, *464*, 59–65. [CrossRef]
37. Zhu, B.; Wang, X.; Li, L. Human gut microbiome: The second genome of human body. *Protein Cell* **2010**, *1*, 718–725. [CrossRef]
38. Forslund, K.; Hildebrand, F.; Nielsen, T.; Falony, G.; Le Chatelier, E.; Sunagawa, S.; Prifti, E.; Vieira-Silva, S.; Gudmundsdottir, V.; Krogh Pedersen, H.; et al. Disentangling type 2 diabetes and metformin treatment signatures in the human gut microbiota. *Nature* **2015**, *528*, 262–266. [CrossRef]
39. Jang, H.R.; Gandolfo, M.T.; Ko, G.J.; Satpute, S.; Racusen, L.; Rabb, H. Early exposure to germs modifies kidney damage and inflammation after experimental ischemia-reperfusion injury. *Am. J. Physiol.-Ren. Physiol.* **2009**, *297*, F1457–F1465. [CrossRef]
40. Noel, S.; Martina-Lingua, M.N.; Bandapalle, S.; Pluznick, J.; Hamad, A.R.A.; Peterson, D.A.; Rabb, H. Intestinal Microbiota-Kidney Cross Talk in Acute Kidney Injury and Chronic Kidney Disease. *Nephron Exp. Nephrol.* **2014**, *127*, 139–143. [CrossRef]
41. Mills, S.; Stanton, C.; Lane, J.; Smith, G.; Ross, R. Precision Nutrition and the Microbiome, Part I: Current State of the Science. *Nutrients* **2019**, *11*, 923. [CrossRef]
42. Noce, A.; Marchetti, M.; Marrone, G.; Di Renzo, L.; Di Lauro, M.; Di Daniele, F.; Albanese, M.; Di Daniele, N.; De Lorenzo, A. Link between gut microbiota dysbiosis and chronic kidney disease. *Eur. Rev. Med. Pharmacol. Sci.* **2022**, *26*, 2057–2074. [CrossRef] [PubMed]
43. Vaziri, N.D. CKD impairs barrier function and alters microbial flora of the intestine. *Curr. Opin. Nephrol. Hypertens.* **2012**, *21*, 587–592. [CrossRef] [PubMed]
44. Vaziri, N.D.; Wong, J.; Pahl, M.; Piceno, Y.M.; Yuan, J.; DeSantis, T.Z.; Ni, Z.; Nguyen, T.-H.; Andersen, G.L. Chronic kidney disease alters intestinal microbial flora. *Kidney Int.* **2013**, *83*, 308–315. [CrossRef] [PubMed]
45. Wesson, D.E. The Continuum of Acid Stress. *Clin. J. Am. Soc. Nephrol.* **2021**, *16*, 1292–1299. [CrossRef]
46. Macfarlane, B.J.; Bezwoda, W.R.; Bothwell, T.H.; Baynes, R.D.; Bothwell, E.J.; MacPhail, A.P.; Lamparelli, R.D.; Mayet, F. Inhibitory effect of nuts on iron absorption. *Am. J. Clin. Nutr.* **1988**, *47*, 270–274. [CrossRef]
47. Helfrich, A. Determination of phytic acid and its degradation products by ion-pair chromatography (IPC) coupled to inductively coupled plasma-sector field-mass spectrometry (ICP-SF-MS). *J. Anal. At. Spectrom.* **2004**, *19*, 1330–1334. [CrossRef]
48. Wyatt, C.J.; Triana-Tejas, A. Soluble and Insoluble Fe, Zn, Ca, and Phytates in Foods Commonly Consumed in Northern Mexico. *J. Agric. Food Chem.* **1994**, *42*, 2204–2209. [CrossRef]
49. Liang, J.; Han, B.-Z.; Nout, M.R.; Hamer, R.J. Effects of soaking, germination and fermentation on phytic acid, total and in vitro soluble zinc in brown rice. *Food Chem.* **2008**, *110*, 821–828. [CrossRef]
50. Moe, S.M.; Zidehsarai, M.P.; Chambers, M.A.; Jackman, L.A.; Radcliffe, J.S.; Trevino, L.L.; Donahue, S.E.; Asplin, J.R. Vegetarian Compared with Meat Dietary Protein Source and Phosphorus Homeostasis in Chronic Kidney Disease. *Clin. J. Am. Soc. Nephrol.* **2011**, *6*, 257–264. [CrossRef]
51. Moorthi, R.N.; Armstrong, C.L.; Janda, K.; Ponsler-Sipes, K.; Asplin, J.R.; Moe, S.M. The Effect of a Diet Containing 70% Protein from Plants on Mineral Metabolism and Musculoskeletal Health in Chronic Kidney Disease. *Am. J. Nephrol.* **2014**, *40*, 582–591. [CrossRef]
52. Vorland, C.J.; Lachcik, P.J.; Aromeh, L.O.; Moe, S.M.; Chen, N.X.; Gallant, K.M.H. Effect of dietary phosphorus intake and age on intestinal phosphorus absorption efficiency and phosphorus balance in male rats. *PLoS ONE* **2018**, *13*, e0207601. [CrossRef] [PubMed]
53. Mannon, E.C.; O'Connor, P.M. Alkali supplementation as a therapeutic in chronic kidney disease: What mediates protection? *Am. J. Physiol.-Ren. Physiol.* **2020**, *319*, F1090–F1104. [CrossRef] [PubMed]
54. Melamed, M.L.; Horwitz, E.J.; Dobre, M.A.; Abramowitz, M.K.; Zhang, L.; Mitch, W.E.; Hostetter, T.H. Effects of Sodium Bicarbonate in CKD Stages 3 and 4: A Randomized, Placebo-Controlled, Multicenter Clinical Trial. *Am. J. Kidney Dis.* **2020**, *75*, 225–234. [CrossRef] [PubMed]
55. Raphael, K.L.; Greene, T.; Wei, G.; Bullshoe, T.; Tuttle, K.; Cheung, A.K.; Beddhu, S. Sodium Bicarbonate Supplementation and Urinary TGF-β1 in Nonacidotic Diabetic Kidney Disease. *Clin. J. Am. Soc. Nephrol.* **2020**, *15*, 200–208. [CrossRef] [PubMed]
56. Dubey, A.K.; Sahoo, J.; Vairappan, B.; Haridasan, S.; Parameswaran, S.; Priyamvada, P.S. Correction of metabolic acidosis improves muscle mass and renal function in chronic kidney disease stages 3 and 4: A randomized controlled trial. *Nephrol. Dial. Transplant.* **2020**, *35*, 121–129. [CrossRef]
57. Mahajan, A.; Simoni, J.; Sheather, S.J.; Broglio, K.R.; Rajab, M.; Wesson, D.E. Daily oral sodium bicarbonate preserves glomerular filtration rate by slowing its decline in early hypertensive nephropathy. *Kidney Int.* **2010**, *78*, 303–309. [CrossRef] [PubMed]

58. Phisitkul, S.; Khanna, A.; Simoni, J.; Broglio, K.; Sheather, S.; Rajab, M.H.; Wesson, D.E. Amelioration of metabolic acidosis in patients with low GFR reduced kidney endothelin production and kidney injury, and better preserved GFR. *Kidney Int.* **2010**, *77*, 617–623. [CrossRef]
59. Gadola, L.; Noboa, O.; Márquez, M.N.; Rodriguez, M.J.; Nin, N.; Boggia, J.; Ferreiro, A.; García, S.; Ortega, V.; Musto, M.L.; et al. Calcium citrate ameliorates the progression of chronic renal injury. *Kidney Int.* **2004**, *65*, 1224–1230. [CrossRef]
60. Tanner, G.A. Potassium citrate/citric acid intake improves renal function in rats with polycystic kidney disease. *J. Am. Soc. Nephrol.* **1998**, *9*, 1242–1248. [CrossRef]
61. Torres, V.E.; Mujwid, D.K.; Wilson, D.M.; Holley, K.H. Renal cystic disease and ammoniagenesis in Han:SPRD rats. *J. Am. Soc. Nephrol.* **1994**, *5*, 1193–1200. [CrossRef]
62. Wesson, D.E.; Simoni, J. Acid retention during kidney failure induces endothelin and aldosterone production which lead to progressive GFR decline, a situation ameliorated by alkali diet. *Kidney Int.* **2010**, *78*, 1128–1135. [CrossRef] [PubMed]
63. Nath, K.A.; Hostetter, M.K.; Hostetter, T.H. Increased Ammoniagenesis as a Determinant of Progressive Renal Injury. *Am. J. Kidney Dis.* **1991**, *17*, 654–657. [CrossRef]
64. Clark, E.C.; Nath, K.A.; Hostetter, M.K.; Hostetter, T.H. Role of ammonia in tubulointerstitial injury. *Miner. Electrolyte Metab.* **1990**, *16*, 315–321. [PubMed]
65. Wesson, D.E.; Dolson, G.M. Endothelin-1 increases rat distal tubule acidification in vivo. *Am. J. Physiol.-Ren. Physiol.* **1997**, *273*, F586–F594. [CrossRef]
66. Khanna, A.; Simoni, J.; Hacker, C.; Duran, M.J.; Wesson, D.E. Increased endothelin activity mediates augmented distal nephron acidification induced by dietary protein. *Trans. Am. Clin. Climatol. Assoc.* **2005**, *116*, 239–256. [CrossRef]
67. Qunibi, W.Y.; Hootkins, R.E.; McDowell, L.L.; Meyer, M.S.; Simon, M.; Garza, R.O.; Pelham, R.W.; Cleveland, M.V.; Muenz, L.R.; He, D.Y.; et al. Treatment of hyperphosphatemia in hemodialysis patients: The Calcium Acetate Renagel Evaluation (CARE Study). *Kidney Int.* **2004**, *65*, 1914–1926. [CrossRef]
68. Hervás, J.G.; Prados, D.; Cerezo, S. Treatment of hyperphosphatemia with sevelamer hydrochloride in hemodialysis patients: A comparison with calcium acetate. *Kidney Int.* **2003**, *63*, S69–S72. [CrossRef]
69. Chen, N.; Wu, X.; Ding, X.; Mei, C.; Fu, P.; Jiang, G.; Li, X.; Chen, J.; Liu, B.; La, Y.; et al. Sevelamer carbonate lowers serum phosphorus effectively in haemodialysis patients: A randomized, double-blind, placebo-controlled, dose-titration study. *Nephrol. Dial. Transplant.* **2014**, *29*, 152–160. [CrossRef]
70. Chiang, S.-S.; Chen, J.-B.; Yang, W.-C. Lanthanum carbonate (Fosrenol®) efficacy and tolerability in the treatment of hyperphosphatemic patients with end-stage renal disease. *Clin. Nephrol.* **2005**, *63*, 461–470. [CrossRef]
71. Goraya, N.; Simoni, J.; Jo, C.-H.; Wesson, D.E. Treatment of metabolic acidosis in patients with stage 3 chronic kidney disease with fruits and vegetables or oral bicarbonate reduces urine angiotensinogen and preserves glomerular filtration rate. *Kidney Int.* **2014**, *86*, 1031–1038. [CrossRef]
72. Wesson, D.E.; Kitzman, H.; Montgomery, A.; Mamun, A.; Parnell, W.; Vilayvanh, B.; Tecson, K.M.; Allison, P. A population health dietary intervention for African American adults with chronic kidney disease: The Fruit and Veggies for Kidney Health randomized study. *Contemp. Clin. Trials Commun.* **2020**, *17*, 100540. [CrossRef]
73. Khor, B.-H.; Tallman, D.A.; Karupaiah, T.; Khosla, P.; Chan, M.; Kopple, J.D. Nutritional Adequacy of Animal-Based and Plant-Based Asian Diets for Chronic Kidney Disease Patients: A Modeling Study. *Nutrients* **2021**, *13*, 3341. [CrossRef] [PubMed]
74. Kopple, J.D.; Shapiro, B.B.; Feroze, U.; Kim, J.C.; Zhang, M.; Li, Y.; Martin, D.J. Hemodialysis treatment engenders anxiety and emotional distress. *Clin. Nephrol.* **2017**, *88*, 205–217. [CrossRef] [PubMed]
75. Gibson, E.L.; Held, I.; Khawnekar, D.; Rutherford, P. Differences in Knowledge, Stress, Sensation Seeking, and Locus of Control Linked to Dietary Adherence in Hemodialysis Patients. *Front. Psychol.* **2016**, *7*, 1864. [CrossRef] [PubMed]
76. Lambert, K.; Mullan, J.; Mansfield, K. An integrative review of the methodology and findings regarding dietary adherence in end stage kidney disease. *BMC Nephrol.* **2017**, *18*, 318. [CrossRef]
77. Bakris, G.L.; Pitt, B.; Weir, M.R.; Freeman, M.W.; Mayo, M.R.; Garza, D.; Stasiv, Y.; Zawadzki, R.; Berman, L.; Bushinsky, D.A. Effect of Patiromer on Serum Potassium Level in Patients With Hyperkalemia and Diabetic Kidney Disease. *JAMA* **2015**, *314*, 151–161. [CrossRef]
78. Agarwal, R.; Rossignol, P.; Romero, A.; Garza, D.; Mayo, M.R.; Warren, S.; Ma, J.; White, W.B.; Williams, B. Patiromer versus placebo to enable spironolactone use in patients with resistant hypertension and chronic kidney disease (AMBER): A phase 2, randomised, double-blind, placebo-controlled trial. *Lancet* **2019**, *394*, 1540–1550. [CrossRef]
79. Rastogi, A.; Hanna, R.M.; Mkrttchyan, A.; Khalid, M.; Yaqoob, S.; Shaffer, K.; Dhawan, P.; Nobakht, N.; Kamgar, M.; Goshtaseb, R.; et al. Sodium zirconium cyclosilicate for the management of chronic hyperkalemia in kidney disease, a novel agent. *Expert Rev. Clin. Pharmacol.* **2021**, *14*, 1055–1064. [CrossRef]
80. Rieg, J.D.; Chavez, S.D.L.M.; Rieg, T. Novel developments in differentiating the role of renal and intestinal sodium hydrogen exchanger 3. *Am. J. Physiol. Integr. Comp. Physiol.* **2016**, *311*, R1186–R1191. [CrossRef]
81. Spencer, A.G.; Greasley, P.J. Pharmacologic inhibition of intestinal sodium uptake. *Curr. Opin. Nephrol. Hypertens.* **2015**, *24*, 410–416. [CrossRef]
82. Linz, B.; Hohl, M.; Reil, J.C.; Böhm, M.; Linz, D. Inhibition of NHE3-mediated Sodium Absorption in the Gut Reduced Cardiac End-organ Damage Without Deteriorating Renal Function in Obese Spontaneously Hypertensive Rats. *J. Cardiovasc. Pharmacol.* **2016**, *67*, 225–231. [CrossRef] [PubMed]

83. Pergola, P.E.; Rosenbaum, D.P.; Yang, Y.; Chertow, G.M. A Randomized Trial of Tenapanor and Phosphate Binders as a Dual-Mechanism Treatment for Hyperphosphatemia in Patients on Maintenance Dialysis (AMPLIFY). *J. Am. Soc. Nephrol.* **2021**, *32*, 1465–1473. [CrossRef] [PubMed]
84. Markham, A. Tenapanor: First Approval. *Drugs* **2019**, *79*, 1897–1903. [CrossRef] [PubMed]
85. Wesson, D.E.; Mathur, V.; Tangri, N.; Stasiv, Y.; Parsell, D.; Li, E.; Klaerner, G.; Bushinsky, D.A. Long-term safety and efficacy of veverimer in patients with metabolic acidosis in chronic kidney disease: A multicentre, randomised, blinded, placebo-controlled, 40-week extension. *Lancet* **2019**, *394*, 396–406. [CrossRef]
86. Sarafidis, P.; Ortiz, A.; Ferro, C.J.; Halimi, J.-M.; Kreutz, R.; Mallamaci, F.; Mancia, G.; Wanner, C. Sodium—Glucose co-transporter-2 inhibitors for patients with diabetic and nondiabetic chronic kidney disease: A new era has already begun. *J. Hypertens.* **2021**, *39*, 1090–1097. [CrossRef]
87. Herrington, W.G.; Preiss, D.; Haynes, R.; Von Eynatten, M.; Staplin, N.; Hauske, S.J.; George, J.T.; Green, J.B.; Landray, M.J.; Baigent, C.; et al. The potential for improving cardio-renal outcomes by sodium-glucose co-transporter-2 inhibition in people with chronic kidney disease: A rationale for the EMPA-KIDNEY study. *Clin. Kidney J.* **2018**, *11*, 749–761. [CrossRef]
88. Sen, T.; Heerspink, H.J. A kidney perspective on the mechanism of action of sodium glucose co-transporter 2 inhibitors. *Cell Metab.* **2021**, *33*, 732–739. [CrossRef]
89. Sattar, N.; Lee, M.M.Y.; Kristensen, S.L.; Branch, K.R.H.; Del Prato, S.; Khurmi, N.S.; Lam, C.S.P.; Lopes, R.D.; McMurray, J.J.V.; Pratley, R.E.; et al. Cardiovascular, mortality, and kidney outcomes with GLP-1 receptor agonists in patients with type 2 diabetes: A systematic review and meta-analysis of randomised trials. *Lancet Diabetes Endocrinol.* **2021**, *9*, 653–662. [CrossRef]
90. Nauck, M.A.; Quast, D.R.; Wefers, J.; Meier, J.J. GLP-1 receptor agonists in the treatment of type 2 diabetes—State-of-the-art. *Mol. Metab.* **2020**, *46*, 101102. [CrossRef]
91. Greco, E.V.; Russo, G.; Giandalia, A.; Viazzi, F.; Pontremoli, R.; De Cosmo, S. GLP-1 Receptor Agonists and Kidney Protection. *Medicina* **2019**, *55*, 233. [CrossRef]
92. Agarwal, R.; Kolkhof, P.; Bakris, G.; Bauersachs, J.; Haller, H.; Wada, T.; Zannad, F. Steroidal and non-steroidal mineralocorticoid receptor antagonists in cardiorenal medicine. *Eur. Heart J.* **2021**, *42*, 152–161. [CrossRef] [PubMed]
93. Barrera-Chimal, J.; Girerd, S.; Jaisser, F. Mineralocorticoid receptor antagonists and kidney diseases: Pathophysiological basis. *Kidney Int.* **2019**, *96*, 302–319. [CrossRef] [PubMed]
94. Patel, V.; Joharapurkar, A.; Jain, M. Role of mineralocorticoid receptor antagonists in kidney diseases. *Drug Dev. Res.* **2021**, *82*, 341–363. [CrossRef] [PubMed]
95. Singh, A.K.; Carroll, K.; Perkovic, V.; Solomon, S.; Jha, V.; Johansen, K.L.; Lopes, R.D.; Macdougall, I.C.; Obrador, G.T.; Waikar, S.S.; et al. Daprodustat for the Treatment of Anemia in Patients Undergoing Dialysis. *N. Engl. J. Med.* **2021**, *385*, 2325–2335. [CrossRef] [PubMed]
96. Mima, A. Hypoxia-inducible factor-prolyl hydroxylase inhibitors for renal anemia in chronic kidney disease: Advantages and disadvantages. *Eur. J. Pharmacol.* **2021**, *912*, 174583. [CrossRef]
97. Block, G.A.; Bushinsky, D.A.; Cheng, S.; Cunningham, J.; Dehmel, B.; Drueke, T.B.; Ketteler, M.; KewalRamani, R.; Martin, K.J.; Moe, S.M.; et al. Effect of Etelcalcetide vs Cinacalcet on Serum Parathyroid Hormone in Patients Receiving Hemodialysis with Secondary Hyperparathyroidism. *JAMA* **2017**, *317*, 156–164. [CrossRef]
98. Friedl, C.; Zitt, E. Role of etelcalcetide in the management of secondary hyperparathyroidism in hemodialysis patients: A review on current data and place in therapy. *Drug Des. Dev. Ther.* **2018**, *12*, 1589–1598. [CrossRef]
99. Kopple, J.D.; Bernard, D.; Messana, J.; Swartz, R.; Bergström, J.; Lindholm, B.; Lim, V.; Brunori, G.; Leiserowitz, M.; Bier, D.M.; et al. Treatment of malnourished CAPD patients with an amino acid based dialysate. *Kidney Int.* **1995**, *47*, 1148–1157. [CrossRef]
100. Feinstein, E.I.; Collins, J.F.; Blumenkrantz, M.J.; Roberts, M.; Kopple, J.D. Nutritional hemodialysis. In *Progress in Artificial Organs*, 1st ed.; ISAO Press: Cleveland, OH, USA, 1984; Volume 1, pp. 421–426.
101. Raskin, N.H.; Fishman, R.A. Pyridoxine-Deficiency Neuropathy Due to Hydralazine. *N. Engl. J. Med.* **1965**, *273*, 1182–1185. [CrossRef]
102. Levy, L.; Higgins, L.J.; Burbridge, T.N. Isoniazid-induced vitamin B6 deficiency. Metabolic studies and preliminary vitamin B6 excretion studies. *Am. Rev. Respir. Dis.* **1967**, *96*, 910–917. [CrossRef]
103. Bastl, C.; Finkelstein, F.O.; Sherwin, R.; Hendler, R.; Felig, P.; Hayslett, J.P. Renal extraction of glucagon in rats with normal and reduced renal function. *Am. J. Physiol.-Ren. Physiol.* **1977**, *233*, F67–F71. [CrossRef] [PubMed]
104. Descombes, E.; Hanck, A.B.; Fellay, G. Water soluble vitamins in chronic hemodialysis patients and need for supplementation. *Kidney Int.* **1993**, *43*, 1319–1328. [CrossRef]
105. Kopple, J.D.; Mercurio, K.; Blumenkrantz, M.J.; Jones, M.R.; Tallos, J.; Roberts, C.; Card, B.; Saltzman, R.; Casciato, D.A.; Swendseid, M.E. Daily requirement for pyridoxine supplements in chronic renal failure. *Kidney Int.* **1981**, *19*, 694–704. [CrossRef]
106. Jennette, J.C.; Goldman, I.D. Inhibition of the membrane transport of folates by anions retained in uremia. *J. Lab. Clin. Med.* **1975**, *86*, 834–843. [PubMed]
107. Obeid, R.; Kuhlmann, M.; Kirsch, C.-M.; Herrmann, W. Cellular Uptake of Vitamin B12 in Patients with Chronic Renal Failure. *Nephron Exp. Nephrol.* **2005**, *99*, c42–c48. [CrossRef]
108. DeLuca, H.F. The kidney as an endocrine organ involved in the function of vitamin D. *Am. J. Med.* **1975**, *58*, 39–47. [CrossRef]
109. Vaziri, N.; Said, H.; Hollander, D.; Barbari, A.; Patel, N.; Dang, D.; Kariger, R. Impaired Intestinal Absorption of Riboflavin in Experimental Uremia. *Nephron Exp. Nephrol.* **1985**, *41*, 26–29. [CrossRef]

110. Said, H.M.; Vaziri, N.D.; Kariger, R.K.; Hollander, D. Intestinal absorption of 5-methyltetrahydrofolate in experimental uremia. *Acta Vitaminol. Et Enzymol.* **1984**, *6*, 339–346.
111. Vaziri, N.D.; Hollander, D.; Hung, E.K.; Vo, M.; Dadufalza, L. Impaired intestinal absorption of vitamin D3 in azotemic rats. *Am. J. Clin. Nutr.* **1983**, *37*, 403–406. [CrossRef]
112. Alqarni, A.M.; Zeidler, M.P. How does methotrexate work? *Biochem. Soc. Trans.* **2020**, *48*, 559–567. [CrossRef]
113. Rhee, C.M.; Ahmadi, S.-F.; Kovesdy, C.P.; Kalantar-Zadeh, K. Low-protein diet for conservative management of chronic kidney disease: A systematic review and meta-analysis of controlled trials. *J. Cachex Sarcopenia Muscle* **2018**, *9*, 235–245. [CrossRef] [PubMed]
114. Hamidianshirazi, M.; Shafiee, M.; Ekramzadeh, M.; Jahromi, M.T.; Nikaein, F. Diet therapy along with Nutrition Education can Improve Renal Function in People with Stages 3-4 chronic kidney disease who do not have diabetes. (A randomized controlled trial). *Br. J. Nutr.* **2022**, 1–36. [CrossRef] [PubMed]
115. Bellizzi, V.; Signoriello, S.; Minutolo, R.; Di Iorio, B.; Nazzaro, P.; Garofalo, C.; Calella, P.; Chiodini, P.; De Nicola, L.; Torraca, S.; et al. No additional benefit of prescribing a very low-protein diet in patients with advanced chronic kidney disease under regular nephrology care: A pragmatic, randomized, controlled trial. *Am. J. Clin. Nutr.* **2022**, *115*, 1404–1417. [CrossRef] [PubMed]
116. Lodebo, B.T.; Shah, A.; Kopple, J.D. Is it Important to Prevent and Treat Protein-Energy Wasting in Chronic Kidney Disease and Chronic Dialysis Patients? *J. Ren. Nutr.* **2018**, *28*, 369–379. [CrossRef]
117. Evangelidis, N.; Sautenet, B.; Madero, M.; Tong, A.; Ashuntantang, G.; Sanabria, L.C.; de Boer, I.H.; Fung, S.; Gallego, D.; Levey, A.S.; et al. Standardised Outcomes in Nephrology—Chronic Kidney Disease (SONG-CKD): A protocol for establishing a core outcome set for adults with chronic kidney disease who do not require kidney replacement therapy. *Trials* **2021**, *22*, 1–8. [CrossRef]
118. Wang, A.Y.-M.; Okpechi, I.G.; Ye, F.; Kovesdy, C.P.; Brunori, G.; Burrowes, J.D.; Campbell, K.; Damster, S.; Fouque, D.; Friedman, A.N.; et al. Assessing Global Kidney Nutrition Care. *Clin. J. Am. Soc. Nephrol.* **2022**, *17*, 38–52. [CrossRef]

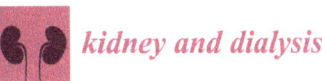

Editorial

Green Nephrology

Raymond Vanholder [1,2]

[1] Nephrology Section, Department of Internal Medicine and Pediatrics, University Hospital, Corneel Heymanslaan 10, 9000 Ghent, Belgium; raymond.vanholder@ugent.be; Tel.: +32-4-75612751

[2] European Kidney Health Alliance (EKHA), Luxemburgstraat 22, 1000 Brussels, Belgium

The greenhouse effect of carbon dioxide, nitrous oxide, and methane release resulted in an exponential rise of land temperatures over the last decades. The parallel warming of the ocean surfaces and the melting of the polar icecap offset the natural buffer against land heating. Global warming results in an unstable climate and many extreme conditions across the globe, with progressively more heatwaves, droughts and forest fires, as well as hurricanes and floods. Drastically lowering greenhouse gas emission is the only option for a sustained effect on this human-caused climate change.

Moreover, the unmanaged worldwide buildup of discarded waste generates tons of plastic ending up in rivers and oceans and, ultimately, in the food chain after ingestion by fish and shellfish. This devastating evolution can be stopped only by measures leading to a circular economy.

Kidney disease occupies a significant place in the environmental challenge: environmental problems aggravate kidney diseases, whereas dialysis especially leaves a huge environmental footprint with regard to water consumption and greenhouse gas and waste production [1–5] (Figure 1). However, the response to this by the nephrological community has remained unenthused, similar to a number of other, be it not all, areas of economic activity.

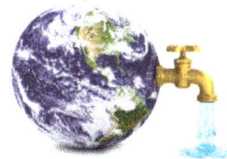

Figure 1. Summary of the main environmental problems related to hemodialysis. Graphic reprinted with permission from Depositphotos™, 2022 (https://depositphotos.com, accessed on 8 July 2022).

A recent policy paper by the European Kidney Health Alliance (EKHA) was drafted by a group of concerned physicians, patients, nurses, engineers and chemists [1]. This text, next to other publications by the EKHA, intends to create awareness among European policy makers of the dimensions of the environmental burden of nephrology [1,6]. It also wants to motivate the nephrological community, both from the manufacturer and provider sides, to take this problem to heart and avoid European nephrology lagging behind compared to other European economic sectors or to the nephrology field in other continents. The publication was written considering the significant boost in environmental action and ample opportunities created by the European Commission with the Green Deal, an overarching plan aiming at a 55% reduction in greenhouse gas emission versus 1990 in the European Union by 2030 and at an energy-neutral Europe by 2050 [7].

Green innovation of nephrology is also the main thematic of EKHA in 2022, and one of the focus points of EKHA's annual European Kidney Forum, held in the European Parliament [8]. Hopefully, these initiatives by EKHA will generate a boost in environmental considerations among professionals involved with kidney care and result in more transparency about undertaken actions. Although the activities mentioned above are essentially aimed at Europe and European policy, the intent of the present editorial is to broaden the scope to a worldwide setting because of the many parallels that can be made with other countries and continents, both regarding desired policy engagement and stakeholder action.

The EKHA publication referred to above [1] contains several tables with recommendations and suggestions on how to cope with the environmental problem in nephrology. Some action points refer to general attention points that are re-emphasizing viewpoints already expressed in previous publications, but the text also contains several suggestions that are novel and should be considered as out-of-the-box. Some suggestions are also specifically directed at policy making, since several action points may be accelerated by transnational coordination and guidance from an overarching level. The most compelling points are summarized in Table 1 of the present publication. Traditional and broadly recognized solutions that are insufficiently applied in nephrology, policy actions, and out-of-the-box thinking should all be combined on a large scale if we want to avoid that kidney care misses the boat of environmental innovation.

Table 1. Main solutions for environmental problems of dialysis [1].

- Established but not systematically applied solutions
    - Decrease water consumption
        - Dialysate regeneration
        - Decrease of dialysate flow
    - Energy neutral practices
        - Solar and wind energy
        - Heat pumps
        - Heat exchangers
    - Waste handling
        - Waste triage
        - Biodegradable plastic
        - Bio-based polymers
        - More durable dialysis machines and electronics
- Less established (out-of-box) solutions
    - Decrease water consumption
        - Water distillation
        - Repurposing of reverse osmosis water
        - Household use (bathing, toilet flush, laundry)
        - Drinking water
        - Spent dialysate as fertilizer
    - Energy neutral practices
        - Spent dialysate as fertilizer
        - Urea fuel cells
    - Waste handling
        - Biodegradable disinfection products
        - Repurposing plastic waste (e.g., to reinforce concrete)
        - Develop safe reuse techniques
- Policy changes
    - Facilitate screening and prevention of CKD and transplantation
    - Facilitate registries and stimulate transparency on environmental burden
    - Promote exchange of best practices
    - Adapt regulations to facilitate recycling of medical material

One of the most important hurdles for the facilitation of green nephrology is the lack of awareness among the general public and policy makers of the ecological burden of nephrology that is further aggravated by the deficient familiarity with kidney health and kidney disease at large. Advocacy efforts by all stakeholders are necessary at all levels (international, national, regional) to increase the knowledge of the humanistic, economical, and social burden of kidney disease. By joining the Decade of the Kidney^{TM} initiative [9], the EKHA, since 2020, further geared up its awareness campaigns on burden of kidney disease, emanating in several initiatives, including a comprehensive review written in language understandable for a lay public and policy makers summarizing all concerns linked to deficient kidney health [6].

The primary step to reduce the environmental burden of kidney care is by the prevention of advanced kidney failure, thus obviating the need for kidney replacement therapies. This implies more streamlined screening, primary and secondary prevention, and more investment in innovative approaches refraining the progression of kidney disease [10]. Of note, heathy lifestyle as primary prevention measure is also eco-friendly [11], e.g., by reducing red meat and processed food consumption and by promoting organic farming products and travel by one's own physical means rather than by fuel-consuming devices.

Among kidney replacement therapies, transplantation causes the lowest environmental burden [12]. Therefore, actions to increase uptake of transplantation are also of the utmost importance [13]. However, less than 40% of Europeans on kidney replacement therapy live with a functioning graft, and the degrees of uptake of transplantation per individual European country differ substantially, suggesting ample room for improvement [14].

With the majority of kidney failure patients on dialysis, especially an environmental optimization of this therapeutic option is imperative and should be pursued from production, transport, and delivery up to the therapeutic application itself and its waste management. Several industrial stakeholders have taken planet-friendly measures [15–17], which, however, seem focused on manufacturing rather than on clinical application. Corrections have been introduced in packaging, transport, and delivery processes, and some of the packaging material is recycled. However, production secrecy seems often an obstacle for a detailed reporting of specific ecologic measures. Along the same line, transnational mapping processes of the exact ecologic burden of clinical dialysis as a whole and per center remains fragmentary [18,19]. Significant quantities of reverse osmosis reject water that usually ends in the drain could easily be used for every-day purposes such as toilet flushes, laundry or bathing [20], and even as drinking water. This should certainly be a primary aim for newly built units but is feasible as well in existing units if an approach that has been well-organized in advance is followed [21].

Dialysate regeneration is another option to reduce water consumption [22–25]. Several compact dialysis systems are currently in use or developed, which next to ecologic benefit due to less water consumption might also allow more flexibility, user-friendliness, and lower cost for individuals and countries or regions adhering to those methods [24,26].

The generation of greenhouse gases [4,20] needs solutions by both manufacturers and providers to make dialysis energy neutral, e.g., by a shift to solar or wind energy, heat pumps, heat exchangers, or dialysate regeneration [27]. Energy consumption can further be reduced by simple actions, such as turning off lights and computers after the end of daily activities [4]. Home dialysis reduces the environmental burden of travel and uses ambient temperature regulation on a small domestic scale, which is usually less energy-consuming than hospital-based or unit-based climatization.

The dialysis concept should be refurbished into a circular model, involving biodegradable or recyclable materials or their repeated use. The current dialysis machines are usually built to be disassembled after a limited lifespan, which interferes with the cradle-to-cradle (circular) concept [19]. Dialysis waste originates from packages, non-contaminated and contaminated disposables, and hardware (electrical and electronic equipment). Corrective actions are indicated, from reduction in used material and careful triage of components before recycling, up to recycling per se, of both contaminated and non-contaminated disposables. However, international, national, and regional regulations often impede the disposal of biohazardous or toxic materials as well as of recycling.

Peritoneal dialysis might be conceived as more environment-friendly in view of the lower water need and (mainly for Continuous Ambulatory Peritoneal Dialysis (CAPD)) lower energy consumption for the dialysis procedure per se. However, this benefit is at least in part offset by a higher need for plastic used for the bags and packaging, which results in more waste, while the production process consumes more water, and more energy is used for production and transport than what is spent for the generation of hemodialysis filters [4].

Out of a conservative reflex, some people may think that most ideas formulated in this and the other referred articles are remote theory. However, these papers contain a large number of practical solutions which are easy to accomplish or could be made possible with some organization, constructive thinking, or research. Initiatives in France [21] and the UK [28,29] mentioned in the referred EKHA publication are real-life initiatives which are currently operational and beyond the stage of theory. If we, as individuals, modify our lifestyle to become energy-neutral and to avoid that life becomes hell for the next generations, we believe such initiatives should also be possible for dialysis units.

Others may suggest that the environmental impact of CKD has already repeatedly been cooked and served in various sauces. However, if one looks for the literature on environment and kidney health, one barely finds papers on this topic and only part of them propose solutions. So, it is fair to propose that there are many areas in nephrology that have been more frequently cooked than green nephrology. It is important to stress that all co-authors were specifically asked to come up with novel ideas, and all of those were included. As a consequence, it is reasonable to state that at least 30% of the entire text and more than half of the section with solutions contain novel ideas [1]. However, even if the publication would be entirely repetitive, the text still collects a large number of proposals for modification, allowing to design a roadmap on how to make progress in the immediate future. The intention of EKHA is to use this text for advocacy purposes with policy makers and major stakeholders on how to support/organize this environmental transition.

In conclusion, in view of the bidirectional relationship between environment and kidneys, it is necessary that the nephrological community takes action without delay. This implies profound shifts in structures, planning, targets and actions of industry, hospitals, medical professionals, and patients alike. Professionals, patients, and insurers as main end-product consumers have a responsibility to enforce this move upon manufacturers and providers. Only with a shift in mentality, it will be possible to overcome the current status quo by finding planet-friendly solutions, which is the only way to forestall the growing environmental burden of kidney care.

Conflicts of Interest: The author declares no conflict of interest.

References

1. Vanholder, R.; Agar, J.; Braks, M.; Gallego, D.; Gerritsen, K.G.F.; Harber, M.; Noruisiene, E.; Pancirova, J.; Piccoli, G.B.; Stamatialis, D.; et al. The European Green Deal and nephrology: A call for action by the European Kidney Health Alliance (EKHA). *Nephrol. Dial. Transplant.* **2022**. [CrossRef] [PubMed]
2. Agar, J.W.M.; Barraclough, K.A. Water use in dialysis: Environmental considerations. *Nat. Rev. Nephrol.* **2020**, *16*, 556–557. [CrossRef] [PubMed]
3. Connor, A.; Mortimer, F.; Tomson, C. Clinical transformation: The key to green nephrology. *Nephron Clin. Pract.* **2010**, *116*, c200–c205; discussion c206. [CrossRef] [PubMed]
4. Piccoli, G.B.; Cupisti, A.; Aucella, F.; Regolisti, G.; Lomonte, C.; Ferraresi, M.; Claudia, D.A.; Ferraresi, C.; Russo, R.; La Milia, V.; et al. Green nephrology and eco-dialysis: A position statement by the Italian Society of Nephrology. *J. Nephrol.* **2020**, *33*, 681–698. [CrossRef] [PubMed]
5. Wu, M.Y.; Lo, W.C.; Chao, C.T.; Wu, M.S.; Chiang, C.K. Association between air pollutants and development of chronic kidney disease: A systematic review and meta-analysis. *Sci. Total Environ.* **2020**, *706*, 135522. [CrossRef]
6. Vanholder, R.; Annemans, L.; Bello, A.K.; Bikbov, B.; Gallego, D.; Gansevoort, R.T.; Lameire, N.; Luyckx, V.A.; Noruisiene, E.; Oostrom, T.; et al. Fighting the unbearable lightness of neglecting kidney health: The decade of the kidney. *Clin. Kidney J.* **2021**, *14*, 1719–1730. [CrossRef]

7. A European Green Deal. Available online: https://ec.europa.eu/info/strategy/priorities-2019-2024/european-green-deal_en (accessed on 3 August 2022).
8. KHA – European Kidney Forum 2022: The Decade of the Kidney™: 10 Years to Bring Innovative and Green Treatments to Kidney Patients in Europe. Available online: https://ekha.eu/european-kidney-forum-2022/ (accessed on 3 August 2022).
9. Decade of the Kidney™. Available online: https://aakp.org/decade-of-the-kidney/ (accessed on 3 August 2022).
10. Vanholder, R.; Annemans, L.; Brown, E.; Gansevoort, R.; Gout-Zwart, J.J.; Lameire, N.; Morton, R.L.; Oberbauer, R.; Postma, M.J.; Tonelli, M.; et al. Reducing the costs of chronic kidney disease while delivering quality health care: A call to action. *Nat. Rev. Nephrol.* **2017**, *13*, 393–409. [CrossRef]
11. Ornish, D. Holy Cow! What's good for you is good for our planet: Comment on "Red Meat Consumption and Mortality". *Arch. Intern. Med.* **2012**, *172*, 563–564. [CrossRef]
12. Grafals, M.; Sanchez, R. The environmental impact of dialysis vs. transplantation [abstract]. *Am. J. Transplant.* **2016**, *16*, C74.
13. Vanholder, R.; Dominguez-Gil, B.; Busic, M.; Cortez-Pinto, H.; Craig, J.C.; Jager, K.J.; Mahillo, B.; Stel, V.S.; Valentin, M.O.; Zoccali, C.; et al. Organ donation and transplantation: A multi-stakeholder call to action. *Nat. Rev. Nephrol.* **2021**, *17*, 554–568. [CrossRef]
14. Stel, V.S.; de Jong, R.W.; Kramer, A.; Andrusev, A.M.; Baltar, J.M.; Barbullushi, M.; Bell, S.; De La Nuez, P.C.; Cernevskis, H.; Couchoud, C.; et al. Supplemented ERA-EDTA Registry data evaluated the frequency of dialysis, kidney transplantation, and comprehensive conservative management for patients with kidney failure in Europe. *Kidney Int.* **2021**, *100*, 182–195. [CrossRef]
15. Protecting Our Planet. Available online: https://www.baxter.com/our-story/corporate-responsibility/protecting-our-planet (accessed on 3 August 2022).
16. Environment. Available online: https://www.freseniusmedicalcare.com/en/about-us/sustainability/environment/ (accessed on 3 August 2022).
17. Sustainability: We Live Responsibly. Available online: https://www.bbraun.com/en/company/sustainability.html# (accessed on 3 August 2022).
18. Connor, A.; Mortimer, F. The green nephrology survey of sustainability in renal units in England, Scotland and Wales. *J. Ren. Care* **2010**, *36*, 153–160. [CrossRef] [PubMed]
19. Piccoli, G.B.; Nazha, M.; Ferraresi, M.; Vigotti, F.N.; Pereno, A.; Barbero, S. Eco-dialysis: The financial and ecological costs of dialysis waste products: Is a 'cradle-to-cradle' model feasible for planet-friendly haemodialysis waste management? *Nephrol. Dial. Transplant.* **2015**, *30*, 1018–1027. [CrossRef] [PubMed]
20. Agar, J.W. Green dialysis: The environmental challenges ahead. *Semin. Dial.* **2015**, *28*, 186–192. [CrossRef]
21. Bendine, G.; Autin, F.; Fabre, B.; Bardin, O.; Rabasco, F.; Cabanel, J.M.; Chazot, C. Haemodialysis therapy and sustainable growth: A corporate experience in France. *Nephrol. Dial. Transplant.* **2020**, *35*, 2154–2160. [CrossRef] [PubMed]
22. Barraclough, K.A.; Agar, J.W.M. Green nephrology. *Nat. Rev. Nephrol.* **2020**, *16*, 257–268. [CrossRef]
23. Agar, J.W. Personal viewpoint: Hemodialysis—Water, power, and waste disposal: Rethinking our environmental responsibilities. *Hemodial. Int. Int. Symp. Home Hemodial.* **2012**, *16*, 6–10. [CrossRef] [PubMed]
24. Agar, J.W. Review: Understanding sorbent dialysis systems. *Nephrology* **2010**, *15*, 406–411. [CrossRef]
25. Burnier, M.; Fouque, D. Global warming applied to dialysis: Facts and figures. *Nephrol. Dial. Transplant.* **2021**, *36*, 2167–2169. [CrossRef] [PubMed]
26. Himmelfarb, J.; Vanholder, R.; Mehrotra, R.; Tonelli, M. The current and future landscape of dialysis. *Nat. Rev. Nephrol.* **2020**, *16*, 573–585. [CrossRef]
27. Agar, J.W. Conserving water in and applying solar power to haemodialysis: 'green dialysis' through wiser resource utilization. *Nephrology* **2010**, *15*, 448–453. [CrossRef] [PubMed]
28. Tennison, I.; Roschnik, S.; Ashby, B.; Boyd, R.; Hamilton, I.; Oreszczyn, T.; Owen, A.; Romanello, M.; Ruyssevelt, P.; Sherman, J.D.; et al. Health care's response to climate change: A carbon footprint assessment of the NHS in England. *Lancet Planet Health* **2021**, *5*, e84–e92. [CrossRef]
29. Sustainable Healthcare Case Studies. Available online: http://map.sustainablehealthcare.org.uk/green-nephrology-projects (accessed on 3 August 2022).

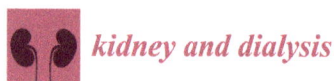 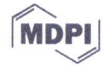

Review

Trace Elements and Their Management in Dialysis Patients—Pathophysiology and Clinical Manifestations

Shu Wakino

Department of Nephrology, Tokushima University Graduate School of Biomedical Sciences, 3-18-15 Kuramoto-cho, Tokushima 770-8503, Japan; shuwakino@tokushima-u.ac.jp

Abstract: Recently, as the number of elderly dialysis patients has been increasing, complications associated with low nutritional status such as infectious disease have had a strong influence on the prognosis of dialysis patients. Nutritional disorders are caused by the inadequate intake of the three major nutrients—proteins, fats, and carbohydrates—as well as vitamin and mineral deficiencies. Minerals are composed of various elements, including small-amount elements and trace elements, which are present in the human body in very small quantities lower than that of iron. In dialysis and predialysis patients, zinc, manganese, and selenium are the three major elements that are significantly depleted as compared to normal subjects; these deficiencies are sometimes symptomatic. Zinc deficiency is manifest as anemia, taste abnormality, and delayed wound healing, while selenium deficiency is associated with impaired cardiac function and immunocompromised condition. Zinc has multiple functions, since various enzymes, including DNA polymerase and RNA polymerase, need zinc as a cofactor, while selenium is a component of selenoproteins, including glutathione peroxidase and thioredoxin reductases, which are major antioxidative stress enzymes. These elements can only be supplemented exogenously and contribute to the sustainable QOL of dialysis patients. On the other hand, as regards other trace elements, including copper, chromium, manganese, lead, arsenic, etc., the association of their deficiency or intoxication with various involvements of dialysis patients were investigated, although all investigations were performed in cross-sectional studies or observational studies. Therefore, the supplementation of these elements is inconclusive, given the scarcity of other intervention studies. More conclusive studies are endorsed for the establishment of proper supplementation strategies.

Keywords: trace elements; dialysis; zinc; selenium

Citation: Wakino, S. Trace Elements and Their Management in Dialysis Patients—Pathophysiology and Clinical Manifestations. *Kidney Dial.* **2023**, *3*, 274–296. https://doi.org/10.3390/kidneydial3030025

Academic Editors: Vladimir Tesar and Ciro Esposito

Received: 18 May 2023
Revised: 25 June 2023
Accepted: 16 August 2023
Published: 21 August 2023

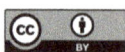

Copyright: © 2023 by the author. Licensee MDPI, Basel, Switzerland. This article is an open access article distributed under the terms and conditions of the Creative Commons Attribution (CC BY) license (https://creativecommons.org/licenses/by/4.0/).

1. Introduction

In recent years, the concept of nutritional management for dialysis patients has been changing, and the number of elderly dialysis patients has been increasing. This is due to the fact that the complications associated with low nutritional status, such as sarcopenia and frailty, have a strong influence on the prognosis of dialysis patients, and concerns about nutritional disorders caused by excessive dietary restriction have become apparent. Nutritional disorders are caused by the inadequate intake of the three major nutrients—proteins, fats, and carbohydrates—as well as vitamin and mineral deficiencies, which cannot be ignored. In this article, we focus on trace elements among minerals, especially zinc and selenium, which have attracted considerable attention in recent years.

2. What Are Trace Elements?

There are currently 118 known elements on earth, and all substances and objects are composed of these elements. The human body is also composed of various elements. In terms of its composition, 60% of the human body is water (H_2O), with the largest content of oxygen, which makes up 90% of the body. Next is C, which makes up organic matter, and H is the third largest by weight, although it is present in large quantities as a molecule because of its small atomic weight of 1. Next is N, which makes up the amino group of amino acids. O, C, H, and N are called macroelements (Figure 1). The largest elements with smaller amounts are Ca and P, which are constituents of bone, and together, they account for 99% of the human body. In contrast, the term mineral is often confused with element. Mineral comes from "mine" and "mineral mine" and is used as a synonym for metal in ordinary daily life but it is used with a different meaning as a term related to nutrition. In other words, proteins, lipids, and carbohydrates are the three major nutrients, and the remaining two become minerals and vitamins, meaning an inorganic substance, which is a general term for elements other than O, C, H, and N, as pointed out earlier. Among them, Ca, P, S, K, Na, Cl, and Mg are contained in relatively large amounts in living organisms and are called small-amount elements among minerals and measured in clinical practice in blood collection tests. In contrast, minerals with lower contents, i.e., Fe and below, are trace elements: Fe, F, Si, Zn, Mn, Cu, Se, I, and Mo. These small-amount elements are called trace elements, and together, they are referred to as the 16 essential elements of minerals. From a nutritional point of view, minerals are not necessarily metals, such as Fe, Zn, and Cu, i.e., substances that are hard at room temperature and have luster. In addition to these metallic elements, F, Se, and I are minerals, although they are nonmetallic elements.

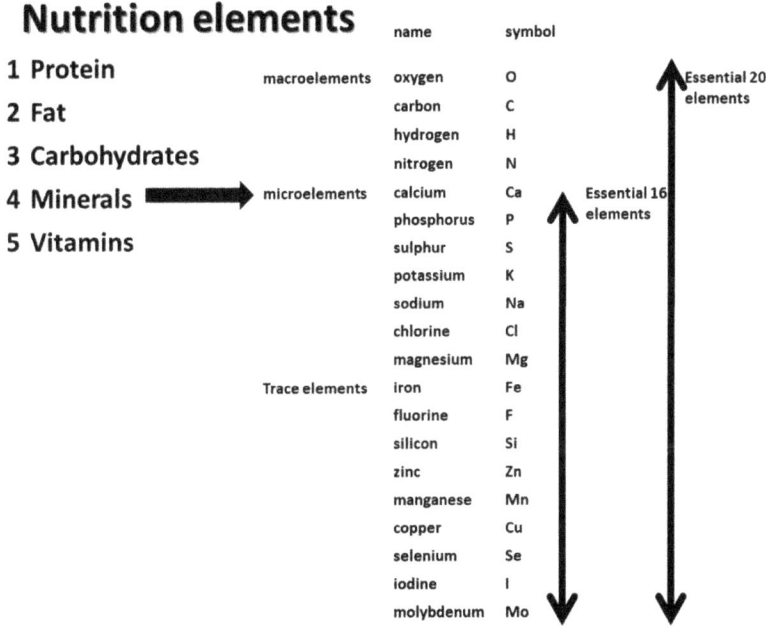

Figure 1. Nutrition elements. Five nutritional elements in which minerals are included. Minerals comprise macroelements, microelements, and trace elements.

Trace elements or minerals are important for four reasons. First, they are structural materials that form the bones and teeth; Ca, P, and Mg are known to make up bones, and F makes up teeth. Secondly, they are activators of enzymes in the body; Zn, Mn, Cu, Mg, and Ca are examples of this, and I makes up part of the thyroid hormones. I is part of the thyroid hormones, and some proteins (selenoproteins and heme proteins) are part of functional proteins. Thirdly, Na, K, and Cl are ions in body fluids, both intracellularly and extracellularly, that maintain the function of various organs. Finally, minerals do not contain calories, and they can only be obtained from food because they cannot be synthesized in the body.

3. Deficiency of Trace Elements

The importance of these minerals and trace elements is due to the fact that minerals and trace elements are decreasing in the Earth's soils; data presented at the Earth Summit in Rio de Janeiro in 1992 indicate that the amount of minerals in the world's soils has decreased over the past 100 years. This is probably due to the abuse of chemical fertilizers. As a result, trace elements in soils and crops have been depleted, with the end result that mineral intakes have decreased and requirements are not being met. Apart from dietary intake, deficiency and excess of trace elements are known to occur in renal failure and dialysis. The blood concentrations of trace elements in renal failure, hemodialysis, and peritoneal dialysis patients are higher than those in normal subjects for many trace metals, including Cr, Mo, and Si, and nonessential elements, such as cobalt, Ni, vanadium, strontium, and Cd. This is because these elements are mainly excreted by the kidneys. In contrast, there are some elements that become deficient, the most common of which are zinc and selenium (Table 1).

Table 1. Trace elements and their concentrations in predialysis, hemodialysis, and peritoneal dialysis patients. ↑ represents "higher than normal", ↓ "lower than normal", and → "the same as normal", and ? "no data available".

Trace Element	Normal Range	Predialysis	Hemodialysis	Peritoneal Dialysis	Deficiency Symptoms
Zinc (Zn)	60–121 mg/dL	↓	↓	↓	Growth retardation, wound-healing delay, taste disorder, and sexual dysfunction
Manganese (Mn)	0.31–1.04 mg/dL	↓	↓ or →	→	Anemia and glucose intolerance
Selenium (Se)	18–40 mg/mL	↓	↓	↓	Cardiac dysfunction, immune disorders, and carcinogenesis
Copper (Cu)	68–128 mg/dL	→	→ or ↑	→	Hemolysis, leukocytosis, and metabolic acidosis
Cobalt (Co)	0.04–0.40 mg/L	→	↑	↑	Cardiac dysfunction and impairment of gluconeogenesis
Chromium (Cr)	0.04–0.35 mg/dL	↑	↑	↑	Liver dysfunction, renal dysfunction, and carcinogenesis
Molybdenum (Mo)	0.27–1.17 mg/L	→	↑	?	Amino acid metabolism disorder, arthropathy, and hypercalcemia
Vanadium (V)	0.10–1.0 mg/L	→	↑	?	Bone disease, dyslipidemia, anemia, and hypertension
Silicon (Si)	0.14–0.20 mg/L	↑	↑	↑	Erythema, bone disease, neuropathy, and Wegener granulomatosis
Nickel (Ni)	0.2–0.8 mg/dL	↑	↑	↑	Cardiac ischemia, anemia, and bone disease
Strontium (Sr)	15–30 mg/L	→	↑	↑	Osteomalacia
Bromine (Br)	2.19–5.00 mg/L	→	↑	↑	Sleep disorders
Cadmium (Cd)	2.19–5.00 mg/L	↑	↑	↑	Growth defects, hypertension, and hyperparathyroidism
Rubidium (Rb)	0.095–0.272 mg/L	→	↑	→	Depression and central nervous system dysfunction

4. Zinc Deficiency in Dialysis Patients

4.1. Zinc and Zinc Deficiency

Zn is at the center of the activity of various enzymes and acts as an essential factor in their activity. Zinc is taken up by insulin-secreting beta cells in the pancreas to regulate insulin secretion. It is also a component of retinol-binding protein, which is a protein that transports vitamin A in the blood. It is an activator of enzymes involved in DNA synthesis and RNA synthesis and is therefore involved in cell division. Therefore, it is involved in wound healing. In recent years, zinc has been attracting attention because of its importance for the maintenance of taste bud cells on the tongue, which detect taste. It is also involved in the synthesis of the male sex hormone, testosterone. Zinc is involved in a wide variety of enzymatic reactions in the body, and Al-p, which is also measured in blood tests, is well-known. RNA polymerase and DNA polymerase are particularly important, as they are involved in DNA replication and transcription and are deeply involved in cell division and cell regeneration. The resulting symptoms of zinc deficiency are manifold. The skin is an important tissue for wound healing, tissue regeneration, and metabolism. Vitamin A is also important, and its deficiency causes dermatitis and stomatitis. Hair root cells also actively divide, and hair loss is observed. The intestinal epithelium is also actively regenerates and divides, and a zinc deficiency causes a loss of appetite. Laboratory findings include low blood zinc levels and low levels of alkaline phosphatase, the enzyme primarily responsible for its activity. Zinc deficiency anemia is also observed. Last year, the Japanese Society of Clinical Nutrition developed diagnostic criteria for zinc deficiency (Figure 2). A suspected case is defined as one in which one or more of the clinical symptoms and low alkaline phosphatase levels are observed, other diseases are ruled out, blood levels are less than 60 µg/dL, and symptoms improve with supplementation [1].

Diagnostic criteria for zinc deficiency
Edited by Japanese Society of Clinical Nutrition in 2018

1. Symptoms/More than one of the following symptoms
    1) Physical findings or symptoms
        dermatitis, oral ulcer, hair loss, **refractory decubitus, appetite loss, growth retardation (impaired weight gain or short status), hypogonadism, immune compromise, taste loss, infertility**
    2) Laboratory test
        Decrease in serum alkaline phosphatase

2. Other diseases were ruled out than zinc deficiency

3. Serum Zinc concentrations
    3-1: 60mg/dL>: zinc deficiency
    3-2: 80 mg/dL> and >60mg/dL: potential Zinc deficiency

4. Correction of symptoms by Zinc Supplementation

Definite diagnosis: 1 and 2 and 3-1 and 4=Zinc deficiency
            1 and 2 and 3-2 and 4=potential Zinc deficiency
Probable diagnosis: 1 and 2 and 3 before the Zinc supplementation,
            Zinc supplementation can be applied to this condition.

Figure 2. Diagnostic criteria for zinc deficiency. The criteria were edited by the Japanese Society of Clinical Nutrition in 2018 [1]. Reprinted with permission from [1], in 2018 from Hiroko Kodama.

4.2. Zinc Deficiency in Dialysis Patients

Zinc deficiency occurs in a variety of pathological conditions, among which dialysis patients are the most common. The causes of zinc deficiency in dialysis patients are (1) elimination by dialysis, (2) dietary restriction, (3) hypoproteinemia, (4) decreased absorption in the small intestine, (5) increased consumption due to increased oxidative stress, and (6) adsorption by adsorbents and ion exchange resins. It is known that cation exchange resins used for the correction of hyperpotassemia adsorb mineral ions other than K. A 2009 study on the effect of zinc supplementation demonstrated that the serum zinc levels of zinc-supplemented individuals and non-zinc-supplemented individuals were 63.29 ± 9.92 mg/dL and 68.07 ± 12.57 mg/dL, respectively, demonstrating that supplementation improved anemia [2].

Several symptoms associated with anemia in dialysis patients have been documented regarding zinc deficiency. In one study, patients on HD with low serum zinc levels (<65 µg/dL) were randomly assigned to two groups: a polaprezinc group (who received daily polaprezinc containing 34 mg/day of zinc) ($n = 35$) and a control group (no supplementation) ($n = 35$) for 12 months. In the polaprezinc group, erythropoiesis-stimulating agent dosage and erythropoiesis resistance (ERI) were significantly decreased at 10 months and 9 months, respectively, as compared with the baseline value. Multiple stepwise regression analysis revealed that the change in the serum zinc level was an independent predictor of lowered ERI. In conclusion, zinc supplementation reduces ERI in patients undergoing HD and may be a novel therapeutic strategy for patients with renal anemia and low serum zinc levels [3]. It has also been reported that Zinc sulfate ameliorates pruritus in patients on maintenance hemodialysis [4]. In the study, a double-blind, randomized, placebo-controlled trial was conducted on 40 adults with end-stage renal disease (ESRD) who were on maintenance hemodialysis. Patients were randomized to receive either zinc sulfate (440 mg/day) or placebo for two consecutive months. The authors reported that zinc sulfate was more effective than the placebo for the relief of pruritus. The main mechanism of this effect is considered to be an inhibitory effect exerted by zinc on histamine release from mast cells. Two other RCTs showed that zinc supplementation was more effective at reducing itching than placebo or hydroxyzine [5,6]. Zinc deficiencies and high serum histamine levels have also been observed in itching patients with ESRD. The sense of taste is also affected by zinc, which plays an important role in the proliferation and maintenance of sensory neuron cells in taste buds in the tongue. The role in the sense of taste has long been recognized among HD patients in non-Asian countries. Two studies examined the effects of Zn replacement on hypogeusia, which refers to diminished sensitivity to detect a specific taste quality or class of compounds [7,8]. In a recent study, the authors divided patients on hemodialysis into two groups based on serum zinc concentration. Salt taste acuity and preference were determined by a sensory test using varying concentrations of NaCl solution, and dietary sodium intake was estimated using 3-day dietary recall surveys. They found that the mean salt recognition threshold and salt taste preference were significantly higher in the zinc-deficient group than in the non-zinc-deficient group. They also reported that there was a significant positive correlation between salt taste preference and dietary sodium intake in the zinc-deficient group. In addition, interdialytic weight gain was significantly higher in the zinc-deficient group than in the non-zinc-deficient group [9]. Finally, Zinc plays an important role in regulating every phase of the wound-healing process, ranging from membrane repair, oxidative stress, coagulation, inflammation, immune defense, tissue re-epithelialization, and angiogenesis to fibrosis/scar formation. Several clinical studies have stressed the importance of zinc in skin ulcer treatment. Although not in the case of dialysis patients, a randomized, double-blind, placebo-controlled trial was conducted regarding the treatment of diabetic foot ulcers [10]. The authors demonstrated that 220 mg zinc sulfate supplementation for 12 weeks had beneficial effects on parameters of ulcer size and metabolic profiles among diabetic foot ulcer patients. A more recent study investigated the relationship between zinc deficiency and clinical outcome in patients with critical limb ischemia [11]. However, in a retrospective observational study of a de novo infrainguinal bypass grafting operation, the authors found that patients in the Zn deficiency group were more likely to have undergone hemodialysis and that graft patency, limb salvage, amputation-free survival, and complete wound-healing rates were significantly lower in the Zn-deficient group. Finally, another report showed that zinc deficiency is related to mortality in dialysis patients [12]. Zinc plays an important role in immune systems and the treatment and prevention of infectious disease. A clinical study reported that in long-term dialysis patients, the serum level of zinc was an independent predictor of future hospitalization due to infectious diseases and of overall mortality. The authors enrolled 111 patients on maintenance dialysis and measured serum levels of selenium, copper, and zinc. Patients were followed for 2 years or until death or withdrawal. Multivariate Cox regression analysis indicated that zinc deficiency (HR, 0.979; 95% CI, 0.966–0.992; p = 0.002) were more likely to be hospitalized for infectious diseases. Multivariate Cox regression also indicated low serum levels of zinc independently predict overall mortality. The survival effects of Zn supplementation are considered to be due to its anti-inflammatory and antioxidative effects. Recently, two meta-analyses including intervention studies conducted in both Western and non-Western countries revealed that Zn replacement results in the reduction in serum CRP levels, as well as MDA concentration, a serum oxidative stress marker [13,14]. More recently, it was demonstrated that Zn sulfate supplementation has favorable effects on CRP, fasting blood glucose, and renal function in Zn-deficient diabetic hemodialysis patients [15].

4.3. Treatment of Zinc Deficiency

A list of these trials is presented in Table 2 [3,15–28]. Zinc preparations such as zinc acetate (Novelzine®) and polaprezinc (Promax®) have been used for zinc supplementation. In Japan, a Zn acetate hydrate tablet containing 50 mg of Zn (Nobelpharma Co., Ltd., Tokyo, Japan) is administered orally after each meal (three times daily) (150 mg/day) for the treatment Zinc deficiency. However, in light of the aging population in recent years, the problem is overwhelmingly one of reduced zinc intake due to dietary restrictions and reduced dietary intake. Therefore, dietary supplementation is the best option. Foods rich in zinc include oysters, pork, and beef. Although these foods contain protein, the dietary intake of the elderly is low, so restricting protein intake because of renal failure is likely to result in a deficiency. Another important issue is that the supplementation dose does not always have effects in clinical practice. Therefore, Zn concentration should be evaluated according to serum protein or albumin concentration, since most Zn is bound to albumin or α2-microglobulin in the blood. In addition, Zn is present in the intracellular space of the whole body. Additional evaluation methods need to be explored.

Table 2. Clinical trials of zinc.

Mode	Number	Treatment Route	Combination	Evaluation	Se Concentration	Outcome	Ref.
HD	40 dialysis HBV non-responder Zn: $n = 28$ Control: $n = 12$	60 mg zinc aspartate after each dialysis session for 8 weeks	None	HBV antibody formation Titer of HVB antibody		HBV antibody formation Zn: 6 out of 28 patients Control: 2 out of 12 patients Antibody titer Zn: 0–2364 IE/L Control: 0–1110 IE/L	[16]
HD	Randomized, double-blind, before–after trial $n = 20$ (15 women, 5 men)	Zn: 7.7 pmol zinc sulfate (2200 μg) daily Control: cornstarch placebo capsule daily 90 days	None	Serum Zn concentration PCR (protein catabolic rate)	12.2 μmol/L (80 μg/dL) on day 0 to 15.3 μmol/L (100 μg/dL) on day 90	A significant positive correlation ($r = 0.61$) between PCR and serum zinc concentrations	[17]
HD	Zn group: 34 zinc-deficient HD patients. Control group: 16 sex- and age-matched normal volunteers	Zn: zinc (20 mg/day) Control: placebo 3 months	None	Levels of Zn malondialdehyde (MDA) osmotic fragility of red blood cells	Zn: 12.5 ± 1.0 to 18.8 ± 3.0 μmol/L Control: from 12.3 ± 1.0 to 12.1 ± 1.4 μmol/L	Increase in Zn concentration; Improvement of osmotic fragility; Decrease in the level of MDA	[18]
HD	Randomized, double-blind, before–after trial	Supplementation of Zn: 7.7 μmol zinc sulfate/day (50 mg elemental zinc/day) Control: cornstarch placebo capsule 90 days	None	Serum zinc, dietary intake, HDL, LDL, and TC	Zn: 0.79 μg/mL to 0.96 μg/mL	Increase in serum total cholesterol and LDL; No change in HDL; Increase in reported energy intake; No change in dietary intake of zinc, cholesterol, total fat, or saturated fat	[19]
HD	$n = 55$ hemodialysis patients (32 men and 23 women)	Zinc supplementation group ($n = 28$): 220 mg zinc sulfate capsule Control group ($n = 27$): placebo capsule (220 mg corn starch) 42 days	None	Serum zinc C-reactive protein levels	Zn group: 57.4 ± 2.4 μg/dL to 88.4 ± 4.8 μg/dL	Decrease in serum C-reactive protein: 13.5 ± 3.8 mg/L to $10.5 +/- 3.5$ mg/L	[20]

Table 2. *Cont.*

Mode	Number	Treatment Route	Combination	Evaluation	Se Concentration	Outcome	Ref.
HD	Double-blind zinc-deficient HD subjects Total: $n = 53$ (25 female and 28 male)	Zn group ($n = 27$): 220 mg zinc sulfate (50 mg elemental zinc) Control group ($n = 26$): starch placebo 42 days	None	Serum concentration of zinc, total cholesterol, HDL and LDL cholesterol, and triglycerides	Zn group: 0.53 ± 0.36 µg/mL to 0.86 µg/mL ± 0.42 µg/mL Control group: 0.52 ± 0.25 µg/mL to 0.64 ± 0.29 µg/mL	Increase in serum total cholesterol, serum LDL, and HDL cholesterol serum triglyceride	[21]
HD	Double-blind, randomized, controlled trial Total: $n = 60$	Zn group ($n = 30$): 100 mg/day zinc Control group ($n = 30$): placebo 2 months	None	Paraoxonase (PON) enzyme activity Lipid profile apolipoprotein AI (Apo-AI) and B (Apo-B) levels	Not measured	No change in serum levels of TC, TG, or LDL or Apo-B levels Increase in serum levels of HDL, Apo-AI, and PON activity	[22]
HD	Double-blind, randomized, clinical trial Total: $n = 97$ ESRD patients with Zn deficiency	Zn group ($n = 50$): 50 mg/day Zn Control group ($n = 47$): placebo 6 weeks	None	Serum Zn Homocysteine (hCys) level	Zn group: 56.9 ± 13.9 to 120.8 ± 26 µg/dL Control group: 60.9 ± 9.8 to 63.9 ± 13.2 µg/dL	Decrease in serum hCys	[23]
HD	Double-blind, randomized, controlled trial 65 HD patients	Group A: placebo Group B: zinc (100 mg/day) 2 months.	None	Serum Zn concentration, total antioxidant capacity (TAC), whole blood glutathione peroxidase (GSH) level, superoxide dismutase (SOD) activity, and malondialdehyde (MDA) level	The levels of serum zinc were increased	Increase in TAC, GSH, and SOD activity Decrease in MDA	[24]
HD	Long-term HD patients with low plasma Zn concentrations (<80 mg/dL)	Zn group ($n = 40$): daily oral Zn No supplements ($n = 25$) Control ($n = 38$): age- and sex-matched healthy individuals 8 weeks	None	Plasma concentrations of Zn and Cu, Cu/Zn ratios, oxidative stress, and proinflammatory cytokines percentages of CD4 and CD19 lymphocytes CD4/CD8 ratios	The levels of serum Zn were increased	Decrease in Cu, Cu/Zn ratios, oxidative stress status, and inflammatory responses Increase in percentages of CD4 and CD19 lymphocytes and CD4/CD8 ratios	[25]

Table 2. Cont.

Mode	Number	Treatment Route	Combination	Evaluation	Se Concentration	Outcome	Ref.
HD	Randomized, double-blind, and placebo-controlled trial 60 HD patients	Supplemented group (n = 30; male/female: 19/11): 100 mg/day elemental Zn Control group (n = 30; male/female: 17/13): placebo 60 days	None	serum zinc serum Leptin anthropometric measurements	Supplemented group: male, 81.7 ± 11 µg/dL to 105.5 ± 18 µg/dL; female, 75.5 ± 11 µg/dL to 106.3 ± 16 µg/dL Control group: male, 85.8 ± 16 µg/dL to 83.6 ± 9.6 µg/dL; female, 80.7 ± 18.8 µg/dL to 86.5 ± 12.7 µg/dL	Decrease in leptin in women; Increase in BMI and body weight in men; Increase in albumin and Hb; Negative association between serum zinc and leptin levels	[26]
HD	Prospective clinical trial study Pediatric HD patients between 5 and 18 years old Total: n = 60	Group I (n = 40): 50–100 mg zinc sulfate (equivalent to 11–22 mg elemental zinc) Group II (n = 20): placebo (cornstarch) twice daily 90 days	None	serum zinc serum leptin anthropometric measurements	Group I: 53.2 ± 8.15 µg/dL to 90.75 ± 12.2 µg/dL Group II: 55.45 ± 9.1 µg/dL to 55.35 ± 9.15 µg/dL	Decrease in leptin; Increase in BMI and body weight; Negative association between serum zinc and leptin levels	[27]
HD	Patients on HD with low serum zinc levels (<65 µg/dL) Total: n = 70	Polaprezinc group (n = 35): polaprezinc, 34 mg/day of zinc Control group (n = 35): no supplementation 12 months	Epoetin alph	ERI (erythropoietin responsiveness index); Weekly ESA dose (units)/dry weight (kg)/hemoglobin (g/dL)	Polaprezinc group: 53 ± 6 µg/dL to 80 ± 18 µg/dL Control group: 55 ± 5 µg/dL to 56 ± 10 µg/dL	Decrease in ESA dosage and ERI; No changes in Hb; No Change in serum iron or TSAT; Decrease in ferritin; Decrease in copper	[3]
HD	RCT Zn-deficient diabetic HD patients Total: n = 46	Zn supplement group (n = 21): 220 mg/day Zn sulfate capsule (containing 50 mg Zn) Control group (n = 25): placebo capsule (220 mg corn starch) 8 weeks	None	serum levels of copeptin, high-sensitive C-reactive protein (hs-CRP) glycemic control anthropometric parameters renal function	Zn supplement group: 55.9 ± 8.0 µg/dL to 90.6 ± 15.7 µg/dL Control group: 68.26 ± 6.2 µg/dL to 68.5 ± 6.5 µg/dL	Decrease in serum copeptin, hs-CRP, BUN, Cr, and FBG levels; Increase in BMI and body weight; No change in QUICKI (quantitative insulin sensitivity check index), HOMA-IR (homeostasis model assessment—insulin resistance), or serum insulin	[15]

Table 2. Cont.

Mode	Number	Treatment Route	Combination	Evaluation	Se Concentration	Outcome	Ref.
HD	Before–after trial Patients with serum Zn < 60 µg/dL Total: $n = 21$	Zinc acetate hydrate 50 mg 6 months	None	erythropoietin resistance index (ERI) ERI = dose (IU) of erythropoiesis-stimulating agent (ESA)/week/body weight (kg)/hemoglobin content (g/dL)	52.4 ± 7.6 µg/dL to 84.1 ± 16.3 µg/dL	Decrease in ERI and ESA dose; No change in Hb	[28]

Zn: zinc, HD: hemodialysis, PCR: protein catabolic rate, BMI: body mass index, ESA: erythropoiesis-stimulating agent, Hb: hemoglobin.

5. Selenium and Selenium Deficiency

5.1. Selenium and Selenium Deficiency

Selenium (Se) is also an important trace element for the maintenance of life. Its functions are described as follows: (1) it promotes the immune system, especially to maintain cellular immunity; (2) it inhibits cancer; (3) it is a constituent of glutathione peroxidase, a representative antioxidant enzyme, and has antioxidant effects; and (4) it is involved in the synthesis and degradation of thyroid hormones. Selenium is a mineral and a trace element but not a metal element. Selenium is a homologous element of sulfur; therefore, selenoamino acids exist in place of amino acids containing sulfur, including selenomethionine and selenocysteine. t-RNA that carries these amino acids, and selenoamino acids are incorporated into proteins, i.e., selenoproteins. In humans, 25 types of selenoproteins have been found (Table 3), major of which are the glutathione peroxidase family, thioredoxin reductase, and iodothyronine deiodinase.

Table 3. The lists of Selenoproteins.

Glutathione peroxidase (GPx)	GPx1 Gpx2 GPx3 Gpx4 Gpx6	The biochemical function of glutathione peroxidase (GPx) is to reduce lipid hydroperoxides to their corresponding alcohols and to reduce free hydrogen peroxide to water.
Thioredoxin reductases (Txnrd)	TrxR1 TrxR2 TrxR3	Thioredoxin reductases (TrxR) are the enzymes that catalyze the reduction of thioredoxin; hence, they are a central component in the thioredoxin system. Together with thioredoxin (Trx) and NADPH, this system's most general description is as a system for reducing disulfide bonds in cells. They contribute to the antioxidant effects.
Iodothyronine deiodinase (DIO)	DIO1 DIO2 DIO3	Iodothyronine deiodinase (DIO) an important enzyme in the activation and deactivation of thyroid hormones. Thyroxine (T_4), the precursor of 3,5,3'-triiodothyronine (T_3), is transformed into T_3 by deiodinase activity.
Selenoprotein	SelH SelI SelK SelM Sel15 SelN SelO SelP SelR SelS SelT SelV SelW	Selenoproteins (Sels) are composed of 13 proteins that contain selenium in the molecule. Selenoprotein P is the most common selenoprotein found in the plasma. It is unusual because in humans, it contains 10 s residues.

The American Society for Parenteral and Enteral Nutrition has defined symptoms of selenium deficiency as cardiomyopathy, myalgia, myositis, hemolysis, cellular immune disorders, nail and hair abnormalities, large cell changes in red blood cells, and anemia. Nail and skin abnormalities are also observed due to the involvement of selenium in DNA synthesis. In 2017, diagnostic criteria for selenium deficiency were developed (Figure 3) [29]. The presence of any one clinical symptom can be recognized by changes such as whitening, deformity, dermatitis, and alopecia in the nails and skin; cardiomyopathy and abnormalities of the conduction system in myocardial disorders; muscle weakness and myalgia in the lower extremities in muscular disorders; and macrocytic anemia in blood data. Laboratory findings may include abnormal thyroid hormones, abnormal muscle enzymes, and liver abnormalities. Electrocardiogram changes may also be present. If one or more of these symptoms and laboratory findings is present, other diseases can be ruled out, the serum selenium level is low, and the patient is considered suspicious and should be considered for supplementation. If the symptoms improve with supplementation, the case is confirmed. The standard serum concentration is 10 μg/dL or 100 pg/mL in adults.

Diagnostic criteria for selenium deficiency
Edited by Japanese Society of Clinical Nutrition in 2018

1. Symptoms/More than one of the following symptoms
    1) nail and skin   pale nail, neil deformity, dermatitis, hair loss, hair color change
    2) myocardium   cardiomyopathy, ischemic heart disease, arrythmia, palpitation
    3) muscle tissue   myopathy of lower extremity, muscle weakness, gait disturbance
    4) hemotological disorder   macrocytic anemia
    5) laboratory findings   low T3, increase in ALT and AST, increase in CPK
    6) electrocardiogram findings   ST depression, inverted T
2. Other diseases were ruled out than selenium deficiency

3. Serum selenium concentrations
    0-5 years old: Serum selenium concentrations ≦ 6.0 μg/dL
    6-14 years old: Serum selenium concentrations ≦ 7.0 μg/dL
    15-18 years old: Serum selenium concentrations ≦ 8.0 μg/dL
    19 years old and over: Serum selenium concentrations ≦ 9.0 μg/dL

4. Correction of symptoms by selenium Supplementation

Definite diagnosis: 1 and 2 and 3 and 4 = selenium deficiency
Probable diagnosis: 1 and 2 and 3 before the selenium supplementation,
    Selenium supplementation can be applied to this condition.

Figure 3. Diagnostic criteria for selenium deficiency. The criteria were edited by the Japanese Society of Clinical Nutrition in 2018 [29]. Reprinted with permission from [29], in 2018 from Hiroko Kodama.

5.2. Selenium Deficiency in Dialysis Patients

Dialysis patients are known to be a risk population for selenium deficiency. Possible causes include decreased selenium intake due to decreased dietary protein intake, decreased selenium-binding proteins, increased selenium requirements, increased urinary excretion, loss from dialyzer membranes, and altered distribution of selenium in the body. There are few case reports of selenium deficiency up to supplementation in dialysis patients. Myocardial symptoms were the main symptoms, with concentrations of less than 2.5 μg/dL and 8 μg/dL, both of which recovered after 3–4 months of supplementation [30,31]. In contrast, a very detailed cohort study of patients on dialysis as a whole was reported in Iwate Prefecture in Japan in 2011 [32]. Blood levels were measured in a multicenter cohort of dialysis patients, and the overall mean was significantly lower in dialysis patients than in healthy controls, with a median value of 10.3 μg/dL. When the cohort was divided into four groups based on serum selenium levels, BMI and serum albumin levels were significantly correlated. The group with the lowest serum selenium concentration had a significantly lower survival rate than the other groups in all-cause and infectious disease mortality [33]. Recently, studies on selenium and life expectancy have been reported in other countries. A study conducted in Alberta, Canada, reported the results of routine measurements of 25 trace elements [34]. Data on 25 trace elements were collected from 1278 multicenter hemodialysis patients. This cohort was followed-up for 2 years to determine which trace elements were associated with death, cardiovascular accidents, systemic infections, and hospitalizations. In 2 years, there were 260 (20%) deaths, 285 (24%) cardiovascular accidents, 117 (10%) systemic infections, and 928 (77%) hospitalizations. When investigating the relationship between 25 trace elements, low selenium levels were significantly associated with death and total hospitalization. Whereas high levels of copper and cadmium were associated with death, low levels of zinc and magnesium and high levels of lead, arsenic, and mercury were not associated with death or hospitalization, contrary to our expectations. In dialysis retrospective observational cohort study conducted in Spain that included 85 patients with ESRD on three modalities of dialysis, selenium was considered to be closely related to death, with a plasma selenium test performed 5–6 years before the study. Patients with low selenium showed an increased risk of all-cause mortality (hazard ratio, 2.952) compared with patients with normal or high selenium [35]. Although these data were observational and other important factors may contribute to the mortality of dialysis patients, these reports from three independent cohorts imply that selenium has some roles in the prognosis of dialysis patients.

In relation to mortality, special attention should be paid in terms of the causal relationship between infection and selenium status. As previously stated, in a hemodialysis cohort study conducted in Iwate prefecture in Japan, complication with infectious disease affected the selenium status, and supplementation of this element was found to help to ameliorate the condition in infectious disease. More recently, the relationship between COVID-19 infection and selenium deficiency was investigated [36]. Chinese cohort surveillance revealed an association between the reported cure rates for COVID-19 and selenium status in one city. Antiviral effects of selenium have been reported previously, and multiple cellular and viral mechanisms involving selenium and selenoproteins may influence viral pathogenicity, including virally encoded selenium-dependent glutathione peroxidases. Furthermore, a meta-analysis consisting of a total of 13 RCTs comparing selenium and placebo for patients with sepsis were reported [37]. The analyses could not detect the association of selenium treatment with a decreased mortality at different time courses. Selenium supplementation did not show a favorable effect on the incidence of renal failure, secondary infection, or duration of mechanical ventilation. However, the study found that selenium therapy was a benefit for sepsis patients, with reduced duration of vasopressor therapy, time in the intensive care unit and hospital, and incidence of ventilator-associated pneumonia.

Cardiovascular complications are also important causes of death in dialysis patients. The relationship between selenium and cardiovascular diseases has been explored since the famous selenium-deficient disease in which Kashan disease was presented with symptoms of dilated cardiomyopathy. A randomized control trial was performed in France in 1989 in which the effects of oral treatment with 500 µg selenium for 3 months and 200 µg for the next 2 months were tested in terms of cardiac function. As compared with the placebo control, the IVS (interventricular septum) in an echocardiogram decreased, although the cardiac function did not change [38]. In another study, a correlation between decreased serum selenium levels and coronary flow reserve was examined as an indicator of endothelial dysfunction and atherosclerosis in HD patients. Serum selenium levels and coronary flow reserve values were significantly lower in hemodialysis patients compared with controls. There was a significant positive correlation between coronary flow reserve and serum levels of selenium. A linear regression analysis showed that serum levels of selenium were independently and positively correlated with coronary flow reserve [39].

The association between selenium and anemia has been shown in hemodialysis patients. A cross-sectional study was performed, and serum selenium levels were determined in 173 hemodialysis patients. The association of serum selenium with the responsiveness to erythropoiesis-stimulating agents, as defined by the ESA resistance index, was analyzed. First, the study showed that 50% of the subjects had lower selenium levels than the population-based reference values. The authors also found that serum selenium levels were significantly and inversely correlated with the erythropoiesis resistance index (ERI) but not transferrin saturation (TSAT) or ferritin levels. Moreover, an independent association between selenium levels and ESA hyporesponsiveness was detected in multiple regression analyses. When patients were divided according to selenium levels and iron status, both low serum selenium (<10.5 µg/dL) and iron deficiency significantly affected the response to ESA. Finally, the association of low serum selenium with ESA hyporesponsiveness persisted after adjustment of confounding variables [40].

Finally, the association between blood trace element levels and sleep quality in patients on maintenance hemodialysis was reported. This cross-sectional and single-center study performed in 2019 examined sleep quality in 121 enrolled HD patients with the use of the

Pittsburgh Sleep Quality Index, which revealed an association between low blood selenium levels and the occurrence of severe sleep disturbances. [41].

5.3. Treatment of Selenium Deficiency in Dialysis Patients

Selenium supplementation in dialysis patients has been attempted for a long time. A lists of these trials is presented in Table 4 [38,42–51]. The treatment protocol has not been well-determined and varies, including intravenous treatment with 400 mg of sodium selenite. In Japan, sodium selenite solution containing of 100 µg of selenium (Fujimoto Co., Ltd., Osaka, Japan) is administered by daily infusion for the treatment selenium deficiency. In almost all studies, serum selenium concentration and glutathione peroxidase (GPx) activity in serum or red blood cells increased, and several biological markers were improved, including oxidative stress. In a more recent studies, selenium tablets or capsules are frequently used in trials. In 2013 one randomized, double-blind, placebo-controlled trial was conducted using selenium (200 µg) or a placebo capsule daily for 12 weeks [47]. The authors observed that the nutritional condition index, subjective global assessment (SGA) score, the systemic inflammation and nutrition condition score, and the malnutrition inflammation score (MIS) decreased significantly in the selenium group compared to the placebo group. Moreover, serum levels of malondialdehyde (MDA), an oxidative stress marker, decreased significantly in the selenium group compared with increasing levels in the placebo group. Selenium supplementation also hindered an increase in IL-6 levels compared with the placebo group. It can be concluded that selenium may be an effective complementary supplement for reducing the severity of malnutrition in HD patients by alleviating oxidative stress and inflammation.

Table 4. Clinical trials of selenium.

Subject	Number	Treatment Route	Combination	Evaluation	Se Concentration	Outcome	Ref.
HD	Se group: $n = 39$ Control group: $n = 15$	500 µg oral administration for 3 months and 200 µg for the next 2 months	None	Serum GPx, GPx in RBC, and muscle volume IVS in echocardiogram	3.83 µg/dL to 9.0–8.0 µg/dL	Increase in serum GPx and GPx in RBC; Increase in muscle volume; Decrease in IVS	[38]
HD	Se group: $n = 6$	50 µg intravenous administration for 5 weeks and 100 µg for the next 15 weeks	Intravenous Zn gluconate for 20 weeks	Serum GPx, GPx in RBC, serum TBARs, and serum Zn	0.45 µmol/L to 0.89 µmol/L	Increase in serum GPx and GPx in RBC; Decrease in serum TBARS; No change in serum Zn	[42]
HD	Se group: $n = 10$ Placebo group: $n = 5$	500 µg oral administration for 3 months and 200 µg for the next 3 months	None	Serum Se fT3 and TSH	Se group: 7.68 µg/dL Placebo group: 5.30 µg/L	Increase in serum Se; Increase in fT3; Decrease in TSH	[43]
HD	Se group: $n = 12$	400 mg Intravenous sodium selenite after HD for 8 weeks	None	Serum Se and α-tocopherol, Se and α-tocopherol in RBC Serum ascorbic acid, serum retinol, serum glutathione, GPx, SOD activity in RBC, and serum MDA	Serum Se: increased to 8.37 µg/dL 4 weeks after the treatment Se in RBC: increased to 15.9 µg/dL 4 weeks after the treatment	GPx activity: increase in serum levels and no change in RBC; Decrease in MDA; No change in CAT or SOD activity	[44]

Table 4. Cont.

Subject	Number	Treatment Route	Combination	Evaluation	Se Concentration	Outcome	Ref.
HD	Total: $n = 793$ Divided into 3 groups Three-affiliation prospective, randomized, single-blind study	Oral selenite Se 28 μg, Oral selenate Se 28 μg Control oral Se 7 μg 14 days	Energy intake of 35 kcal/kg/day	Serum GPx, GPx in RBC, and Se in RBC	Selenite group: 1.4 μmol/L Selenate group: 1.5 μmol/L Control group: 1.2 μmol/L	No differences in serum GPx, GPx in RBC, or Se in RBC	[45]
HD	4 groups $n = 15$ in each group	Erythropoietin (EPO) 2000 × 3/week Se-rich yeast 300 μg × 3/week	1. Placebo 2. EPO 3. Se-rich yeast 4. EPO + Se-rich yeast	Serum GPx and GPx activity in RBC	Increased to 120, 110, and 150 ng/mL in Se concentration in serum, blood, and RBC. Se concentration in serum and blood plateaued. Se in RBC increased to 200–250 ng/mL.	Increase in GPx activity in RBC in groups 3 and 4; No change in serum GPx	[46]
HD	Total: $n = 80$ Se group: $n = 29$ Placebo group: $n = 36$ Randomized, double-blind, placebo-controlled study	200 μg/day oral administration for 12 weeks	None	Primary; SGA Secondary: MDA, IL-6, high-sensitivity CRP, homocysteine, transferrin, ferritin, MIS, and Hb	Not measured	Decrease in SGA and MIS; Decrease in MDA; No change in IL-6, high-sensitivity CRP, homocysteine, transferrin, ferritin, or Hb	[47]
HD	Total: $n = 150$ Three groups $n = 50$ in each group Randomized, double-blind, active-control study	Se capsule 1. standard supplementation (SS) (vitamins) 2. Low supplementation (LS) SS + vitamin E 250 IU + Zn 25 mg + Se 5 μg 3. Moderate supplementation (MS) SS + vitamin E 250 IU + Zn 50 mg + Se 75 μg	Standard supplementation; biotin 300 μg, folic acid 1 mg, nicotinamide 20 mg, thiamine 1.5 mg Cyanocobalamin 6 μg, riboflavin 1.7 mg, pyridoxine 10 mg, ascorbic acid 100 mg	Primary: incidence of low Se and low Zn after 90 days Secondary: incidence of low Se and low Zn after 180 days Low Zn: Zn < 815 μg/L Low Se: Se < 121 μg/L	Day 90: SS: Se, 13.1 μg/dL LS: Se, 14.0 μg/dL MS: Se, 14.6 μg/dL Day 180: SS: Se, 13.5 μg/dL LS: Se, 13.5 μg/dL MS: Se, 13.0 μg/dL	Primary and secondary outcomes: No difference among three groups; No difference in sodium sensitivity or intradialytic body weight gain	[48]
HD	Total: $n = 68$ Se and NAC (N-acetylcysteine) treatment 4 groups each $n = 17$ 12 weeks	Group A: placebo Group B: NAC 600 μg/day Group C: Se 200 μg/day Group D: Se 200 μg/day+ NAC 600 μg/day	NAC N-acetylcysteine	Free tri-iodothyronine (FT3), free thyroxine (FT4), thyroid-stimulating hormone (TSH), and reverse T3 (rT3)	Not measured	Decrease in rT3 levels in groups B, C, and D; No change in FT3, FT4, and TSH between the groups; Good effects on nonthyroidal illness syndrome (NTIS)	[49]

Table 4. Cont.

Subject	Number	Treatment Route	Combination	Evaluation	Se Concentration	Outcome	Ref.
HD	53 diabetic HD patients Randomized, double-blind, placebo-controlled trial	Selenium group (n = 26): 200 μg selenium per day Placebo group (n = 27) for 24 weeks	None	Carotid intima-media thickness, FPG, insulin, HOMA-IR, QUICKI, triglycerides, VLDL-C, total-C, LDL-C, HDL-C, CRP, total nitrites, TAC, GSH (total glutathione), and MDA	Not measured	Decrease in serum insulin levels, insulin resistance, total cholesterol, LDL cholesterol, and CRP; Increase in insulin sensitivity, HDL cholesterol, and GSH; No change in carotid intima-media thickness	[50]
HD	Total: n = 78 Intervention: n = 40 Placebo: n = 38 Double-blind clinical trial	400 μg Oral selenium vs. placebo tablets three times after each hemodialysis session for 3 months	None	Blood Se levels, serum triglyceride, total cholesterol, weight, and physical activities (five times sit to stand test)	Intervention: 40 to 65 μg/L Placebo: 45 to 42 μg/L	Increase in Se concentration and physical activity in intervention group; No change in triglycerides, total cholesterol, or body weight in either group	[51]

HD, hemodialysis; Se, selenium; RBC, red blood cell; Zn, zinc; IVS, interventricular septum; TBARS, thiobarbituric acid reactive substances; GPx, glutathione peroxidase; T3, tri-iodothyronine; SOD, superoxide dismutase; TAC, total antioxidant capacity; GSH, total glutathione; MDA, malondialdehyde; MIS, malnutrition–inflammation score; Hb, hemoglobin; SGA, subjective global assessment.

5.4. Several Controversies about Selenium Supplementation

5.4.1. Optimal Serum Concentration of Selenium

A therapeutic threshold should be established with respect to the effectiveness of serum selenium concentrations. A U-shaped phenomenon is observed for the optimal selenium concentration. Thus, selenium should not be supplemented at overdosage levels. A previous study, selenium therapy had no effects on subjects with normal selenium concentration, and only half of the subjects exhibited an increase in GPx activity [52]. On the other hand, anticancer effects were not evident in patients with very low concentrations of selenium.

5.4.2. The Tissue Distribution of Selenium

As selenium functions are incorporated in the selenoprotein enzyme, the actual physiological effects may not be evaluated by the serum concentration. To overcome this problem, the activity of GP_X in blood cells can be utilized as an alternative for the assessment of systemic selenium condition. In this regard, the normal range of serum concentration should be carefully considered.

5.4.3. Gene Polymorphism of Selenoprotein

Some SNPs or mutation on selenoproteins have been reported so far, which reduce the therapeutic effects of supplementation treatment. In these patients, supplementation is of little clinical relevance.

5.4.4. The Unique Bioavailability of Selenium

The unique characteristics of selenium bioavailability make its assessment complicated. Selenium is incorporated in selenoproteins and mobilized by a specific genetic code. In this regard, the adequate evaluation of selenium function is complex.

As selenium deficiency has some significance in the QOL and mortality of patients in end-stage renal disease, an appropriate method for assessment of selenium condition including measurement of serum concentration and cellular activity of GPx should be developed in the future. Considering its role of survival effects, supplementation should be limited to severely compromised patients, including sepsis, SIRS, severe heart failure, or end-stage kidney disease patients. Moreover, the supplementation regimen should be carefully determined because overdose treatment has either no effects or adverse effects. Selenium is an essential and vital element that contributes to mortality, and its supplementation can open a novel path to nutrition support therapy. As selenium plays a pivotal role in the cardiovascular system and defense against infectious disease, clinical trials targeted at the patients with acute heart failure, septic shock, or acute kidney injury are optimal to confirm the efficacy of selenium intervention.

6. Copper

Plasma Copper (Cu) levels can be of clinical relevance in relation to Zn deficiency. In HD patients, as described above, the plasma Zn concentration decreases, and improper Zn supplementation can lead to Cu deficiency, since Zn antagonizes the uptake of divalent cations, including iron (Fe) and Cu, in erythrocyte precursors. Cu is required for Fe transfer from cells to blood, ensuring dietary Fe absorption and systemic Fe distribution [53]. Cu/Zn superoxide dismutase (Cu/Zn-SOD), an antioxidant enzyme, is decreased in Cu-deficient subjects, which may accelerate oxidation reactions and shorten the life span of erythrocytes. In these mechanisms, Cu deficiency may lead to refractory anemia in HD patients, and its correction can improve erythropoietin non-responsive anemia in HD patients [54].

On the other hand, elevated levels of serum Cu have been reported to trigger oxidative stress and activate inflammation [55]. The disruption of Cu and Zn homeostasis increases the risk of adverse outcomes. Significant negative associations between the Cu/Zn ratio and peripheral T-lymphocyte subsets (CD3 and CD4) and B-lymphocytes CD19 exist in CAPD patients, suggesting that variations in the Cu/Zn ratio can indicate oxidative stress and inflammation status in CAPD patients [56]. Zn supplementation significantly increases plasma Zn concentration, decreases Cu concentration and the Cu/Zn ratio, and decreases C-reactive protein and proinflammatory cytokine concentrations in HD patients [25].

7. Chromium

Chromium (Cr) levels in dialysis patients are regarded to be of clinical importance. One cohort study revealed higher concentrations of Cr than normal control in patients with ESKD [34]. In particular, in PD patients, Cr toxicity has been of clinical interest, and the consideration and measurement of dialysate fluid of PD may be necessary in the future [57]. The role of Cr can be either beneficial or harmful, depending on the ionic form. It is well established that Cr (VI) ions can easily enter cells and are associated with oxidative stress due to the reduction to Cr (III) in vivo [58]. In contrast, the more commonly found Cr (III) ion is much less dangerous or may actually be beneficial [58]. Serum Cr concentration is negatively associated with malnutrition in HD patients [59]. A prospective observational study is required to determine its toxicity to PD or HD patients.

8. Manganese

Serum manganese (Mn) levels are reported to be low in hemodialysis patients [60]. The main mechanisms for this deficiency include that Mn absorption is possibly decreased in the iron deficiency state [61], providing an additional rationale for Mn deficiency in HD patients, who are often iron deficient. Another mechanism deduced that dietary sources of Mn include meat, fish, nuts, and dried fruit [62], and the intake of these materials is often restricted in hemodialysis patients. However, a recent study reported that in Canada, there was no evidence that low Mn concentrations exist in hemodialysis patients [63]. Similar results were reported in a Spanish cohort [64]. Several previous reports have revealed the clinical consequences of Mn deficiency in hemodialysis patients. A low blood Mn level was independently associated with lower hemoglobin levels and anemia in patients undergoing hemodialysis [65]. This association was also observed in data and sample information of 110 hemodialysis patients downloaded from the UC San Diego

Metabolomics Workbench public repository. Patients with scarce response to erythropoiesis-stimulating agents (ESAs) were shown to be characterized by reduced Mn-to-nickel and Mn-to-antimony (Sb) ratios, which showed that Mn plays a role in the mechanisms underlying the human response to ESAs [66]. Low intake of Mn has also been reported to be related to malnutrition and systemic inflammation [67]. However, data on Mn deficiency in hemodialysis patients are still lacking, without any Mn supplementtation study, and whether its deficiency contributes to ill health in hemodialysis patients remains unknown, with no strong argument in favor of Mn supplementation.

9. Lead

Lead (Pb) is a heavy metal that is widespread and easy to extract and work with. Because of these characteristics, it has been used for thousands of years, and Pb toxicity has been extensively documented. Pb toxicity was previously reported in hemodialysis patients. An 18-month cross-sectional and prospective study included 927 patients on maintenance hemodialysis and revealed that a high blood Pb level is associated with increased risk for all-cause, cardiovascular-cause, and infection-cause 18-month mortality [68]. Similarly, blood Pb concentrations were associated with residual renal function and hyperparathyroidism and were related to an increased hazard ratio for all-cause 18-month mortality in peritoneal dialysis patients [69]. More recent cohort studies conducted in Canada and Spain also reported that excessive Pb concentrations were common [63,64], but the improvement in environmental condition reduced the lead intoxication in dialysis patients, and a higher concentration of Pb was not associated with higher risk of clinical outcomes such as mortality and hospitalization [34]. In general subjects, Pb accumulation affects hematopoiesis and bone formation, as well as the nervous and cardiovascular systems. Pb toxicity may present nonspecific symptoms, including colicky abdominal pain, nausea, constipation, arthralgias and myalgias, headaches and inability to concentrate, and peripheral neuropathy, especially affecting the wrist and finger extensors [70,71]. Similarly, in hemodialysis patients, several studies have delineated the clinical significance of Pb toxicity. Blood Pb levels were positively associated with carpal tunnel syndrome in patients on maintenance hemodialysis [72]. A nationwide analysis linking drinking water supply records to patient data showed that in hemodialysis patients, even low levels of Pb that were commonly encountered in community water systems throughout the United States were associated with lower hemoglobin levels and higher ESA use [73]. These data endorsed the further investigation of Pb toxicity among dialysis patients. Pb tends to be accumulated in bone, and Pb toxicity is associated with bone remodeling. Secondary hyperparathyroidism in dialysis patients can result in increased release of Pb from bone stores. Under this mechanism, blood Pb concentration was shown to be effectively suppressed by calcitriol therapy [74].

10. Arsenic

Arsenic (As) is a metalloid element that is naturally present in the Earth. In human beings, As accumulates in multiple tissues, including the peripheral nervous system, skin, gastrointestinal system, bone marrow, and kidneys, and is predominantly cleared from urines [75]. Chronic As poisoning predominantly affects the skin and nervous system. Symmetrical polyneuropathy and cognitive changes are common neurologic sequelae [76,77]. Underweight or malnourished humans, especially those lacking selenium, might also be at increased risk [76], suggesting that hemodialysis patients may be at higher-than-average risk of toxicity. Several previous studies have reported increased serum concentrations of As in dialysis patients [63,64]. However, scace data of clinical significance have been reported on increased As concentration in dialysis patients. One recent study reported that high serum As was associated with cardiovascular risk factors in patients undergoing continuous ambulatory peritoneal dialysis [78]. However, there is an argument that As and its compounds occur in both organic and inorganic forms. Inorganic As compounds are highly toxic, while organic As from food is considered nontoxic. Because only total As concentrations are measured in plasma samples of the hemodialysis patients, it is difficult to determine whether the excessive plasma As concentrations could have adverse health effects on these patients.

11. Other Trace Elements

Previous reports have measured the serum or tissue concentrations of other trace elements than were described above. In a Canadian cohort, the concentrations of several trace elements in hemodialysis patients were measured and evaluated based on the 5th and 95th percentile plasma concentrations from healthy reference populations. In terms of other trace elements, excessive plasma concentrations of cobalt, vanadium, cadmium, barium, antimony, nickel, and molybdenum were common, as were low platinum, tungsten, and beryllium concentrations [63]. Using this cohort, the clinical significances were analyzed by prospective study for 2 years of followup. Higher concentrations of mercury were not independently associated with higher risk of clinical outcomes including mortality or hospitalization. Cadmium levels in the highest decile were associated with higher risk of death [34]. In a Spanish cohort, it was reported that hemodialysis patients showed significantly higher concentrations of nickel as compared with normal controls [64]. Prior to these recent surveillance studies, a systemic review and metanalysis of 128 eligible studies was reported, and levels of cadmium and vanadium were higher [60]. Tissue concentrations of these trace elemtns were also measured to evaluate trace element deficiency or accumulation. In scalp hair of hemodialysis patients, the concentrations of beryllium, molybdenum, iodine, vanadium, and cobalt were significantly higher than those in healthy subjects, while mercury, germanium, and bromine levels were significantly lower than those in the former group. No significant differences were observed for lithium, aluminum, cadmium, boron, or nickel [79]. Significant bone accumulation of aluminium and vanadium occurred in the hemodialyzed azotemic individuals [80].

The abnormalities of several trace elements were investigated in a specific function. High cadmium levels might play a role in coronary artery calcification development in hemodialysis patients [81]. The relationship between serum nickel and homocysteine concentration was reported in hemodialysis patients, and nickel might also be involved in the regulation of the methionine-folate cycle in humans [82]. Finally, a multicenter study indicated that patients from particular dialysis centers are at an increased risk for strontium accumulation [83], and an association between osteomalacia and increased bone strontium concentrations in dialysis patients was reported [84]. However, all these clinical data were obtained in a cross-sectional or observational study, and a cause-and-effect relationship has not been demonstrated. Moreover, the methods of measurement were not the same between past and the recent studies, and the soil, drinking water, and dialysate water contents of trace elements varied among areas or countries. Confirmation of these clinical data awaits further investigation.

12. Conclusions

The major causes of death in dialysis patients are heart failure and infections, which may be closely related to poor nutrition. Although not specific to any one nutrient, trace element deficiency or toxicity is also a factor that cannot be ignored. For example, it has been reported that selenium deficiency is associated with infection and cardiac dysfunction and that its deficiency may affect the life expectancy of hemodialysis patients. However, in most trace elements other than Zn or Se, only association or observation studies have been reported, and there has been no consensus with respect to supplementation of these elements. Additional investigations are necessary to confirm the efficacy of intervention in the future.

Funding: This research received no external funding.

Institutional Review Board Statement: Ethical review and approval were waived for this study because this article is a review.

Informed Consent Statement: Patient consent was waived because this article is review.

Data Availability Statement: No new data were created or analyzed in this study. Data sharing is not applicable to this article.

Conflicts of Interest: The author declares no conflict of interest.

References

1. Kodama, H.; Itakura, H.; Omori, H.; Sasaki, M.; Sando, K.; Kamura, T.; Fuse, Y.; Hosoi, T.; Yoshida, H. Clinical guidelines for zinc deficiency. *J. Jpn. Soc. Clin. Nutr.* **2018**, *40*, 120–167.
2. Fukushima, T.; Horike, H.; Fujiki, S.; Kitada, S.; Sasaki, T.; Kashihara, N. Zinc deficiency anemia and effects of zinc therapy in maintenance hemodialysis patients. *Ther. Apher. Dial.* **2009**, *13*, 213–219. [CrossRef]
3. Kobayashi, H.; Abe, M.; Okada, K.; Tei, R.; Maruyama, N.; Kikuchi, F.; Higuchi, T.; Soma, M. Oral zinc supplementation reduces the erythropoietin responsiveness index in patients on hemodialysis. *Nutrients* **2015**, *7*, 3783–3795. [CrossRef]
4. Najafabadi, M.M.; Faghihi, G.; Emami, A.; Monghad, M.; Moeenzadeh, F.; Sharif, N.; Jazi, A.H.D. Zinc sulfate for relief of pruritus in patients on maintenance hemodialysis. *Ther. Apher. Dial.* **2012**, *16*, 142–145. [CrossRef] [PubMed]
5. Mapar, M.A.; Pazyar, N.; Siahpoosh, A.; Latifi, S.M.; SS, B.M.; Khazanee, A. Comparison of the efficacy and safety of zinc sulfate vs.placebo in the treatment of pruritus of hemodialytic patients: A pilot randomized, triple-blind study. *G Ital. Dermatol. Venereol.* **2015**, *150*, 351–355.
6. Amerian, M.; Nezakati, E.; Ebrahimi, H.; Zolfaghari, P.; Yarmohammadi, M.; Sohrabi, M.B. Comparative effects of zinc sulfate and hydroxyzine in decreasing pruritus among hemodialysis patients: A cross-over clinical trial. *J. Maz. Univ. Med. Sci.* **2019**, *29*, 81–90.
7. Atkin-Thor, E.; Goddard, B.W.; O'Nion, J.; Stephen, R.L.; Kolff, W.J. Hypogeusia and zinc depletion in chronic dialysis patients. *Am. J. Clin. Nutr.* **1978**, *31*, 1948–1951. [CrossRef] [PubMed]
8. Sprenger, K.B.; Bundschu, D.; Lewis, K.; Spohn, B.; Schmitz, J.; Franz, H.E. Improvement of uremic neuropathy and hypogeusia by dialysate zinc supplementation by dialysate zinc supplementation: A double-blind study. *Kidney Int. Suppl.* **1983**, *16*, S315–S318.
9. Kim, S.M.; Kim, M.; Lee, E.K.; Kim, S.B.; Chang, J.W.; Kim, H.W. The effect of zinc deficiency on salt taste acuity, preference, and dietary sodium intake in hemodialysis patients. *Hemodial. Int.* **2016**, *20*, 441–446. [CrossRef]
10. Momen-Heravi, M.; Barahimi, E.; Razzaghi, R.; Bahmani, F.; Gilasi, H.R.; Asemi, Z. The effects of zinc supplementation on wound healing and metabolic status in patients with diabetic foot ulcer: A randomized, double-blind, placebo-controlled trial. *Wound Repair Regen.* **2017**, *25*, 512–520. [CrossRef]
11. Koyama, A.; Tsuruoka, T.; Fujii, T.; Sugimoto, M.; Banno, H.; Komori, K. Zinc Deficiency and Clinical Outcome After Infrainguinal Bypass Grafting for Critical Limb Ischemia. *Circ. Rep.* **2020**, *2*, 167–173. [CrossRef] [PubMed]
12. Yang, C.-Y.; Wu, M.-L.; Chou, Y.-Y.; Li, S.-Y.; Deng, J.-F.; Yang, W.-C.; Ng, Y.-Y. Essential trace element status and clinical outcomes in long-term dialysis patients: A two-year prospective observational cohort study. *Clin. Nutr.* **2012**, *31*, 630–636. [CrossRef] [PubMed]
13. Wang, L.-J.; Wang, M.-Q.; Hu, R.; Yang, Y.; Huang, Y.-S.; Xian, S.-X.; Lu, L. Effect of Zinc Supplementation on Maintenance Hemodialysis Patients: A Systematic Review and Meta-Analysis of 15 Randomized Controlled Trials. *BioMed. Res. Int.* **2017**, *2017*, 1024769. [CrossRef] [PubMed]
14. Mousavi, S.M.; Djafarian, K.; Mojtahed, A.; Varkaneh, H.K.; Shab-Bidar, S. The effect of zinc supplementation on plasma C-reactive protein concentrations: A systematic review and meta-analysis of randomized controlled trials. *Eur. J. Pharmacol.* **2018**, *834*, 10–16. [CrossRef] [PubMed]
15. Hosseini, R.; Montazerifar, F.; Shahraki, E.; Karajibani, M.; Mokhtari, A.M.; Dashipour, A.R.; Ferns, G.A.; Jalali, M. The Effects of Zinc Sulfate Supplementation on Serum Copeptin, C-Reactive Protein and Metabolic Markers in Zinc-Deficient Diabetic Patients on Hemodialysis: A Randomized, Double-Blind, Placebo-Controlled Trial. *Biol. Trace Elem. Res.* **2022**, *200*, 76–83. [CrossRef] [PubMed]
16. Brodersen, H.-P.; Holtkamp, W.; Larbig, D.; Beckers, B.; Thiery, J.; Lautenschläger, J.; Probst, H.-J.; Ropertz, S.; Yavari, A. Zinc supplementation and hepatitis B vaccination in chronic haemodialysis patients: A multicentre study. *Nephrol. Dial. Transpl.* **1995**, *10*, 1780.
17. Jern, N.A.; Vanbeber, A.D.; Gorman, M.A.; Weber, C.G.; Liepa, G.U.; Cochran, C.C. The effects of zinc supplementation on serum zinc concentration and protein catabolic rate in hemodialysis patients. *J. Ren. Nutr.* **2000**, *10*, 148–153. [CrossRef]
18. Candan, F.; Gültekin, F.; Candan, F. Effect of vitamin C and zinc on osmotic fragility and lipid peroxidation in zinc-deficient haemodialysis patients. *Cell Biochem. Funct.* **2002**, *20*, 95–98. [CrossRef]
19. Chevalier, C.A.; Liepa, G.; Murphy, M.D.; Suneson, J.; VanBeber, A.D.; Gorman, M.A.; Cochran, C. The effects of zinc supplementation on serum zinc and cholesterol concentrations in hemodialysis patients. *J. Ren. Nutr.* **2002**, *12*, 183–189. [CrossRef]
20. Rashidi, A.A.; Salehi, M.; Piroozmand, A.; Sagheb, M.M. Effects of zinc supplementation on serum zinc and C-reactive protein concentrations in hemodialysis patients. *J. Ren. Nutr.* **2009**, *19*, 475–478. [CrossRef]
21. Roozbeh, J.; Hedayati, P.; Sagheb, M.M.; Sharifian, M.; Jahromi, A.H.; Shaabani, S.; Jalaeian, H.; Raeisjalali, G.A.; Behzadi, S. Effect of zinc supplementation on triglyceride, cholesterol, LDL, and HDL levels in zinc-deficient hemodialysis patients. *Ren. Fail.* **2009**, *31*, 798–801. [CrossRef] [PubMed]

22. Rahimi-Ardabili, B.; Argani, H.; Ghorbanihaghjo, A.; Rashtchizadeh, N.; Naghavi-Behzad, M.; Ghorashi, S.; Nezami, N. Paraoxonase enzyme activity is enhanced bey zinc supplementation in hemodialysis patients. *Ren. Fail.* **2012**, *34*, 1123–1128. [CrossRef] [PubMed]
23. Pakfetrat, M.; Shahroodi, J.R.; Zolgadr, A.A.; Larie, H.A.; Nikoo, M.H.; Malekmakan, L. Effects of zinc supplement on plasma homocysteine level in end-stage renal disease patients: A double-blind randomized clinical trial. *Biol. Trace Elem. Res.* **2013**, *153*, 11–15. [CrossRef] [PubMed]
24. Mazani, M.; Argani, H.; Rashtchizadeh, N.; Ghorbanihaghjo, A.; Hamdi, A.; Estiar, M.A.; Nezami, N. Effects of zinc supplementation on antioxidant status and lipid peroxidation in hemodialysis patients. *J. Ren. Nutr.* **2013**, *23*, 180–184. [CrossRef] [PubMed]
25. Guo, C.H.; Wang, C.L. Effects of zinc supplementation on plasma copper/zinc ratios, oxidative stress, and immunological status in hemodialysis patients. *Int. J. Med. Sci.* **2013**, *10*, 79–89. [CrossRef] [PubMed]
26. Argani, H.; Mahdavi, R.; Ghorbani-Haghjo, A.; Razzaghi, R.; Nikniaz, L.; Gaemmaghami, S.J. Effects of zinc supplementation on serum zinc and leptin levels, BMI, and body composition in hemodialysis patients. *J. Trace Elem. Med. Biol.* **2014**, *28*, 35–38. [CrossRef] [PubMed]
27. Sherbini, N.S.; El-Shazly, A.N.; Elhady, S.A.; El-Mashad, G.M.; Sabry, J.H. Effect of zinc supplementation on body mass index and serum levels of zinc and leptin in pediatric hemodialysis patients. *Int. J. Nephrol. Renov. Dis.* **2015**, *8*, 159–163. [CrossRef]
28. Sato, E.; Sato, S.; Degawa, M.; Ono, T.; Lu, H.; Matsumura, D.; Nomura, M.; Moriyama, N.; Amaha, M.; Nakamura, T. Effects of Zinc Acetate Hydrate Supplementation on Renal Anemia with Hypozincemia in Hemodialysis Patients. *Toxins* **2022**, *14*, 746. [CrossRef]
29. Kodama, H.; Asagiri, M.; Etani, Y.; Koyama, H.; Soh, H.; Ida, S.; Tanaka, Y.; Takayanagi, M.; Funakoshi, M.; Yoshida, M. Clinical guidelines for selenium deficiency. *J. Jpn. Soc. Clin. Nutr.* **2019**, *40*, 239–283.
30. Mochizuki, H.; Yokota, S.; Kaneko, K.; Koh, H.; Ishi, J.; Katsuta, M. A case of SEP complicated with dilated cardiomyopathy probably due to selenium deficiency. *J. Jpn. Soc. Dial. Ther.* **2001**, *34*, 1095–1099. [CrossRef]
31. Nishida, H.; Abe, H.; Iida, Y.; Toriyama, C. A case of left ventricular hypofunction due to selenium-arginine depletion associated with short bowel syndrome and dialysis. *Jpn. J. Intern. Med.* **2016**, *106*, 828–833.
32. Fujishima, Y.; Ohsawa, M.; Itai, K.; Kato, K.; Tanno, K.; Turin, T.C.; Onoda, T.; Endo, S.; Okayama, A.; Fujioka, T. Serum selenium levels are inversely associated with death risk among hemodialysis patients. *Transplant* **2011**, *26*, 3331–3338. [CrossRef] [PubMed]
33. Fujishima, Y.; Ohsawa, M.; Itai, K.; Kato, K.; Tanno, K.; Turin, T.C.; Onoda, T.; Endo, S.; Okayama, A.; Fujioka, T. Serum selenium levels in hemodialysis patients are significantly lower than those in healthy controls. *Blood Purif.* **2011**, *32*, 43–47. [CrossRef] [PubMed]
34. Tonelli, M.; Wiebe, N.; Bello, A.; Field, C.J.; Gill, J.S.; Hemmelgarn, B.R.; Holmes, D.T.; Jindal, K.; Klarenbach, S.W.; Manns, B.J.; et al. Concentrations of Trace Elements and Clinical Outcomes in Hemodialysis Patients: A Prospective Cohort Study. *Clin. J. Am. Soc. Nephrol.* **2018**, *13*, 907–915. [CrossRef] [PubMed]
35. Ruiz, A.A.; Jiménez, E.M.; Bermejo-Barrera, P.; Lozano, R.; Seijas, V.M.-E. Selenium and All-cause Mortality in End-Stage Renal Disease. Retrospective Observational Cohort Study. *J. Ren. Nutr.* **2020**, *30*, 484–492. [CrossRef] [PubMed]
36. Zhang, J.; Taylor, E.W.; Bennett, K.; Saad, R.; Rayman, M.P. Association between regional selenium status and reported outcome of COVID-19 cases in China. *Am. J. Clin. Nutr.* **2020**, *111*, 1297–1299. [CrossRef] [PubMed]
37. Li, S.; Tang, T.; Guo, P.; Zou, Q.; Ao, X.; Hu, L.; Tan, L. A meta-analysis of randomized controlled trials: Efficacy of selenium treatment for sepsis. *Medicine* **2019**, *98*, e14733. [CrossRef] [PubMed]
38. Saint-Georges, M.D.; Bonnefont, D.J.; Bourely, B.A.; Jaudon, M.C.; Cereze, P.; Chaumeil, P.; Gard, C.; D'Auzac, C.L. Correction of selenium deficiency in hemodialyzed patients. *Kidney Int. Suppl.* **1989**, *27*, S274–S277.
39. Atakan, A.; Macunluoglu, B.; Kaya, Y.; Ari, E.; Demir, H.; Asicioglu, E.; Kaspar, C. Decreased serum selenium levels are correlated with diminished coronary flow reserve among hemodialysis patients. *Biol. Trace Elem. Res.* **2013**, *155*, 333–338. [CrossRef]
40. Yasukawa, M.; Arai, S.; Nagura, M.; Kido, R.; Asakawa, S.; Hirohama, D.; Yamazaki, O.; Tamura, Y.; Fujimaki, M.; Kobayashi, S.; et al. Selenium Associates with Response to Erythropoiesis-Stimulating Agents in Hemodialysis Patients. *Kidney Int. Rep.* **2022**, *7*, 1565–1574. [CrossRef]
41. Xu, S.; Zou, D.; Tang, R.; Li, S.; Chen, W.; Wen, L.; Liu, Y.; Liu, Y.; Zhong, X. Levels of trace blood elements associated with severe sleep disturbance in maintenance hemodialysis patients. *Sleep Breath* **2021**, *25*, 2007–2013. [CrossRef]
42. Richard, M.J.; Ducros, V.; Forêt, M.; Arnaud, J.; Coudray, C.; Fusselier, M.; Favier, A. Reversal of selenium and zinc deficiencies in chronic hemodialysis patients by intravenous sodium selenite and zinc gluconate supplementation. *Biol. Trace Elem. Res.* **1993**, *39*, 149–159. [CrossRef] [PubMed]
43. Napolitano, G.; Bonomini, M.; Bomba, G.; Bucci, I.; Todisco, V.; Albertazzi, A.; Monaco, F. Thyroid function and plasma selenium in chronic uremic patients on hemodialysis treatment. *Biol. Trace Elem. Res.* **1996**, *55*, 221–230. [CrossRef] [PubMed]
44. Koenig, J.; Fischer, M.; Bulant, E.; Tiran, B.; Elmadfa, I.; Druml, W. Antioxidant status in patients on chronic hemodialysis therapy: Impact of parenteral selenium supplementation. *Wien. Klin. Wochenschr.* **1997**, *109*, 13–19. [PubMed]
45. Temple, K.A.; Smith, A.M.; Cockram, D.B. Selenate-supplemented nutritional formula increases plasma selenium in hemodialysis patients. *J. Ren. Nutr.* **2000**, *10*, 16–23. [CrossRef]

46. Zachara, B.A.; Koterska, D.; Manitius, J.; Sadowski, L.; Dziedziczko, A.; Salak, A.; Wasowicz, W. Selenium supplementation on plasma glutathione peroxidase activity in patients with end-stage chronic renal failure. *Biol. Trace Elem. Res.* **2004**, *97*, 15–30. [CrossRef]
47. Salehi, M.; Sohrabi, Z.; Ekramzadeh, M.; Fallahzadeh, M.K.; Ayatollahi, M.; Geramizadeh, B.; Hassanzadeh, J.; Sagheb, M.M. Selenium supplementation improves the nutritional status of hemodialysis patients: A randomized, double-blind, placebo-controlled trial. *Nephrol. Dial. Transpl.* **2013**, *28*, 716–721. [CrossRef]
48. Tonelli, M.; Network, F.T.A.K.D.; Wiebe, N.; Thompson, S.; Kinniburgh, D.; Klarenbach, S.W.; Walsh, M.; Bello, A.K.; Faruque, L.; Field, C.; et al. Alberta Kidney Disease Network. Trace element supplementation in hemodialysis patients: A randomized controlled trial. *BMC Nephrol.* **2015**, *16*, 52. [CrossRef]
49. Shahreki, E.; Kaykhaei, M.A.; Mosallanezhad, Z.; Adineh, Z.; Mokhtari, A.M.; Mohammadi, M.; Hosseini, R.; Bazi, A. Effects of Selenium and/or N-Acetyl-Cysteine Supplementation on Nonthyroidal Illness Syndrome in Hemodialysis Patients: A Factorial Randomized Controlled Trial. *Pharmacology* **2022**, *107*, 480–485. [CrossRef]
50. Salimian, M.; Soleimani, A.; Bahmani, F.; Tabatabaei, S.M.H.; Asemi, Z.; Talari, H.R. The effects of selenium administration on carotid intima-media thickness and metabolic status in diabetic hemodialysis patients: A randomized, double-blind, placebo-controlled trial. *Clin. Nutr. ESPEN* **2022**, *47*, 58–62. [CrossRef]
51. Atapour, A.; Vahdat, S.; Hosseini, M.; Mohamadian, H. Effect of Selenium on Triglyceride and Total Cholesterol, Weight Gain, and Physical Activity on Hemodialysis Patients: A Randomized Double-Blinded Controlled Trial. *Int. J. Prev. Med.* **2022**, *13*, 63. [PubMed]
52. Hurst, R.; Armah, C.N.; Dainty, J.R.; Hart, D.J.; Teucher, B.; Goldson, A.J.; Broadley, M.R.; Motley, A.K.; Fairweather-Tait, S.J. Establishing optimal selenium status: Results of a randomized, double-blind, placebo-controlled trial. *Am. J. Clin. Nutr.* **2010**, *91*, 923–931. [CrossRef] [PubMed]
53. Takahashi, A. Role of Zinc and Copper in Erythropoiesis in Patients on Hemodialysis. *J. Ren. Nutr.* **2022**, *32*, 650–657. [CrossRef] [PubMed]
54. Higuchi, T.; Matsukawa, Y.; Okada, K.; Oikawa, O.; Yamazaki, T.; Ohnishi, Y.; Fujita, T.; Fukuda, N.; Soma, M.; Matsumoto, K. Correction of copper deficiency improves erythropoietin unresponsiveness in hemodialysis patients with anemia. *Intern. Med.* **2006**, *45*, 271–273. [CrossRef] [PubMed]
55. Gaetke, L.M.; Chow-Johnson, H.S.; Chow, C.K. Copper: Toxicological relevance and mechanisms. *Arch. Toxicol.* **2014**, *88*, 1929–1938. [CrossRef] [PubMed]
56. Guo, C.-H.; Chen, P.-C.; Yeh, M.-S.; Hsiung, D.-Y.; Wang, C.-L. Cu/Zn ratios are associated with nutritional status, oxidative stress, inflammation, and immune abnormalities in patients on peritoneal dialysis. *Clin. Biochem.* **2011**, *44*, 275–280. [CrossRef] [PubMed]
57. Feldman, L.; Beberashvili, I.; Hamad, R.A.; Yakov-Hai, I.; Abramov, E.; Wasser, W.; Gorelik, O.; Rozenberg, R.; Efrati, S. Serum Chromium Levels Are Higher in Peritoneal Dialysis than in Hemodialysis Patients. *Perit. Dial. Int.* **2019**, *39*, 330–334. [CrossRef]
58. Jomova, K.; Valko, M. Advances in metal-induced oxidative stress and human disease. *Toxicology* **2011**, *283*, 65–87. [CrossRef]
59. Hsu, C.-W.; Weng, C.-H.; Lee, C.-C.; Yen, T.-H.; Huang, W.-H. Association of serum chromium levels with malnutrition in hemodialysis patients. *BMC Nephrol.* **2019**, *20*, 302. [CrossRef]
60. Tonelli, M.; Wiebe, N.; Hemmelgarn, B.; Klarenbach, S.; Field, C.; Manns, B.; Thadhani, R.; Gill, J. Alberta Kidney Disease Network. Trace elements in hemodialysis patients: A systematic review and meta-analysis. *BMC Med.* **2009**, *7*, 25. [CrossRef]
61. Aschner, J.L.; Aschner, M. Nutritional aspects of manganese homeostasis. *Mol. Aspects Med.* **2005**, *26*, 353–362. [CrossRef] [PubMed]
62. Keen, C.; Zidenburg-Cherr, S. *Encyclopedia of Food Science, Food Technology, and Nutrition*; Academic Press: London, UK, 1993.
63. Tonelli, M.; Wiebe, N.; Bello, A.; Field, C.J.; Gill, J.S.; Hemmelgarn, B.R.; Holmes, D.T.; Jindal, K.; Klarenbach, S.W.; Manns, B.J.; et al. Alberta Kidney Disease Network. Concentrations of Trace Elements in Hemodialysis Patients: A Prospective Cohort Study. *Am. J. Kidney Dis.* **2017**, *70*, 696–704. [CrossRef]
64. Gómez de Oña, C.; Martínez-Morillo, E.; Gago González, E.; Vidau Argüelles, P.; Fernández Merayo, C.; Álvarez Menéndez, F.V. Variation of trace element concentrations in patients undergoing hemodialysis in the north of Spain. *Scand. J. Clin. Lab. Invest.* **2016**, *76*, 492–499. [CrossRef] [PubMed]
65. Liu, Y.; Hu, J.; Tang, R.; Guo, H.; Chen, Q.; Qiu, J.; Liu, Y.; Tan, R.; Zhong, X. Association between the blood manganese (Mn) and hemoglobin in patients undergoing maintenance hemodialysis. *J. Trace Elem. Med. Biol.* **2022**, *71*, 126947. [CrossRef]
66. Vignoli, A.; Tenori, L.; Luchinat, C. An omics approach to study trace metals in sera of hemodialysis patients treated with erythropoiesis stimulating agents. *Metallomics* **2022**, *14*, mfac028. [CrossRef] [PubMed]
67. Chen, J.; Peng, H.; Zhang, K.; Xiao, L.; Yuan, Z.; Chen, J.; Wang, Z.; Wang, J.; Huang, H. The insufficiency intake of dietary micronutrients associated with malnutrition-inflammation score in hemodialysis population. *PLoS ONE* **2013**, *8*, e66841. [CrossRef] [PubMed]
68. Lin, J.L.; Lin-Tan, D.T.; Hsu, C.W.; Yen, T.H.; Chen, K.H.; Hsu, H.H.; Ho, T.C.; Hsu, K.H. Association of blood lead levels with mortality in patients on maintenance hemodialysis. *Am. J. Med.* **2011**, *124*, 350–358. [CrossRef] [PubMed]
69. Lin, J.L.; Lin-Tan, D.T.; Chen, K.H.; Hsu, C.W.; Yen, T.H.; Huang, W.H.; Huang, Y.L. Blood lead levels association with 18-month all-cause mortality in patients with chronic peritoneal dialysis. *Nephrol. Dial. Transplant.* **2010**, *25*, 1627–1633. [CrossRef]
70. Feldman, R.G. Urban lead mining: Lead intoxication among deleaders. *N. Engl. J. Med.* **1978**, *298*, 1143–1145. [CrossRef]

71. Thomson, R.M.; Parry, G.J. Neuropathies associated with excessive exposure to lead. *Muscle Nerve* **2006**, *33*, 732–741. [CrossRef]
72. Huang, W.H.; Hu, C.C.; Yen, T.H.; Hsu, C.W.; Weng, C.H. Blood lead level: An overlooked risk of carpal tunnel syndrome in hemodialysis patients. *Ren. Fail.* **2019**, *41*, 786–793. [CrossRef] [PubMed]
73. Danziger, J.; Mukamal, K.J.; Weinhandl, E. Associations of Community Water Lead Concentrations with Hemoglobin Concentrations and Erythropoietin-Stimulating Agent Use among Patients with Advanced CKD. *J. Am. Soc. Nephrol.* **2021**, *32*, 2425–2434. [CrossRef]
74. Lu, K.C.; Wu, C.C.; Ma, W.Y.; Chen, C.C.; Wu, H.C.; Chu, P. Decreased blood lead levels after calcitriol treatment in hemodialysis patients with secondary hyperparathyroidism. *Bone* **2011**, *49*, 1306–1310. [CrossRef] [PubMed]
75. Ford, M.; Goldfrank, L.; Flomenbaum, N.; Lewin, N.; Howland, M.; Hoffman, R.; Nelson, L. (Eds.) Arsenic. In *Goldfrank's Toxicological Emergencies*; McGraw-Hill: New York, NY, USA, 2002; pp. 1183–1199.
76. Schoen, A.; Beck, B.; Sharma, R.; Dube, E. Arsenic toxicity at low doses: Epidemiological and mode of action considerations. *Toxicol, Appl, Pharmacol.* **2004**, *198*, 253–267. [CrossRef] [PubMed]
77. Morton, W.E.; Caron, G.A. Encephalopathy: An uncommon manifestation of workplace arsenic poisoning? *Am. J. Ind. Med.* **1989**, *15*, 1–5. [CrossRef] [PubMed]
78. Xiang, S.; Jin, Q.; Xu, F.; Yao, Y.; Liang, W.; Zuo, X.; Ye, T.; Ying, C. High serum arsenic and cardiovascular risk factors in patients undergoing continuous ambulatory peritoneal dialysis. *J. Trace Elem. Med. Biol.* **2019**, *52*, 1–5. [CrossRef]
79. Ochi, A.; Ishimura, E.; Tsujimoto, Y.; Kakiya, R.; Tabata, T.; Mori, K.; Shoji, T.; Yasuda, H.; Nishizawa, Y.; Inaba, M. Trace elements in the hair of hemodialysis patients. *Biol. Trace Elem. Res.* **2011**, *143*, 825–834. [CrossRef] [PubMed]
80. Navarro, J.A.; Granadillo, V.A.; Salgado, O.; Rodríguez-Iturbe, B.; García, R.; Delling, G.; Romero, R.A. Bone metal content in patients with chronic renal failure. *Clin. Chim. Acta* **1992**, *211*, 133–142. [CrossRef]
81. Oruc, M.; Mercan, S.; Bakan, S.; Kose, S.; Ikitimur, B.; Trabulus, S.; Altiparmak, M.R. Do trace elements play a role in coronary artery calcification in hemodialysis patients? *Int. Urol. Nephrol.* **2023**, *55*, 173–182. [CrossRef]
82. Katko, M.; Kiss, I.; Karpati, I.; Kadar, A.; Matyus, J.; Csongradi, E.; Posta, J.; Paragh, G.; Balla, J.; Kovacs, B.; et al. Relationship between serum nickel and homocysteine concentration in hemodialysis patients. *Biol. Trace. Elem. Res.* **2008**, *124*, 195–205. [CrossRef]
83. Schrooten, I.; Elseviers, M.M.; Lamberts, L.V.; De Broe, M.E.; D'Haese, P.C. Increased serum strontium levels in dialysis patients: An epidemiological survey. *Kidney Int.* **1999**, *56*, 1886–1892. [CrossRef]
84. D'Haese, P.C.; Schrooten, I.; Goodman, W.G.; Cabrera, W.E.; Lamberts, L.V.; Elseviers, M.M.; Couttenye, M.M.; De Broe, M.E. Increased bone strontium levels in hemodialysis patients with osteomalacia. *Kidney Int.* **2000**, *57*, 1107–1114. [CrossRef] [PubMed]

Disclaimer/Publisher's Note: The statements, opinions and data contained in all publications are solely those of the individual author(s) and contributor(s) and not of MDPI and/or the editor(s). MDPI and/or the editor(s) disclaim responsibility for any injury to people or property resulting from any ideas, methods, instructions or products referred to in the content.

Review

Chronic Kidney Disease—Mineral and Bone Disorder (CKD-MBD), from Bench to Bedside

Kosaku Nitta [1,*], Norio Hanafusa [2], Kenichi Akiyama [1], Yuki Kawaguchi [2] and Ken Tsuchiya [2]

1. Department of Nephrology, Tokyo Women's Medical University, Tokyo 162-8666, Japan
2. Department of Blood Purification, Tokyo Women's Medical University, Tokyo 162-8666, Japan
* Correspondence: knitta@twmu.ac.jp

Abstract: Chronic kidney disease—mineral and bone disorder (CKD-MBD) is a systemic disorder that increases the risk of morbidity and mortality in dialysis patients. CKD-MBD is highly prevalent in dialysis patients, and appropriate treatment is important for improving their outcomes. Inorganic phosphate, fibroblast growth factor 23, parathyroid hormone, and calciprotein particles are markers for critical components and effectors of CKD-MBD, and higher circulating levels of these markers are linked to cardiovascular diseases. In this short review, we focus on the pathogenesis and management of CKD-MBD in CKD patients, especially those on dialysis therapy, and discuss the prospects for improving the management in CKD patients, including those on dialysis.

Keywords: CKD-MBD; hemodialysis; phosphate; cakciprotein particle; vascular calcification; mortality

1. Introduction

Abnormalities of bone and mineral metabolism in patients with chronic kidney disease (CKD) were previously regarded as a disorder of the bones and parathyroid glands [1]. However, these abnormalities are now recognized as a systemic disorder that affects a wide variety of systems, including cardiovascular (CV) organs, and is referred to as CKD—mineral and bone disorder (MBD) [2,3]. Abnormal serum levels of phosphate (P), calcium (Ca), and parathyroid hormone (PTH) are associated with increased risk of morbidity and mortality in hemodialysis (HD) patients [4], and various evidence has confirmed that hyperphosphatemia is closely related to higher risk of CV events and death [5]. A growing body of evidence has recently shown that increased serum fibroblast growth factor (FGF)-23 levels are associated with left ventricular hypertrophy, vascular calcification (VC), infection, anemia, and inflammation in HD patients [6]. Because serum levels of PTH and FGF-23 are increased in response to phosphate loading, lowering serum P and reducing P loading is crucial in the management of CKD-MBD in HD patients [7].

CKD-MBD involves biochemical abnormalities, bone disorders, and VC, all of which can cause CV events, bone fractures, and other serious complications, ultimately leading to death in CKD patients, including those on dialysis [2,3]. Notably, the concept of CKD-MBD continues to develop and the scope of this disorder is expanding to encompass a wide range of diseases, due to advances in our understanding of the pathogenesis of CKD-MBD.

2. P Imbalance and CKD-MBD

The control of serum P is recognized to be important in the treatment of CKD-MBD because of both the role of P overload in the development of the disorder and the independent association between hyperphosphatemia and CV disease (CVD) [8]. Good management of P metabolism likely reduces the risk of VC [9], secondary hyperparathyroidism (SHPT) [10], and decreased FGF-23 production [11], thus slowing the progression of CKD-MBD and reducing CV mortality risk. However, an obstacle to effective P control for the treatment of CKD-MBD is the lack of P management strategies that can be used to maintain P concentrations within the normal range of <5.5 mg/dL, in dialysis patients [3].

Phosphate binders (PBs) have recently been used as a pharmacological treatment for hyperphosphatemia. However, PBs bind only a portion of dietary phosphate and require patients to take many pills with meals [12,13]. In addition, proper adherence to PBs is challenging [14]. The effectiveness of PBs and dietary P restriction are further limited by maladaptive upregulation of P absorption [15,16].

New strategies for P management should take into account the latest understanding of P adsorption, namely, that the paracellular P absorption pathway is the dominant route of intestinal P absorption [17]. A novel P absorption inhibitor, tenapanor, has recently been developed. It directly targets the intestinal sodium/hydrogen exchanger isoform 3 (NHE3), leading to reduced sodium absorption [18]. In clinical trials, tenapanor has also been shown to reduce serum P concentrations and to be generally well tolerated [19,20]. It may offer a novel treatment approach for CKD-MBD.

3. CKD-MBD: As a Risk Factor for CV Mortality

CKD-MBD is a common comorbidity and a main cause of CV mortality in patients on dialysis [2]. Along with declines in kidney function, progressive disruption in Ca and P metabolism is associated with abnormalities in circulating hormone concentrations such as PTH and FGF-23 and decreases in calcitriol (Figure 1) [21].

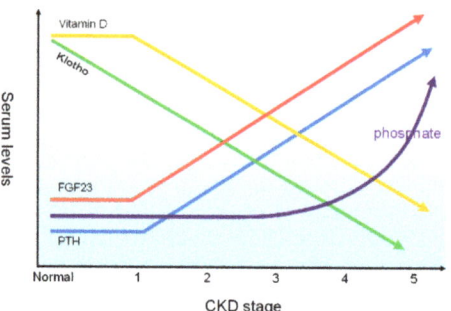

Figure 1. Changes in biochemical markers of MBD during the progression of CKD. Reproduced with permission from John, GB et al., Am J Kidney Dis, published by Elsevier, 2011.

Various components of CKD-MBD such as hyperphosphatemia, VC, and elevated FGF-23 concentrations are known to be significantly associated with increased CV morbidity and mortality [3]. CVD accounted for 45% of deaths among Japanese dialysis patients in 2021 [22]. Traditional risk factors for CV mortality, such as hypertension and diabetes, do not explain the higher CV morbidity and mortality in dialysis patients [23], and established treatment strategies for these risk factors have not seen significant advancements. Better control of P may be necessary to improve clinical outcomes and quality of life in dialysis patients and reduce mortality risk [24].

Therapeutic approaches for CKD-MBD that may decrease CV mortality include improving dialysis modalities [25], decreasing inflammation [26], and better managing serum P concentrations [27]. In particular, hyperphosphatemia is a major modifiable target [28]. An abnormal P concentration has been identified as an independent risk factor for CV morbidity and mortality in dialysis patients [29]. A linear correlation has been found between progression of coronary calcification and increasing serum P concentrations [30].

4. The Pathogenesis and Associations of VC with CKD-MBD

Among the three components of CKD-MBD, VC has recently been in the spotlight, with various research seeking to clarify its pathogenesis in CKD patients [31]. VC is a common complication in CKD patients and is associated with increased CV morbidity and mortality [32,33]. VC was previously regarded as a passive and degenerative process of Ca deposition in the vessel wall, but it is now recognized as an actively regulated cellular process [34]. Table 1 shows the risk factors for VC in dialysis patients. Over the past decade, basic research has revealed that VC is mediated by complex cellular mechanisms including transdifferentiation of vascular smooth muscle cells (VSMCs) into osteoblast-like cells, apoptosis of VSMCs, degradation of the extracellular matrix, formation and release of calcifying matrix vesicles, and formation and maturation of calciprotein particles (CPPs) [35]. Among these factors, CPPs have attracted research interest in the fields of nephrology and CKD-MBD and are now suggested to be a critical mediator of VC [36,37]. CPPs contain Ca, inorganic P, fetuin-A, and other proteins and increase in response to an increasing P and Ca burden, inducing inflammatory responses in leukocytes, monocytes, renal tubular cells, and VSMCs (Figure 2) [37,38]. When VSMCs are exposed to high CPP conditions, CPPs enter the intracellular space through scavenger receptor A or act on the cells through certain Toll-like receptors and induce intracellular Ca overload, resulting in apoptosis, altered autophagy, and calcification of the extracellular matrix [39,40]. CPPs are now considered one of the strong drivers for uremic VC.

Table 1. Risk factors for vascular calcification.

Clinical	<ul><li>Age</li><li>Duration of Dialysis</li><li>Kidney Function/Uremia</li><li>Diabetes</li><li>Known Coronary Artery Disease</li><li>Abnormal Bone</li></ul>
Biochemical	<ul><li>Hyperphosphatemia</li><li>Hypercalcemia</li><li>High Parathyroid Hormone</li><li>Low Fetuin-A</li><li>Increased Aldosterone</li><li>Oxidative Stress</li><li>Low Pyrophosphate</li><li>Decreased MGP</li><li>Decreased BMP-7</li></ul>
Medications	<ul><li>Calcium-Containing Phosphate Binders</li><li>High-Dose Vitamin D</li><li>Coumadin (Decreases Active MGP)</li></ul>

MGP, matrix Gla protein; BMP, bone morphogenic protein.

For VC, another important consideration is imbalance between inducers and inhibitors of calcification. In CKD, inducers of calcification such as P and Ca loading are accumulated, while calcification inhibitors such as fetuin-A, pyrophosphate, and magnesium (Mg) are decreased in the circulation, thereby accelerating the VC process [41].

Unfortunately, treatment of VC remains challenging in the clinical settings. However, basic studies have provided some ideas for preventing progression of VC in CKD patients. In an experimental study, dietary P restriction or treatment with PBs prevented or halted the progression of uremic VC [42]. Oxidative stress, which is high in CKD patients, including the dialysis population, plays an important role in the pathogenesis of VC, and treatment with antioxidants slows the progression of VC in uremic rodents [43]. Mg ions, which were recently reassessed as a potentially attractive therapeutic option in CKD, inhibited the formation and maturation of CPPs and prevented inflammation and VC in CKD [44]. VC is considered a largely irreversible biochemical phenomenon, so it is very difficult to achieve regression of VC once it has formed in the blood vessel wall, although some therapeutic interventions have been reported to reverse VC [45]. Therefore, at present, prevention of VC is a reasonable and feasible strategy in CKD patients, including dialysis population.

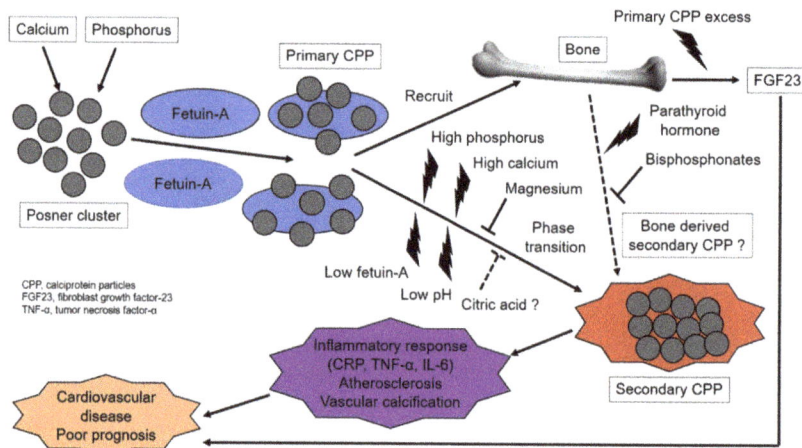

Figure 2. Role of CPP in CKD-MBD.

5. Biomarkers of CKD-MBD Assessment

With progression of CKD, the glomerular filtration rate is reduced, leading to P retention [46]. In earlier CKD stages, PTH and FGF-23 concentrations steadily increase, while P concentrations are stable [22]. Abnormalities in mineral metabolism (e.g., SHPT, decreased vitamin D) are seen in CKD patients before hyperphosphatemia develops [47]. Increased PTH [48,49], increased FGF-23 [50], hypocalcemia [51], and low vitamin D concentrations [52] have all been found to be associated with increased risk of CVD. Inhibition of calcitriol production due to increased FGF-23 [53] has been associated with coronary artery calcification [54] and myocardial fibrosis [55].

In CKD stages 4 and 5, P concentrations begin to increase despite the elevations in FGF-23 and PTH levels, indicating that compensatory mechanisms are no longer sufficient to maintain P balance and prevent hyperphosphatemia [22]. CKD patients with poorly managed P metabolism have almost 30% greater mortality risk than those who achieve and continuously maintain normal P concentration [5]. In addition, hyperphosphatemia is directly linked to hypertension, a major CVD risk factor present in up to 90% of CKD patients [56]. Therefore, P control has the potential to be a major therapeutic target for reducing mortality in CKD patients.

FGF-23 and PTH concentrations are key regulators of P metabolism and their concentrations increase in response to P retention [57,58]. Elevated FGF-23 concentrations are the earliest mineral metabolism abnormality observed in CKD patients [22]. P retention stimulates progressive increases in FGF-23 concentrations [53]., which directly target the heart to promote left ventricular hypertrophy and congestive heart failure [59]. Higher FGF-23 concentrations are independently associated with a greater risk of CV events, particularly congestive heart failure [50]. Elevated PTH concentrations are associated with various negative effects including increased bone resorption [60], decreased cardiac index and mean arterial pressure via impaired myocardial energy production [61], and genesis of cardiac fibrosis [62].

6. Management of CKD-MBD

CKD-MBD is a multifactorial disease. Despite of the great efforts to improve the management of patients with CKD-MBD, several unmet needs still remain. The management of CKD-MBD is based on several strategies to prevent the adverse complications associated with SHPT. The current KDIGO guideline recommends treatment of SHPT based on repeated measures of the biochemical markers including serum P, Ca and PTH [63]. Abnormal P/Ca metabolism is a major characteristic of CKD-MBD, which is associated with clinically significant VC and increased mortality risk [3]. In Japan, the target range of serum Ca concentrations was decided according to the results of an analysis of data from the Japanese Society for Dialysis Therapy (JSDT) patient registry, which collected data on patients treated in accordance with the 2008 JSDT guideline [64].

After the 2008 JSDT guideline was issued [64], awareness of CKD-MBD increased in Japan, and new drugs have been considered for the treatment of CKD-MBD, such as cinacalcet hydrochloride, lanthanum carbonate and iron-containing PBs.

Based on the analysis of data from 128,125 dialysis patients who could be monitored from the end of 2006 to the end of 2009 [4], the target range for serum P range was set at 3.5–6.0 mg/dL. The dialysis serum P range was set at 3.5–5.5 mg/dL in the KDOQI clinical practice guideline, while the 2009 CKD-MBD KDIGO guidelines [3] recommended that the serum P concentration be lowered if higher than the reference level.

The target range for serum Ca concentration is 8.4–10.0 mg/dL in the JSDT guideline [64]. The KDOQI guideline states that serum Ca levels should be 8.4–9.5 mg/dL, while KDIGO guidelines states that the target should be within the normal range [3].

The JSDT guideline clearly recommends that control of serum P should be given the highest priority, followed by control of serum Ca, and then PTH. Previous studies have shown that prognosis is improved more by appropriate control of serum P and Ca levels compared with control of PTH alone [65–67]. In Japan, the serum levels of P and corrected Ca should be controlled first, and then the dose of vitamin D receptor activators (VDRAs) or cinacalcet hydrochloride should be adjusted to maintain serum PTH levels within the target range (60–240 pm/mL).

Various PBs are available and can be used when tailored to individual patients (Table 2). When PBs are prescribed, patient adherence must be confirmed. Moreover, it is important to bear in mind that certain drugs are more effective when taken at specific times. For instance, sevelamer hydrochloride, bixalomer and sucroferric oxyhydrate (SFOH) should be taken before a meal, and $CaCO_3$, lanthanum carbonate and ferric citrate hydrate (FCH) should be taken immediately after a meal.

Drugs for CKD-MBD-related drugs should be considered from perspective of not only serum P/Ca control but also prognosis. A number of observational cohort studies of dialysis patients indicate that administration of VDRA is associated with lower all-cause and CV mortality risk, independent of control of serum P, Ca, or PTH levels [68–72]. One the options for SHPT treatment is to combine low-dose VDRAs with calcimimetics [73].

Cinacalcet hydrochloride is expected to prevent progression of VC and improve prognosis because it can simultaneously lower serum P/Ca/PTH levels. Analysis of the combined results of four safety survey studies showed that the risk for vascular disease-related hospitalization was reduced in patients taking cinacalcet hydrochloride [74]. Moreover, a large-scale observational study revealed that cinacalcet hydrochloride was associated with reduced risk all-cause and cardiovascular mortality [75]. Recently, the Evaluation of Cinacalcet HCl Therapy to Lower cardioVascular Events (EVOLVE) study, a double-blind randomized controlled study, showed that cinacalcet hydrochloride did not significantly reduce the risk of death or major CV events in dialysis patients with moderate-to-severe SHPT [76].

Isakova et al. reported that the risk of mortality was lower in patients treated with PBs than in those not treated with PBs [77]. An appropriate upper limit for $CaCO_3$ administration is around 3 g/day, considering the importance of avoiding excessive Ca load [78]. Reduction of $CaCO_3$ should be considered when hypercalcemia is likely to occur, there is marked VC, adynamic bone disease is suspected, or the blood PTH level is constantly low [78]. In addition, switching to Ca-free PBs is reasonable.

Table 2. Comparison of phosphate binders in chronic kidney disease.

Phosphate Binder	Pros	Cons
Calcium-based: calcium acetate calcium carbonate calcium citrate	• Increases calcium and can correct hypocalcemia • Low cost • Moderate pill burden	• Hypercalcemia and/or positive calcium balance • Cardiovascular calcification
Sevelamer-based: sevelamer carbonate sevelamer hydrochloride	• No systemic absorption • Potentially less vascular calcification (calcium-free) • Lowers LDL cholesterol • Improvement in metabolic acidosis with carbonate variant	• Adverse GI effects • High pill burden • High cost • Binds fat-soluble vitamins • Metabolic acidosis with the hydrochloride variant
Iron-based: sucroferric oxyhydroxide	• Lower pill burden • Minimal systemic absorption, no iron overload • Greater efficacy • Increased GI motility which might be beneficial in constipated and PD patients	• High cost
Iron-based: ferric citrate	• Noninferior to sevelamer, well tolerated, beneficial effect on renal anemia	• Systemic absorption with potential for iron overload
Lanthanum carbonate	• Twice as potent as calcium and sevelamer	• High cost • Systemic absorption and potential tissue deposition/toxicity • GI intolerance, nausea • Difficult to chew

GI, gastrointestinal; LDL, low-density lipoprotein; PD, peritoneal dialysis. Reproduced with permission from Rastogi, A. et al., J Ren Nutr, published by Elsevier, 2021.

The tight links among iron deficiency, renal anemia, and CKD-MBD has opened the door to the use of iron-containing PBs with the aim of iron supplementation and subsequent improvement in blood hemoglobin levels, CVD, and survival [79]. Although the efficacy and safety of ferric citrate hydrate (FCH) and sucroferric oxyhydroxide (SFOH) were found to be similar to those of sevelamer, there have been no head-to-head studies with lanthanum carbonate [80,81]. Clinical data for 1 year in a small patient cohort suggested improved adherence with SFOH, and a large randomized controlled trial is now needed to confirm these possible advantages. Cost-effectiveness in comparison with other PBs and the safety of long-term treatment will determine the future use of both FCH and SFOH.

7. Conclusions

CKD-MBD is highly prevalent complication in CKD patients, including those on dialysis, and contribute to increased risk of CV mortality. It is important to understand that P retention triggers increases in CPPs and serum FGF-23 and PTH, but these increases may be associated with CVD. Dietary restriction of P is complicated by inorganic P in food additives, and the use of many medications makes control of P difficult for dialysis patients with CKD-MBD. Dialysis can only remove ~900 to 1200 mg of P per day. PBs, including iron-containing ones, constitute the major pharmacological treatment for hyperphosphatemia and VC. When PBs are insufficient to maintain a normal P concentration, combination of low-dose VDRAs with cinacalcet hydrochloride is useful for treating CKD-MBD in dialysis patients with SHPT. Tenapanor is a novel P absorption inhibitor that acts on the primary absorption pathway, providing a new approach to treating hyperphosphatemia. Further research is necessary to determine whether tenapanor is effective in reducing the CVD risk in dialysis patients.

Author Contributions: K.N. wrote the draft of the manuscript and N.H., Y.K., K.A. and K.T. revised the manuscript. All authors have read and agreed to the published version of the manuscript.

Funding: This research received no external funding.

Institutional Review Board Statement: Not applicable.

Informed Consent Statement: Not applicable.

Data Availability Statement: Not applicable.

Acknowledgments: We would like to express our sincere thanks to all the doctors and medical staff to collect data in Departments of Nephrology and Blood Purification.

Conflicts of Interest: The authors have no conflict of interest to declare.

References

1. Llach, F.; Fernandez, E. Overview of renal bone disease: Causes of treatment failure, clinical observations, the changing pattern of bone lesions, and future therapeutic approach. *Kidney Int. Suppl.* **2003**, *87*, S113–S119. [CrossRef] [PubMed]
2. Moe, S.; Drueke, T.; Cunningham, J.; Goodman, W.; Martin, K.; Olgaard, K.; Ott, S.; Sprague, S.; Lameire, N.; Eknoyan, G.; et al. Definition, evaluation, and classification of renal osteodystrophy: A position statement from Kidney Disease: Improving Global Outcomes (KDIGO). *Kidney Int.* **2006**, *69*, 1945–1953. [CrossRef] [PubMed]
3. Kidney Disease: Improving Global Outcomes (KDIGO) CKDMBD Work Group. KDIGO clinical practice guideline for the diagnosis, evaluation, prevention, and treatment of Chronic Kidney Disease-Mineral and Bone Disorder (CKD-MBD). *Kidney Int. Suppl.* **2009**, *113*, S1–S130.
4. Taniguchi, M.; Fukagawa, M.; Fujii, N.; Hamano, T.; Shoji, T.; Yokoyama, K.; Nakai, S.; Shigematsu, T.; Iseki, K.; Tsubakihara, Y. Serum phosphate and calcium should be primarily and consistently controlled in prevalent hemodialysis patients. *Ther. Apher. Dial.* **2013**, *17*, 221–228. [CrossRef] [PubMed]
5. Block, G.A.; Hulbert-Shearon, T.E.; Levin, N.W.; Port, F.K. Association of serum phosphorus and calcium × phosphate product with mortality risk in chronic hemodialysis patients: A national study. *Am. J. Kidney. Dis.* **1998**, *31*, 607–617. [CrossRef]
6. Richter, B.; Faul, C. FGF23 actions on target tissues-with and without Klotho. *Front. Endocrinol.* **2018**, *2*, 189. [CrossRef]
7. Komaba, H.; Fukagawa, M. Phosphate-a poison for humans? *Kidney Int.* **2016**, *90*, 753–763. [CrossRef]
8. Block, G.A.; Klassen, P.S.; Lazaraus, J.M.; Ofsthun, N.; Lowrie, E.G.; Chertow, G.M. Mineral metabolism, mortality, and morbidity in maintenance hemodialysis. *J. Am. Soc. Nephrol.* **2004**, *15*, 2208–2218. [CrossRef]
9. Raggi, P.; Boulay, A.; Chasan-Taber, S.; Amin, N.; Dillon, M.; Burke, S.K.; Chertow, G.M. Cardiac calcification in adult hemodialysis patients. A link between end-stage renal disease and cardiovascular disease? *J. Am. Coll. Cardiol.* **2002**, *39*, 695–701. [CrossRef]
10. De Francisco, A.L.; Cobo, M.A.; Setien, M.A.; Rodrigo, E.; Fresnedo, G.F.; Unzueta, M.T.; Amado, J.A.; Ruiz, J.C.; Arias, M.; Rodriguez, M. Effect of serum phosphate on parathyroid hormone secretion during hemodialysis. *Kidney Int.* **1998**, *54*, 2140–2145. [CrossRef]
11. Rodelo-Haad, C.; Rodriguez, M.E.; Martin-Malo, A.; VictoriaPendon-Ruiz de Mier, M.; Aguera, M.L.; Munoz-Castaneda, J.R.; Soriano, S.; Caravaca, F.; Alvarez-Lara, M.A.; Felsenfeld, A.; et al. Phosphate control in reducing FGF23 levels in hemodialysis patients. *PLoS ONE* **2018**, *13*, e0201537. [CrossRef]
12. Daugirdas, J.T.; Finn, W.F.; Emmett, M.; Chertow, G.M.; Frequent Hemodialysis Network Trial Group. The phosphate binder equivalent dose. *Semin. Dial.* **2011**, *24*, 41–49. [CrossRef]
13. Martin, P.; Wang, P.; Robinson, A.; Poole, L.; Dragone, J.; Smyth, M.; Pratt, R. Comparison of dietary phosphate absorption after single doses of lanthanum carbonate and sevelamer carbonate in healthy volunteers: A balance study. *Am. J. Kidney Dis.* **2011**, *57*, 700–706. [CrossRef]
14. Chiu, Y.-W.; Teitelbaum, I.; Misra, M.; de Leon, E.M.; Adzize, T.; Mehrotra, R. Pill burden, adherence, hyperphosphatemia, and quality of life in maintenance dialysis patients. *Clin. J. Am. Soc. Nephrol.* **2009**, *4*, 1089–1096. [CrossRef]
15. Giral, H.; Caldas, Y.; Sutherland, E.; Wilson, P.; Breusegem, S.; Barry, N.; Blaine, J.; Jiang, T.; Wang, X.X.; Levi, M. Regulation of rat intestinal Na-dependent phosphate transporters by dietary phosphate. *Am. J. Physiol. Ren. Physiol.* **2009**, *297*, F1466–F1475. [CrossRef]
16. Schiavi, S.C.; Tang, W.; Bracken, C.; O'Brien, S.P.; Song, W.; Boulanger, J.; Ryan, S.; Phillips, L.; Liu, S.; Arbeeny, C.; et al. Npt2b deletion attenuates hyperphosphatemia associated with CKD. *J. Am. Soc. Nephrol.* **2012**, *23*, 1691–1700. [CrossRef]
17. Davis, G.R.; Zerwekh, J.E.; Parker, T.F.; Krejs, G.J.; Pak, C.Y.; Fordtran, J.S. Absorption of phosphate in the jejunum of patients with chronic renal failure before and after correction of vitamin D deficiency. *Gastroenterology* **1983**, *85*, 908–916. [CrossRef]
18. King, A.L.; Siegel, M.; He, Y.; Nie, B.; Wang, J.; Koo-McCoy, S.; Minassian, N.A.; Jafri, Q.; Pan, D.; Kohler, J.; et al. Inhition of sodium/hydrogen exchanger 3 in the gastrointestinal tract by tenapanor reduces paracellular phosphate permeability. *Sci. Transl. Med.* **2018**, *10*, eaam6474.
19. Block, G.A.; Rosenbaum, D.P.; Yan, A.; Chertow, G.M. Efficacy and safety of Tenapanor in patients with hyperphosphatemia receiving maintenance hemodialysis. A randomized phase 3 trial. *J. Am. Soc. Nephrol.* **2019**, *30*, 641–652. [CrossRef]

20. Pergola, P.E.; Rosenbaum, D.P.; Yang, Y.; Chertow, G.M. A randomized trial of Tenapanor and phosphate binders as a dual-mechanism treatment for hyperphosphatemia in patients on maintenance dialysis (AMPLIFY). *J. Am. Soc. Nephrol.* **2012**, *32*, 1465–1473. [CrossRef]
21. Isakova, T.; Wahl, P.; Vargas, G.S.; Gutierrez, O.M.; Scialla, J.; Xie, H.; Appleby, D.; Nessel, L.; Bellovich, K.; Chen, J.; et al. Fibroblast growth factor 23 is elevated before parathyroid hormone and phosphate in chronic kidney disease. *Kidney Int.* **2011**, *79*, 1370–1378. [CrossRef] [PubMed]
22. Nitta, K.; Nakai, S.; Masakane, I.; Hanafusa, N.; Goto, S.; Taniguchi, M.; Hasegawa, T.; Wada, A.; Hamano, T.; Hoshino, J.; et al. Annual dialysis data report of the 2018 JSDT Renal Registry: Dementia, performance status, and exercise habits. *Ren. Replace. Ther.* **2021**, *7*, 41. [CrossRef]
23. Cheung, A.K.; Sarnak, M.J.; Yan, G.; Dwyer, J.T.; Heyka, R.J.; Rocco, M.V.; Teehan, B.P.; Levey, A.S. Atherosclerotic cardiovascular disease risks in chronic hemodialysis patients. *Kidney Int.* **2000**, *58*, 353–362. [CrossRef]
24. Kestenbaum, B.; Sampson, J.N.; Rudser, K.D.; Patterson, D.J.; Seliger, S.L.; Young, B.; Sherrard, D.J.; Andress, D.L. Serum phosphate levels and mortality risk among people with chronic kidney disease. *J. Am. Soc. Nephrol.* **2005**, *16*, 520–528. [CrossRef] [PubMed]
25. Maduell, F.; Moreso, F.; Pons, M.; Ramos, R.; Mora-Macia, J.; Carreras, J.; Soler, J.; Torres, F.; Campistol, J.M.; Matinez-Castelao, A.; et al. High- efficacy postdilution online hemodiafiltration reduces all-cause mortality in hemodialysis patients. *J. Am. Soc. Nephrol.* **2013**, *24*, 487–497. [CrossRef]
26. Panichi, V.; Rizza, G.M.; Paoletti, S.; Bigazzi, R.; Aloisi, M.; Barsotti, G.; Rindi, P.; Donati, G.; Antonelli, A.; Panicucci, E.; et al. Chronic inflammation and mortality in haemodialysis: Effect of different renal replacement therapies. Results from the RISCAVID study. *Nephrol. Dial. Transplant.* **2008**, *23*, 2337–2343. [CrossRef]
27. Lopes, M.B.; Karaboyas, A.; Bieber, B.; Pisoni, R.L.; Walpen, S.; Fukagawa, M.; Christensson, A.; Evenepoel, P.; Pegoraro, M.; Robinson, B.M.; et al. Impact of longer term phosphorus control on cardiovascular mortality in hemodialysis patients using an area under the curve approach: Results from the DOPPS. *Nephrol. Dial. Transplant.* **2020**, *35*, 1794–1801. [CrossRef]
28. Major, R.W.; Cheng, M.R.I.; Grant, R.A.; Shantikumar, S.; Xu, G.; Oozeerally, I.; Brunskill, N.J.; Gray, L.J. Cardiovascular disease risk factors in chronic kidney disease: A systematic review and meta-analysis. *PLoS ONE* **2018**, *13*, e0192895. [CrossRef]
29. McGovern, A.P.; de Lusignan, S.; van Vlymen, J.; Liyanage, H.; Tomson, C.R.; Gallagher, H.; Rafig, M.; Jones, S. Serum phosphate as a risk factor for cardiovascular events in people with and without chronic kidney disease: A large community based cohort study. *PLoS ONE* **2013**, *8*, e74996. [CrossRef]
30. Shang, D.; Xie, Q.; Ge, X.; Yan, H.; Tian, J.; Kuang, D.; Hao, C.-M.; Zhu, T. Hyperphosphatemia as an independent risk factor for coronary artery calcification progression in peritoneal dialysis patients. *BMC Nephrol.* **2015**, *16*, 107. [CrossRef]
31. Edmonston, D.; Wolf, M. FGF23 at the crossroads of phosphate, iron economy and erythropoiesis. *Nat. Rev. Nephrol.* **2020**, *16*, 7–19. [CrossRef]
32. Yamada, S.; Giachelli, C.M. Vascular calcification in CKD-MBD: Roles for phosphate, FGF23, and Klotho. *Bone* **2017**, *100*, 87–93. [CrossRef]
33. Blacher, J.; Guerin, A.P.; Pannier, B.; Marchais, S.J.; London, G.M. Arterial calcifications, arterial stiffness, and cardiovascular risk in end-stage renal disease. *Hypertension* **2001**, *38*, 938–942. [CrossRef]
34. Raggi, P.; Bellasi, A.; Gamboa, C.; Ferramosca, E.; Ratti, C.; Block, G.A.; Muntner, P. All-cause mortality in hemodialysis patients with heart valve calcification. *Clin. J. Am. Soc. Nephrol.* **2011**, *6*, 1990–1995. [CrossRef]
35. Voelkl, J.; Lang, F.; Eckardt, K.U.; Amann, K.; Kuro-O, M.; Pasch, A.; Pieske, B.; Alesutan, I. Signaling pathways involved in vascular smooth muscle cell calcification during hyperphosphatemia. *Cell. Mol. Life. Sci.* **2019**, *76*, 2077–2091. [CrossRef] [PubMed]
36. Durham, A.L.; Speer, M.Y.; Scatena, M.; Giachelli, C.M.; Shanahan, C.M. Role of smooth muscle cells in vascular calcification: Implications in atherosclerosis and arterial stiffness. *Cardiovasc. Res.* **2018**, *114*, 590–600. [CrossRef] [PubMed]
37. Kutikhin, A.G.; Feenstra, L.; Kostyunin, A.E.; Yuzhalin, A.E.; Hillebrands, J.L.; Krenning, G. Calciprotein particles: Balancing mineral homeostasis and vascular pathology. *Arterioscler. Thromb. Vasc. Biol.* **2021**, *41*, 1607–1624. [CrossRef] [PubMed]
38. Akiyama, K.; Kimura, T.; Shiizaki, K. Biological and Clinical Effects of Calciprotein Particles on Chronic Kidney Disease-Mineral and Bone Disorder. *Int. J. Endocrinol.* **2018**, *27*, 5282389. [CrossRef] [PubMed]
39. Koppert, S.; Buscher, A.; Babler, A.; Ghallab, A.; Buhl, E.M.; Latz, E.; Hengstler, J.G.; Smith, E.R.; Jahnen-Dechent, W. Cellular clearance and biological activity of calciprotein particles depend on their maturation state and crystallinity. *Front. Immunol.* **2018**, *4*, 1991. [CrossRef]
40. Viegas, C.S.B.; Santos, L.; Macedo, A.L.; Matos, A.A.; Silva, A.P.; Neves, P.L.; Staes, A.; Gevaert, K.; Morais, R.; Vermeer, C.; et al. Chronic kidney disease circulating calciprotein particles and extracellular vesicles promote vascular calcification: A role for GRP (Gla-Rich Protein). *Arterioscler. Thromb. Vasc. Biol.* **2018**, *38*, 575–587. [CrossRef]
41. Gungor, O.; Kocyigit, I.; Yilmaz, M.I.; Sezer, S. Role of vascular calcification inhibitors in preventing vascular dysfunction and mortality in hemodialysis patients. *Semin. Dial.* **2018**, *31*, 72–81. [CrossRef]
42. Yamada, S.; Tatsumoto, N.; Tokumoto, M.; Noguchi, H.; Ooboshi, H.; Kitazono, T.; Tsuruya, K. Phosphate binders prevent phosphate-induced cellular senescence of vascular smooth muscle cells and vascular calcification in a modified, adenine-based uremic rat model. *Calcif. Tissue Int.* **2015**, *96*, 347–358. [CrossRef]

43. Yamada, S.; Taniguchi, M.; Tokumoto, M.; Toyonaga, J.; Fujisaki, K.; Suehiro, T.; Noguchi, H.; Iida, M.; Tsuruya, K.; Kitazono, T. The antioxidant tempol ameliorates arterial medial calcification in uremic rats: Important role of oxidative stress in the pathogenesis of vascular calcification in chronic kidney disease. *J. Bone Miner. Res.* **2012**, *27*, 474–485. [CrossRef]
44. Ter Braake, A.D.; Smit, A.E.; Bos, C.; van Herwaarden, A.E.; Alkema, W.; van Essen, H.W.; Bravenboer, N.; Vervloet, M.G.; Hoenderop, J.G.J.; de Baaij, J.H.F. Magnesium prevents vascular calcification in Klotho deficiency. *Kidney Int.* **2020**, *97*, 487–501. [CrossRef]
45. Nitta, K.; Akiba, T.; Suzuki, K.; Uchida, K.; Watanabe, R.; Majima, K.; Aoki, T.; Nihei, H. Effects of cyclic intermittent etidronate therapy on coronary artery calcification in patients receiving long-term hemodialysis. *Am. J. Kidney Dis.* **2004**, *44*, 680–688. [CrossRef]
46. Slatopolsky, E.; Robson, A.M.; Elkan, I.; Bricker, N.S. Control of phosphate excretion in uremic man. *J. Clin. Investig.* **1968**, *47*, 1865–1874. [CrossRef]
47. Levin, A.; Bakris, G.L.; Molitch, M.; Smulders, M.; Tian, J.; Williams, L.A.; Andress, D.L. Prevalence of abnormal serum vitamin D, PTH, calcium, and phosphorus in patients with chronic kidney disease: Results of the study to evaluate early kidney disease. *Kidney Int.* **2007**, *71*, 31–38. [CrossRef]
48. De Boer, I.H.; Gorodetskaya, I.; Young, B.; Hsu, C.-Y.; Chertow, G.M. The severity of secondary hyperparathyroidism in chronic renal insufficiency is GFR-dependent, race-dependent, and associated with cardiovascular disease. *J. Am. Soc. Nephrol.* **2002**, *13*, 2762–2769. [CrossRef]
49. Hagstrom, E.; Hellman, P.; Larsson, T.E.; Ingelsson, E.; Berglund, L.; Sundstrom, J.; Melhus, H.; Held, C.; Lind, L.; Michaelsson, K.; et al. Plasma parathyroid hormone and the risk of cardiovascular mortality in the community. *Circulation* **2009**, *119*, 2765–2771. [CrossRef]
50. Scialla, J.J.; Xie, H.; Rashman, M.; Anderson, A.H.; Isakova, T.; Ojo, A.; Zhang, X.; Nessel, L.; Hamano, T.; Grunwald, J.E.; et al. Fibroblast growth factor-23 and cardiovascular events in CKD. *J. Am. Soc. Nephrol.* **2014**, *25*, 349–360. [CrossRef]
51. Yamaguchi, S.; Hamano, T.; Doi, Y.; Oka, T.; Kajimoto, S.; Kubota, K.; Yasuda, S.; Shimada, K.; Matsumoto, A.; Hashimoto, N.; et al. Hidden hypocalcemia as a risk factor for cardiovascular events and all-cause mortality among patients undergoing incident hemodialysis. *Sci. Rep.* **2020**, *10*, 4418. [CrossRef] [PubMed]
52. Kendrick, J.; Targher, G.; Smits, G.; Chonchol, M. 25-hydroxyvitamin D deficiency is independently associated with cardiovascular disease in the Third National Health and Nutrition Examination Survey. *Atherosclerosis* **2009**, *205*, 255–260. [CrossRef] [PubMed]
53. Gutierrez, O.; Isakova, T.; Rhee, E.; Shah, A.; Holmes, J.; Collerone, G.; Juppner, H.; Wolf, M. Fibroblast growth factor-23 mitigates hyperphosphatemia but accentuates calcitriol deficiency in chronic kidney disease. *J. Am. Soc. Nephrol.* **2005**, *16*, 2205–2215. [CrossRef] [PubMed]
54. Watson, K.E.; Abrolat, M.L.; Malone, L.L.; Hoeg, J.M.; Doherty, T.; Detrano, R.; Demer, L.L. Active serum vitamin D levels are inversely correlated with coronary calcification. *Circulation* **1997**, *96*, 1755–1760. [CrossRef] [PubMed]
55. Artaza, J.N.; Norris, K.C. Vitamin D reduces the expression of collagen and key profibrotic factors by inducing an antifibrotic phenotype in mesenchymal multipotent cells. *J. Endocrinol.* **2009**, *200*, 207–221. [CrossRef]
56. Cozzolino, M.; Mangano, M.; Stucchi, A.; Ciceri, P.; Conte, F.; Galassi, A. Cardiovascular disease in dialysis patients. *Nephrol. Dial. Transplant.* **2018**, *33*, iii28–iii34. [CrossRef]
57. Hasegawa, H.; Nagano, N.; Urakata, I.; Yamazaki, Y.; Iijima, K.; Fujita, T.; Yamashita, T.; Fukumoto, S.; Shimada, T. Direct evidence for a causative role of FGF23 in the abnormal renal phosphate handling and vitamin D metabolism in rats with early-stage chronic kidney disease. *Kidney Int.* **2010**, *78*, 975–980. [CrossRef]
58. Centeno, P.; Herberger, A.; Mun, H.-C.; Tu, C.; Nemeth, E.F.; Chang, W.; Conigrave, A.D.; Ward, D.T. Phosphate acts directly on the calcium-sensing receptor to stimulate parathyroid hormone secretion. *Nat. Commun.* **2019**, *10*, 4693. [CrossRef]
59. Faul, C.; Amaral, A.P.; Oskouei, B.; Hu, M.-C.; Sloan, A.; Isakova, T.; Gutierrez, O.M.; Aguillon-Prada, R.; Lincoln, J.; Hare, J.M.; et al. FGF23 induces left ventricular hypertrophy. *J. Cin. Investig.* **2011**, *121*, 4393–4408. [CrossRef]
60. Grey, A.; Mitnick, M.A.; Masiukiewicz, U.; Sun, B.H.; Rudikoff, S.; Jilka, R.L.; Manolagas, S.C.; Insogna, K. A role for interleukin-6 in parathyroid hormone-induced bone resorption in vivo. *Endocrinology* **1999**, *140*, 4683–4690. [CrossRef]
61. Baczynski, R.; Massry, S.G.; Kohan, R.; Magott, M.; Saglikes, Y.; Brautbar, N. Effect of parathyroid hormone on myocardial energy metabolism in the rat. *Kidney Int.* **1985**, *27*, 718–725. [CrossRef]
62. Amann, K.; Ritz, E.; Wiest, G.; Klaus, G.; Mall, G. A role of parathyroid hormone for the activation of cardiac fibroblasts in uremia. *J. Am. Soc. Nephrol.* **1994**, *4*, 1814–1819. [CrossRef]
63. Wang, A.Y.; Akizawa, T.; Bavanandan, S.; Hamano, T.; Liew, A.; Lu, K.C.; Lumlertgul, D.; Oh, K.H.; Zhao, M.H.; Ka-Shun Fung, S.; et al. 2017 Kidney Disease: Improving Global Outcomes (KDIGO) Chronic Kidney Disease-Mineral and Bone Disorder (CKD-MBD) Guideline Update Implementation: Asia Summit Conference Report. *Kidney Int. Rep.* **2019**, *4*, 1523–1537. [CrossRef]
64. Fukagawa, M.; Yokoyama, K.; Koiwa, F.; Taniguchi, M.; Shoji, T.; Kazama, J.J.; Komaba, H.; Ando, R.; Kakuta, T.; Fujii, H.; et al. Clinical practice guideline for the management of chronic kidney disease-mineral and bone disorder. *Ther. Apher. Dial.* **2013**, *17*, 247–288. [CrossRef]
65. Slinin, Y.; Foley, R.N.; Collins, A.J. Calcium, phosphorus, parathyroid hormone, and cardiovascular disease in hemodialysis patients: The USRDS waves 1, 3, 4 study. *J. Am. Soc. Nephrol.* **2005**, *16*, 1788–1793. [CrossRef]

66. Kimata, N.; Albert, J.M.; Akiba, T.; Yamazaki, S.; Kawaguchi, T.; Fukuhara, S.; Akizawa, T.; Saito, A.; Asano, Y.; Kurokawa, K.; et al. Association of mineral metabolism factors with all-cause and cardiovascular mortality in hemodialysis patients: The Japan dialysis outcomes and practice patterns study. *Hemodial. Int.* **2007**, *11*, 340–348. [CrossRef]
67. Danese, M.D.; Belozeroff, V.; Smirnakis, K.; Rothman, K.J. Consistent control of mineral and bone disorder in incident hemodialysis patients. *Clin. J. Am. Soc. Nephrol.* **2008**, *3*, 1423–1429. [CrossRef]
68. Teng, M.; Wolf, M.; Ofsthun, M.N.; Lazarus, J.M.; Hernan, M.A.; Camargo, C.A., Jr.; Thadhani, R. Active injectable vitamin D and hemodialysis survival: A historical cohort study. *J. Am. Soc. Nephrol.* **2005**, *16*, 1115–1125. [CrossRef]
69. Melamed, M.L.; Eustace, J.A.; Plantinga, L.; Jaar, B.G.; Fink, N.E.; Coresh, J.; Klag, M.J.; Powe, N.R. Changes in serum calcium, phosphate, and PTH and the risk of death in incident dialysis patients: A longitudinal study. *Kidney Int.* **2006**, *70*, 351–357. [CrossRef]
70. Tentori, F.; Hunt, W.C.; Stidley, C.A.; Rohrscheib, M.R.; Bedrick, E.J.; Meyer, K.B.; Johnson, H.K.; Zager, P.G. Mortality risk among hemodialysis patients receiving different vitamin D analogs. *Kidney Int.* **2006**, *70*, 1858–1865. [CrossRef]
71. Kovesdy, C.P.; Ahmadzadeh, S.; Anderson, J.E.; Kalantar-Zadef, K. Association of activated vitamin D treatment and mortality in chronic kidney disease. *Arch. Intern. Med.* **2008**, *168*, 397–403. [CrossRef] [PubMed]
72. Naves-Diaz, M.; Alvarez-Hernandez, D.; Passlick-Deetjen, J.; Guinsburg, A.; Marelli, C.; Rodriguez-Puyol, D.; Cannata-Andia, J.B. Oral active vitamin D is associated with improved survival in hemodialysis patients. *Kidney Int.* **2008**, *74*, 1070–1078. [CrossRef] [PubMed]
73. Nakai, K.; Komaba, H.; Fuakagawa, M. Management of mineral and bone disorder in chronic kidney disease: Quo vadis? *Ther. Apher. Dial.* **2009**, *13*, S2–S6. [CrossRef] [PubMed]
74. Cunningham, J.; Danese, M.; Olson, K.; Klassen, P.; Chertow, G.M. Effects of the calcimimetic cinacalcet HCl on cardiovascular disease, fracture, and health-related quality of life in secondary hyperparathyroidism. *Kidney Int.* **2005**, *68*, 1793–1800. [CrossRef] [PubMed]
75. Chertow, G.M.; Pupim, L.B.; Block, G.A.; Correa-Rotter, R.; Drueke, T.B.; Floege, J.; Goodman, W.G.; London, G.M.; Mahaffery, K.W.; Moe, S.M.; et al. Evaluation of Cinacalcet Therapy to Lower Cardiovascular Events (EVOLVE): Rationale and design overview. *Clin. J. Am. Soc. Nephrol.* **2007**, *2*, 898–905. [CrossRef]
76. Block, G.A.; Zaun, D.; Smits, G.; Persky, M.; Brillhart, S.; Nieman, K.; Liu, J.; Peter, W.L.S. Cinacalcet hydrochrolide treatment significantly improves all-cause and cardiovascular survival in a large cohort of hemodialysis patients. *Kidney Int.* **2010**, *78*, 578–589. [CrossRef]
77. Isakova, T.; Gutierrez, O.M.; Chang, Y.; Shah, A.; Tamez, H.; Smith, K.; Thadhani, R.; Wolf, M. Phosphate binders and survival on hemodialysis. *J. Am. Soc. Nephrol.* **2009**, *20*, 388–396. [CrossRef]
78. Goodman, W.G.; Goldin, J.; Kuizon, B.D.; Yoon, C.; Gales, B.; Sider, D.; Wang, Y.; Chung, J.; Emerick, A.; Greaser, L.; et al. Coronary-artery calcification in young adults with end-stage renal disease who are undergoing dialysis. *N. Engl. J. Med.* **2000**, *342*, 1478–1483. [CrossRef]
79. Ketteler, M.; Liangos, O.; Biggar, P.H. Treating hyperphosphatemia–Current and advancing drugs. *Expert Opin. Pharmacother.* **2016**, *17*, 1873–1879. [CrossRef]
80. Yokoyama, K.; Akiba, T.; Fukagawa, M.; Nakayama, M.; Sawada, K.; Kumagai, Y.; Chertow, G.M.; Hirakata, H. Long-term safety and efficacy of a novel iron-containing phosphate binder, JTT-751, in patients receiving hemodialysis. *J. Ren. Nutr.* **2014**, *24*, 261–267. [CrossRef]
81. Koiwa, F.; Yokoyama, K.; Fukagawa, M.; Akizawa, T. Long-term assessment of the safety and efficacy of PA21 Sucroferric oxyhydroxide) in Japanese hemodialysis patients with hyperphosphatemia: An open-label, multicenter, Phase III study. *J. Ren. Nutr.* **2017**, *27*, 346–354. [CrossRef]

Disclaimer/Publisher's Note: The statements, opinions and data contained in all publications are solely those of the individual author(s) and contributor(s) and not of MDPI and/or the editor(s). MDPI and/or the editor(s) disclaim responsibility for any injury to people or property resulting from any ideas, methods, instructions or products referred to in the content.

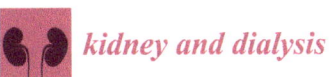

Review

Multifaceted Nutritional Disorders in Elderly Patients Undergoing Dialysis

Katsuhito Mori [1,*], Masafumi Kurajoh [2], Masaaki Inaba [3] and Masanori Emoto [1,2]

1. Department of Nephrology, Graduate School of Medicine, Osaka Metropolitan University, Osaka 545-8585, Japan
2. Department of Metabolism, Endocrinology, and Molecular Medicine, Graduate School of Medicine, Osaka Metropolitan University, Osaka 545-8585, Japan
3. Renal Center, Ohno Memorial Hospital, Osaka 550-0015, Japan
* Correspondence: ktmori@omu.ac.jp; Tel.: +81-6-6645-3806

Abstract: Advances in medicine have resulted in increased longevity, which has consequently led to unexpected geriatric syndromes, such as frailty and sarcopenia. Patients with end-stage kidney disease, especially those receiving dialysis treatment, often show characteristic reductions in body protein and energy storage, termed protein energy wasting (PEW). Therefore, maintenance of nutritional condition has a key role in defending against both geriatric syndromes and PEW, which share several components in elderly individuals undergoing hemodialysis. To counteract the development of an undesirable condition, nutritional evaluation is indispensable. In addition to simple measurements of body mass index, and serum albumin and creatinine, a composite nutritional assessment including a malnutrition inflammation score is useful, although subjective elements are included and a well-trained examiner is required. On the other hand, the geriatric nutritional risk index and nutritional risk index for Japanese hemodialysis patients (NRI-JH) are objective tools, and easy to use in clinical settings. Undernutrition is closely related to infectious events and the results of an infection are often serious in elderly patients, even those with survival, with large medical costs incurred. Together with appropriate nutritional evaluation, it is necessary to clarify the underlying relationship of PEW with infection for improvement of prognosis in affected elderly individuals.

Keywords: nutrition; protein energy wasting (PEW); sarcopenia; frailty; hemodialysis; end-stage kidney disease (ESKD); chronic kidney disease (CKD)

1. Introduction

Malnutrition has factors related to both overnutrition and undernutrition [1]. Obesity is a representative overnutrition-related disorder and profoundly linked to various adverse conditions, such as metabolic syndrome, diabetes, cardiovascular disease (CVD), non-alcoholic fatty liver disease, and chronic kidney disease (CKD), etc. [2]. Great efforts have been made to improve poor outcomes induced by overweight and obesity conditions. At the same time, while advances in public health and medical treatments have extended longevity [3], rapid aging has brought on unexpected geriatric syndromes including frailty [4] and sarcopenia [5], with undernutrition rather than overnutrition considered to be the more serious issue related to those conditions.

CKD has become a major health problem throughout the world and known as not only a risk factor for end-stage kidney disease (ESKD), but also for CVD and death. Increased longevity has highlighted the importance of measures needed to protect against CKD development. In addition to primary diseases, such as diabetes and hypertension, aging accelerates structural and functional deteriorations in the kidneys [6,7], resulting in an increased prevalence of CKD and subsequent ESKD in association with aging [8]. In Japan, more than half of current dialysis patients are aged 70 years or older [9]. In patients with advanced CKD and ESKD, a unique nutritional disorder resistant to various interventions has become recognized as a condition termed protein energy wasting (PEW).

Elderly patients undergoing dialysis suffer from both geriatric syndromes and PEW [10–12]. No definitive medication has yet been developed for these conditions, thus improvement of nutritional status is currently the only treatment option available. Generally, energy restriction for diabetes patients and protein restriction in patients with CKD have been accepted as standard diet therapy protocols, although a paradigm shift from restriction to adequate intake has occurred in recent years [12,13]. The present review was conducted to elucidate how to evaluate nutritional status in patients undergoing hemodialysis, primarily elderly, based on considerations of overlapping of PEW, sarcopenia, and frailty in those individuals. In addition, infection as a serious consequence in this population has received focus as a factor for future medical and economic measures.

2. What Are PEW, Frailty, and Sarcopenia?

2.1. PEW

Nutritional derangement in patients with CKD, in particular ESKD, is characterized by wasting (loss of muscle and fat tissues), regardless of the etiology, with multiple mechanisms thought to be involved in this phenotype [14–17]. While an inadequate diet generally induces undernutrition in this population, increased food intake does not always correct wasting. It is considered that the presence of chronic inflammation manifested by increased pro-inflammatory cytokines may be profoundly linked to wasting coupled with endocrine disorders, such as impaired insulin/insulin growth factor-1 signaling. Moreover, metabolic acidosis and uremic toxins exacerbate and accelerate catabolic pathways, increasing the effects of co-morbidities.

To date, many terms have been proposed for this condition, such as protein-energy malnutrition [18], malnutrition-inflammation complex syndrome [19], uremic malnutrition [20], and uremic cachexia [21]. However, those may not adequately cover the common features seen in CKD and ESKD patients, while the most common term, protein energy wasting (PEW), has been proposed by the International Society of Renal Nutrition and Metabolism (ISRNM) [14,22]. Diagnosis of PEW is based on the following four categories: (1) Serum chemistry, such as low serum albumin and low serum cholesterol; (2) body mass, such as low BMI, unintentional body weight loss, and low body fat; (3) muscle mass, such as reduced muscle mass over time and creatinine appearance; and (4) dietary intake, such as unintentional low levels of dietary protein and energy intake (Table 1). Discussion regarding adaptation of the PEW criteria for Asian patients receiving dialysis is presented later in this review.

Table 1. Comparison of NRI-JH with PEW criteria components in dialysis patients [14,23].

PEW Component		NRI-JH Component	Cut-Off Values	Score
Serum chemistry	Albumin < 3.5 g/dL Transthyretin (prealbumin) < 30 mg/dL Total cholesterol < 100 mg/dL	Albumin	Age ≥ 65 → <3.5 g/dL Age < 65 → <3.7 g/dL	4
		Total cholesterol	<130 mg/dL	1
			≥220 mg/dL	2
Body mass	BMI < 23 kg/m^2 Unintentional weight loss 5% over 3M or 10% over 6M Total body fat percentage < 10%	BMI	<20 kg/m^2	3

Table 1. Cont.

PEW Component		NRI-JH Component	Cut-Off Values	Score
Muscle mass	Reduced muscle mass 5% over 3M or 10% over 6M Reduced mid-arm muscle circumference area Creatinine appearance	Creatinine	Age ≥ 65 → Male < 9.7 mg/dL Female < 8.0 mg/dL Age < 65 → Male < 11.6 mg/dL Female < 9.7 mg/dL	4
Dietary intake	Unintentional low DPI < 0.80 g/kg/day for at least 2M Unintentional low DEI < 25 kcal/kg/day for at least 2M	-	-	

Abbreviations: BMI, body mass index; DPI, dietary protein intake; DEI, dietary energy intake.

2.2. Frailty

Frailty is a vague word originally used to indicate a state in elderly individuals with decreased activities of daily living (ADL) indicating their need for nursing care [24]. However, there is confusion regarding the true meaning and its implications. Apart from impaired ADL, frailty has been used to indicate an age-related state of decreased physiological reserve and increased vulnerability to stressors, resulting in disability, then leading to hospitalization and finally death. Impairment of neurological factors, mechanical performance, and energy metabolism may be involved [25]. Rockwood et al. proposed a frailty index to show accumulation of deficits, such as age-associated disease, non-specific vulnerability, and disabilities [26]. In contrast to an accumulated deficit model, Fried et al. suggested a phenotype model that includes observations of weakness (grip strength), slow gait, unintentional weight loss, low tolerance for physical activity, and self-reported exhaustion, with frailty diagnosed when three or more of those are noted [4].

2.3. Sarcopenia

Sarcopenia is related to anatomical and functional deterioration in skeletal muscle. The term sarcopenia (*sarx* meaning flesh, *penia* meaning loss in Greek) was coined by Rosenberg in the 1980s, and literally meant aging-related loss of skeletal muscle, while some later studies included function of skeletal muscle and physical performance in addition to muscle quantity. As a result, the prevalence of sarcopenia in early reported CKD cases showed great inconsistency, ranging from 4% to 63% [27]. For comparisons among different cohorts, diagnostic criteria with a sense of unity were required. The European Working Group on Sarcopenia in Older People (EWGSOP) was first to present a definition as well as diagnostic criteria, consisting of muscle mass, muscle strength (handgrip strength), and physical performance (gait speed) [28]. Since the establishment of objective assessments (methods, cut-off values, criteria), research regarding sarcopenia has dramatically progressed. However, another problem to emerge is adaptation of the EWGSOP criteria for non-European populations throughout the world, who show differences in these factors as anthropometric characteristics, ethnicity, and culture. As a result, the Asian Working Group on Sarcopenia (AWGS) proposed criteria for Asian populations in 2014 [29] based on concepts similar to those used by EWGSOP. For the purpose of early detection and treatment of patients with sarcopenia, consensus findings of the EWGSOP and AWGS 2014 criteria have recently been presented as EWGSOP2 [30] and AWGS 2019 [31], respectively.

2.4. Conceptual Overlapping among PEW, Frailty, and Sarcopenia

The concepts of age-related frailty and sarcopenia have developed independently of CKD-accelerated PEW [11]. However, aging deepens the relationships, since these disorders share common components. A comprehensive approach may be required to improve prognosis in elderly patients undergoing hemodialysis.

3. Evaluation of Nutritional Status

The term 'malnutrition' is commonly used to indicate a state of undernutrition, although an evaluation of nutritional status is not easily performed. While nutritional screening and assessment classifications are used, they are confusing and often misunderstood [32]. Nutritional screening is a quicker and more simple to use tool for identification of at-risk subjects, and generally does not require any special techniques. On the other hand, nutritional assessment is performed by trained health-care professionals and provides a nutritional diagnosis, with adequate follow-up of the patient after nutritional intervention. Subjective global assessment (SGA) [33] and malnutrition inflammation score (MIS) [34], as described in the following section, are considered as the gold standard methods. However, in clinical settings in Japan, it is very difficult to perform nutritional assessments including SGA and MIS. Therefore, nutritional screening tools are mainly used, which have both advantages and disadvantages, as noted below.

3.1. Anthropometric Indices

3.1.1. BMI

BMI is a simple anthropometric index to indicate body size. In contrast to overnutrition, a serious health problem in general populations [2], it is well-known that higher BMI is paradoxically correlated to better prognosis in patients with CKD, especially those receiving hemodialysis. This phenomenon has been termed 'obesity paradox' [35] or 'reverse epidemiology' [36]. The inverse association between BMI and mortality is highly consistent, beyond race/ethnicity and geographical area [37,38], suggesting that obesity paradox and reverse epidemiology refer to a universal phenomenon.

Although BMI is a popular and convenient index, there are some points regarding body composition to consider. BMI is influenced by water or solid weight. Apart from nutrition, hydration status in patients receiving dialysis treatment is a critical factor for prognosis. Even when BMI apparently increases, fluid retention is known to be a risk factor for CVD mortality [39]. In contrast, solid mass, including muscle mass and fat mass, is more relevant to nutrition. Unfortunately, separate evaluations of those are very difficult to perform [35]. Furthermore, fat mass is roughly divided into subcutaneous fat, which functions as an energy reservoir, and visceral fat mass, which shows metabolic abnormalities and pro-inflammatory characteristics [40]. Increased waist circumference as a surrogate of visceral fat was found to be associated with all-cause and CV mortality in 537 patients with ESKD [41]. Although it remains controversial whether an increase in fat mass, especially visceral fat mass, may have benefits, maintenance of muscle mass is believed to at least provide an advantage for survival [42].

Additionally, it is recognized that obesity paradox or reverse epidemiology is not always observed, even in patients undergoing dialysis, when BMI alone is utilized without consideration of body composition or age [43,44]. Inconsistent findings may be the result of a discordant contribution of increases in undesirable factors, such as fluid or visceral fat, different follow-up periods, or different modalities used for dialysis.

3.1.2. Measurement of Subcutaneous Fat and Fat-Free Mass

Skinfold measurements to determine subcutaneous fat are useful to estimate body fat mass [45]. The biceps skinfold (front side of mid-upper arm), triceps skinfold (TSF) (back side of mid-upper arm), subscapular skinfold (under the shoulder blade), and suprailiac skinfold (above the iliac crest) are measured. It was found that skinfold thickness was lower in patients on dialysis for 5 years or more as compared to those treated for less than 5 years [46], suggesting that fat mass loss is a time-dependent process. The triceps skinfold is considered to provide the most reliable results, since fluid retention is not often observed in the upper arm in dialysis patients. Although a skinfold caliper is not expensive and measurements are easy to perform with that device, a trained clinician should perform that examination to obtain an accurate result.

Measurements of circumferences with the use of a tape measure, such as of the arm, calf, and waist, can also reflect nutritional status to some degree. Waist circumference is known to be correlated with visceral adiposity, thus it is a critical factor for diagnosis of metabolic syndrome in examinations of general population subjects [47], although its significance in patients undergoing dialysis remains a matter of debate, as noted above. Calf circumference is related to protein storage and used for sarcopenia screening [29], while a recently published work showed the usefulness of calf circumference to discriminate sarcopenia in patients undergoing hemodialysis [48]. Measurement of mid-upper arm circumference (MAC) is easy and simple, and the results are found to be useful as an independent predictor of all-cause mortality in patients receiving hemodialysis therapy [49,50]. Nevertheless, it is also necessary to calculate mid-upper arm muscle circumference (MAMC) combined with TSF, performed with the following equation: $MAMC = MAC - (TSF \times 3.14)$ (where MAMC, MAC, and TSF are measured in centimeters) [51], since this can be used to determine muscle tissue reserve. Higher MAMC was shown to be associated with better mental health as well as better survival in hemodialysis patients [52]. Nevertheless, while MAMC has been classically used as an index of muscle mass and calf circumference [53], thigh muscle area assessed by computed tomography, when available, may be better for nutritional evaluation of patients undergoing hemodialysis [54].

3.2. Blood Chemistry Parameters

3.2.1. Albumin

A reduced level of serum albumin has been shown to be a predictor of mortality in patients undergoing hemodialysis [55]. In investigations of other nutritional screening tools, as described below, albumin has been found to be comparable to those in patients undergoing dialysis [56–58].

It is important to note that albumin reflects not only a nutritional disorder but also inflammation. For example, hypoalbuminemia is the result of the combined effects of poor nutritional status and inflammation [59]. Both undernutrition and inflammation reduce protein synthesis, resulting in hypoalbuminemia, while inflammation is associated with protein catabolism [60]. Although a decrease in serum albumin was found to be associated with increased mortality risk in dialysis patients, adjustment for SGA did not decrease that risk, whereas adjustment for inflammation did, suggesting a profound association of the inflammatory process with poor outcome [61]. Therefore, albumin may be more than only an indicator of nutritional status.

A recent study retrospectively examined the association between long-term trajectory of serum albumin and mortality in 421 patients undergoing hemodialysis [62]. In patients who died, serum albumin tended to decrease at 7 to 8 years before death as compared to those who survived, with a difference in albumin trajectory between survivors and non-survivors becoming apparent 3 years before death. This led to the question of whether a change in albumin level is associated with mortality. In association with that, the influence of changes in serum albumin level over time on all-cause or CVD mortality was examined. Time-varying hypoalbuminemia was found to be a predictor of all-cause mortality and CVD death, while an increased albumin level over time was associated with better survival independent of baseline albumin level [63]. In addition, higher dietary protein intake, evaluated using normalized protein catabolic rate (nPCR), which was corrected based on renal urea clearance, during the first 6 months was associated with higher serum albumin level and lower mortality [64]. These findings suggest the importance of periodic measurements of serum albumin.

A number of studies have emphasized various problems associated with an aging society and it is considered that typical guidelines should not be consulted for managing very elderly patients. A recent work examined the association of quality-of-care indicators, including spKt/V, calcium, phosphate, hemoglobin, and albumin, with CVD events and mortality, as those are known to be associated with prognosis in patients receiving hemodialysis. Interestingly, in patients aged 80 years and older, low serum albumin level was the only factor significantly associated with CVD events and all-cause mortality [65]. Albumin measurement may be useful for elderly patients undergoing dialysis treatment.

Although serum albumin level is useful as a nutritional screening tool, it is unclear whether its most diluted concentration during the preparation for hemodialysis is accurate. Therefore, albumin levels before (diluted) and after (concentrated) a hemodialysis session were compared [66]. For prediction of 1- and 5-year mortality, the pre-albumin level was more accurate than post-albumin level. Importantly, among other nutritional factors, such as blood urea nitrogen and BMI, pre-hemodialysis creatinine level, which is described in the following section, was also predictive of mortality.

3.2.2. Pre-Albumin (Transthyretin)

Pre-albumin, also known as transthyretin, is mainly synthesized by the liver according to dietary intake [67] and, when compared to albumin, its half-life is relatively short, thus it is thought to be a more sensitive indicator of nutritional condition than albumin. Reports have noted that serum pre-albumin could be used to predict survival and hospitalization for infection independent of serum albumin in patients undergoing hemodialysis [68,69]. Furthermore, a decrease in serum pre-albumin over time was found to be significantly associated with mortality in patients receiving hemodialysis [70]. Moreover, significant increases in serum pre-albumin as well as albumin were observed in association with oral nutritional supplementation during hemodialysis session over a period of 6 months [71]. These findings suggest that pre-albumin is a good indicator of nutritional status.

3.2.3. Transferrin

Transferrin, a powerful iron chelator that maintains Fe^{3+} in a redox-inactive state and inhibits the generation of free radicals in blood [72], is predominantly expressed in the liver. The synthesis of transferrin increases in association with iron deficiency, although the underlying mechanism is unknown. In the general population, high transferrin levels have been observed in subjects with iron deficiency, pregnancy, or contraceptives use [73], while it is also known to be a surrogate marker of nutritional status and potential indicator of PEW [14]. In clinical settings, serum transferrin level is indirectly evaluated by determination of total iron-binding capacity (TIBC) [74]. TIBC is well correlated to nutritional marker, such as SGA in relation to hemodialysis, with low TIBC in those patients found to be associated with PEW, iron deficiency, inflammation, poor quality of life, and mortality [75]. Therefore, as a component of MIS, TIBC is usually measured, while transferrin can be alternatively used [34].

3.2.4. Creatinine

Serum creatinine is considered to be a surrogate marker of skeletal muscle mass in patients undergoing dialysis [76,77]. Along with albumin, creatinine has been found to be inversely correlated with mortality [50,56]. As compared to other body components, including subcutaneous and visceral fat mass, muscle mass has been shown to be the most critical component of PEW and directly related to sarcopenia [14]. In fact, a lower serum creatinine level was found to be associated with poor prognosis in 119,099 Japanese patients undergoing hemodialysis, although no significant association between BMI and mortality was noted [44]. Furthermore, addition of creatinine to the PEW criteria resulted in more identification in 109 patients on hemodialysis [78].

Low triiodothyronine (T3) syndrome, highly prevalent in patients undergoing dialysis, is characterized by a low free T3 (FT3) level, along with normal concentrations of thyroid stimulating hormone (TSH), the most sensitive and specific test of thyroid function, and free thyrotoxin (FT4) [79]. This syndrome is thought to be a physiologic adaptive response to excessive catabolism, such as PEW and has been reported to be associated with CVD mortality in patients receiving dialysis treatment [80]. We examined the association between low T3 syndrome and clinical factors associated with nutrition and inflammation in 332 hemodialysis patients [81]. The results indicated that serum creatinine, but not albumin or CRP, was significantly associated with FT3/FT4 ratio, a relevant indicator for low T3 syndrome, suggesting that low muscle mass may be a cause of this syndrome. Local T3 generation from T4 occurs in skeletal muscle; therefore, this conclusion is plausible. In addition, serum creatinine may be an indirect marker of dietary protein intake, as creatine levels have been found to be positively associated with nPCR [44].

3.2.5. Lipids (Cholesterol)

Dyslipidemia is caused by a disbalance of lipids, such as high level of total cholesterol (TC), low density lipoprotein cholesterol (LDL-C), and non-high density lipoprotein cholesterol (non-HDL-C), and established as a cardiovascular risk factor in the general population [82]. However, an opposite association of dyslipidemia with mortality is known in patients with advanced CKD [36,83]. As noted above, an unexpected observation regarding the association between BMI and mortality was reported, and termed 'reverse epidemiology'. More precisely, analysis findings revealed a U-shaped curve between TC and mortality in a cohort of Japanese patients undergoing hemodialysis [84], findings that were then reproduced in the study that developed a nutritional risk index for Japanese hemodialysis patients (NRI-JH) as discussed in detail later [23]. Although these seem to be a contradiction, the key factor to interpret this relationship may be PEW, as an inverse association between low TC and high mortality was found to be mainly due to the presence of PEW. On the other hand, the positive association of high TC with high mortality may reflect atherosclerotic CVD-induced death. Indeed, high non-HDL was shown to be an independent predictor of a CVD event in a study that enrolled 45,390 hemodialysis patients [85]. Nevertheless, while low TC is a good candidate for use as a nutritional marker, biphasic aspects should be also considered.

3.2.6. Other Possible Markers Related to the Immune System

As discussed in detail later, a dysfunction of the immune system consisting of innate and adaptive responses is often observed in patients undergoing dialysis [86]. Neutrophils and monocytes play crucial roles as cellular components in the innate immune system, whereas the complement system promotes and modulates the process through classical, lectin, and alternative pathways. Patients undergoing hemodialysis are known to be affected by problems related to membrane biocompatibility. Adhesion of circulating immunoglobulin (IgG) activates the classical pathway by biding to C1q, while properdin, C3b, albumin, and lipopolysaccharide can stimulate an alternative pathway, as well as activation of the lectin pathway by Ficolin-2. During this process, immune cells including neutrophils are recruited, resulting in leukocytopenia. On the other hand, lymphoid cell lineage, including T cells and B cells function as an adaptive immune system. This dysfunction in dialysis patients may be also profoundly associated with inflammation and nutritional disorder. Unfortunately, these factors are not easily measured. In clinical settings, neutrophil to lymphocyte ratio (NLR) may be useful, as it was reported to be positively related to tumor-necrosis factor α in 61 patients receiving dialysis treatment [87]. In addition, higher NLR was found to be associated with increased risk of cardiovascular and all-cause mortality in 170 incident hemodialysis patients [88], and a significant association between NLR and mortality was confirmed in a large cohort study of 108,548 incident hemodialysis patients [89]. In this study, NLR in addition to serum albumin provided a modest benefit to predict mortality, suggesting that NRL together with albumin may be useful as surrogate indicators of nutritional and inflammatory status.

Furthermore, it has been speculated that a strong association exists among inflammation, immune-deficiency, and nutritional disorder, although the underlying mechanisms are largely unknown. Further studies are necessary to establish immune parameters as nutritional markers.

3.3. Evaluation of Dietary Intake

Dietary evaluation is imperative for nutritional management and four dietary assessment methods are commonly used [90]. (1) The 24-h dietary recall is a rapid and convenient method to gather information about recent food intake, and does not require maintaining a diary [91]. However, this is dependent on the memory and cooperation of the patient. For hemodialysis patients, it should be noted that the food intake pattern differs on dialysis and non-dialysis days [92]. (2) Diet records and diaries are used to gather dietary information over a period of several days, usually three or seven. Dietitians give instruction about how to record that information with the use of a special booklet. Although this method includes a real-time record of food intake beyond 24 h, it relies on compliance by the patient to follow the instructions. (3) For an evaluation of dietary protein intake, nPCR or protein nitrogen appearance (nPNA) can be used [93]. Since most patients receiving hemodialysis treatments do not excrete nitrogen into urine, an increase in serum urea nitrogen between consecutive hemodialysis sessions reflects dietary protein intake. This method is objective and does not require a dietary evaluation. However, nPCR (nPNA) can only evaluate protein intake. It is underestimated whether the patients have residual renal function [64]. (4) A food frequency questionnaire (FFQ) can be useful to estimate long-term dietary intake (weeks to months) and daily intake of many different food items can be calculated with its use. Since an FFQ is convenient when used in a self-administered form, it is a feasible method for large epidemiologic studies. However, at individual levels, under- or over-estimation of food intake can occur. Furthermore, the different diet intake patterns on dialysis and non-dialysis days by hemodialysis patients must be considered. To overcome this limitation, the dialysis-FFQ has been developed, which uses a 3-day record for a dialysis day and two subsequent non-dialysis days, with the data gathering supplemented by a person-to-person dietary interview [94].

3.4. Bioelectrical Impedance Analysis

Bioelectrical impedance analysis (BIA) is used to estimate body composition, such as fat-free mass (FFM) and total body water (TBW), which has become established as a portable, inexpensive, and non-invasive method [95–98]. Theoretically, an electric current is not easily conducted through a fat mass, whereas it can be freely transmitted through electrolytes that are abundant in FFM, which includes bone and body cell mass (BCM), with skeletal muscle mass, a major component of the latter. TBW in the human body is comprised of 65% intracellular water and 35% extracellular water, with the proportion of FFM to TBW presumed to be 73% [99]. Using the different levels of conductivity in various body components, the device measures the opposition to a small alternating electric current as it travels through the body. Impedance consists of two components: Resistance (R), caused by total body water, and reactance (Xc), caused by cell membrane capacitance [95–98]. In other words, R represents opposition to electron flow through ionic solutions, while Xc is delay in the flow, which reflects dielectric properties.

Phase angle (PhA), calculated using R and Xc, is a biomarker of cellular health [95,97,98], and seems to reflect cellularity, cell membrane integrity, and distribution of intra-/extra-cellular fluid. Furthermore, PhA is commonly considered to be a predictor for various outcomes in patients receiving hemodialysis [100,101].

For dialysis patients, fluid retention and water shift between intra- and extra-cellular compartments can have profound effects on BIA parameters [98]. Therefore, measurement condition settings are critical. To assess skeletal muscle mass, BIA should be performed following a dialysis session. On the other hand, it is measured both before and after a session to determine dry weight and hydration state.

3.5. SGA and MIS—Comprehensive Nutritional Assessment Tools

As noted previously, SGA is a well-established nutritional assessment tool that is used in a wide range of clinical settings [102,103]. This assessment method is based on medical history and clinical findings. Using SGA as a basis, MIS was developed for patients with CKD and includes BMI, serum albumin, and TIBC in addition to seven SGA components [34]. MIS findings were found to be associated with 5-year mortality as well as quality of life in 809 patients undergoing hemodialysis [104], and also shown to effectively identify patients at risk for PEW [105]. However, both SGA and MIS require subjective assessment and evaluation by a well-trained examiner to obtain consistent results.

3.6. Geriatric Nutritional Risk Index (GNRI)

In contrast to SGA and MIS, GNRI is a simple combined nutritional screening tool originally developed for examinations of elderly patients [106]. This objective tool is based on the calculation of only two components, serum albumin and actual to ideal body weight ratio, and its usefulness was examined in 490 patients undergoing hemodialysis. As compared to MIS, used as the reference standard, GNRI was found to be superior as a nutritional tool [107]. Indeed, our group reported that lower GNRI was a significant predictor of all-cause mortality in 490 hemodialysis patients [108]. Subsequently, GNRI findings were shown to be capable of predicting cardiovascular [109] and infection-related [110] mortality. Moreover, a meta-analysis that included 19 studies (10,739 hemodialysis patients) revealed an inverse association between GNRI and all-cause mortality [odds ratio (OR) 0.90, 95% confidence interval (CI) 0.84–0.97, $p = 0.004$ (per one unit increase) and OR 2.15, 95% CI 1.88–2.46, $p < 0.00001$] [111]. Additionally, the results of this analysis showed similar negative associations of GNRI with CVD events and CVD mortality. Together, these findings suggest that GNRI is not only a useful nutritional screening tool but can also be used as a prognosis indicator for patients undergoing hemodialysis treatment.

3.7. GLIM

Apart from PEW, nutritional improvement is a common challenge in a variety of clinical settings, including treatment for conditions, such as cancer, as well as liver and inflammatory bowel diseases. Since a universal evaluation of nutritional status may be required, the Global Leadership Initiative on Malnutrition (GLIM) criteria have been proposed [112]. The main feature is etiology-independent diagnosis for use in various clinical settings that consists of a two-step approach, including an initial screening to identify at-risk status, followed by a second assessment for diagnosis and grading the severity of nutritional disorders. The usefulness of GLIM was investigated in patients undergoing hemodialysis, which showed low levels of agreement, sensitivity, and accuracy as compared to the well-established SGA and MIS [113]. GLIM, SGA, and MIS findings were each shown to be capable of predicting death in crude analysis. However, a more consistent and stronger association was found with MIS and SGA as compared to GLIM with an adjusted model. Therefore, it is suggested that SGA and MIS may be superior to GLIM for evaluating nutritional status in patients with hemodialysis-related PEW.

3.8. NRI-JH

A diagnosis of PEW consists of four categories, as noted previously, although there have been problems with the adaption of these criteria for Asian patients including Japanese. For example, the cut-off value noted for serum albumin is less than 3.8 g/dL. Since the mean level of serum albumin in Japanese patients undergoing dialysis is 3.6 g/d, a more appropriate reference value should be considered [114]. In addition, age and gender are critical factors for cut-off values, such as for creatinine, as they have a relationship with muscle volume. Therefore, Kanda et al. developed a nutritional risk index for Japanese patients, NRI-JH, for predicting 1-year mortality based on data in the Japanese Society for Dialysis Therapy Renal Data Registry [23]. According to the concept of PEW, NRI-JH is calculated based on serum albumin (serum chemistry), serum total cholesterol (serum chemistry), BMI (body mass), and serum creatinine (muscle mass), with considerations for age and gender (Table 1). In this study, nPCR was examined as dietary protein intake (dietary intake), although no clear association with mortality was shown. Based on risk score, patients were divided into three groups: Low-risk: score 0 to 7, Medium-risk: score

8 to 10, and High-risk: score 11 and higher. In addition to 1-year mortality, a recent study showed a significant association of NRI-JH and long-term all-cause mortality in 3046 patients undergoing hemodialysis [115]. Furthermore, NRI-JH was associated with CVD mortality and infection-related mortality in this study.

Although NRI-JH may not be adequate for a full nutritional assessment, it is an objective tool based on practical measurements and the repeated use of this index may be useful for an evaluation of need for nutritional intervention. Furthermore, inclusion of creatinine in NRI-JH may reflect an aspect of sarcopenia as a surrogate marker of muscle mass.

3.9. Functional Evaluation of Skeletal Muscle

Evaluations of both physical function and body composition are necessary for comprehensive management of patients with nutritional disorders. Measurement of muscle strength is one representative approach. Notably, loss of muscle mass and decrease in muscle strength do not always occur simultaneously [11]. Observational studies suggested that a decline in muscle strength could precede a decrease in muscle loss in healthy elderly subjects [116,117]. The most common measurement of muscle strength is handgrip strength, while another is lower extremity (knee extensor) muscle strength. Handgrip strength assessment is also required for diagnosis of sarcopenia. Although the method for determining handgrip strength is simple, there are measurement variations among the presented reports. The inconsistent results may be due to varying posture, different dynameter devices, the hand used for testing, and intervals between the measurement. Therefore, the development of a standard procedure is required [118].

Previous studies have also noted that handgrip strength could be used to predict mortality in patients receiving dialysis [119,120]. More importantly, other reports noted that hemodialysis patients with low muscle strength showed worse prognosis as compared to those with low muscle mass [121,122]. Additionally, a recent meta-analysis of 14 studies demonstrated that lower handgrip strength had a stronger association with all-cause mortality as compared to higher handgrip strength in patients with CKD including ESKD (hazard ratio = 1.99) [123], although this study did not include the muscle mass data. In contrast to handgrip strength, knee extensor muscle strength, measured with a handheld dynamometer, is not commonly used, although it may have a direct link to physical performance [124]. Indeed, decreased knee extensor muscle strength was shown to be strongly associated with mortality in 190 patients receiving hemodialysis treatments [125].

4. Prevalence of PEW, Frailty, and Sarcopenia in Patients Receiving Dialysis

To counteract nutritional and geriatric syndromes, it is indispensable to understand their prevalence rates, as this information is necessary to evaluate the efficacy of possible intervention for patients affected by these syndromes and to allocate necessary health care resources. Although a meta-analysis is desirable, presently only limited data are available since international diagnostic criteria for each disorder have only been recently accepted or not yet reported.

4.1. Prevalence of PEW in Dialysis Patients

The prevalence of PEW in patients receiving dialysis ranges from 20% to 60% [16], as this is dependent on the availability and use of diagnostic criteria. Evidence-based determination of PEW prevalence is required. On behalf of the ISRNM, a meta-analysis was performed to examine the global prevalence of PEW based on results of 90 studies that included 16,434 dialysis patients from 34 countries [126]. For this study, SGA and MIS results were adopted for diagnosis of PEW. The 25th–75th percentile for PEW prevalence ranged from 28% to 54%, although a very high level of heterogeneity was observed among the studies ($I^2 = 97\%$, $p < 0.001$).

4.2. Prevalence of Frailty in Dialysis Patients

In a study of elderly community-dwelling subjects, frailty was noted in 6.9% [4]. However, limited information is available for dialysis patients [127]. Using the above-mentioned validated scoring system [4], frailty in patients undergoing hemodialysis was thoroughly examined with consideration of body composition [128]. As expected, the 30% prevalence of frailty in those patients was significantly higher than the general elderly population. Notably, a lower level of intracellular water, a marker of muscle mass, was strongly associated with frailty [128], which may also be linked to sarcopenia and PEW. Moreover, a recent meta-analysis provided additional information regarding frailty obtained by seven studies of a total of 2604 patients undergoing hemodialysis [129]. In six of those reports, the Fried phenotype scoring system was used for frailty diagnosis. The pooled prevalence of frailty was 46% (95% CI 34.2–58.3) and a high level of heterogeneity was observed ($I^2 = 96\%$, $p < 0.001$). In this study, advanced age, female gender, and presence of diabetes were found to significantly contribute to risk of frailty.

4.3. Prevalence of Sarcopenia in Dialysis Patients

To elucidate factors related to sarcopenia in dialysis patients, a meta-analysis was recently performed using 30 studies published after 2013 that included a total of 6162 patients [130]. Those results showed that the prevalence of sarcopenia was 28.5% (95% CI 22.9–34.1), although the range was quite wide from 4% to 68%. Intriguingly, age was not found to contribute to the prevalence of sarcopenia, suggesting that this population is highly susceptible to muscle disorders related to factors other than aging.

4.4. Overlap between Nutritional Disorders and Sarcopenia

A considerable overlap of PEW, sarcopenia, and frailty is expected, although scant related information is available. The association of sarcopenia, evaluated using the EWGSOP criteria with nutritional status assessed by SGA score in 170 elderly patients receiving hemodialysis in Brazil, was reported [131]. Interestingly, patients with sarcopenia had lower SGA scores, indicating a worse nutritional status. Moreover, the association of sarcopenia, scored according to the EWGSOP criteria and MIS, was examined in 70 hemodialysis patients in Brazil [132]. MIS was significantly associated with each parameter related to sarcopenia except for gait speed. In addition, in two reports from Asia, an inverse association between sarcopenia and MIS was shown in one [133], while this was non-significant in the other [134], even though the EWGSOP criteria were used in both.

Since these studies did not focus on the overlap between sarcopenia and nutritional status, we directly investigated the relationship between nutritional status assessed by NRI-JH and sarcopenia evaluated by the AWGS 2019 criteria in 315 patients undergoing hemodialysis [135]. The prevalence of medium-/high-risk patients was 31.1%, of whom 64.3% were diagnosed with sarcopenia. Importantly, 84.7% patients considered to be medium-/high-risk fell below the cut-off value for muscle strength related to sarcopenia. These results suggest a profound association of nutritional disorder with sarcopenia and a search for common factors related to both conditions may lead to novel interventions.

5. Mortality Related to PEW, Frailty, and Sarcopenia in Patients Undergoing Dialysis

Nutritional disorders and geriatric syndromes are comprised of multifaceted factors, resulting in a variety of outcomes, including cognitive impairment, falls, fractures, vascular access failure, and poor quality of life, as well as CVD and infection events. Among those, all-cause death may be the clearest outcome. However, there are no meta-analysis results available regarding the relationship of PEW and mortality.

As for frailty, it generally seems to be associated with death as compared to other outcomes, regardless of the evaluation method used [136]. A recent meta-analysis showed that patients with frailty undergoing hemodialysis had a greater risk for all-cause mortality as compared to those without frailty (HR 2.02, 95% CI 1.65–2.48) [129].

As compared to a diagnosis of frailty, the criteria for sarcopenia presented by the EWGSOP and AWGS are clear. A recently conducted meta-analysis of eight studies (2117 dialysis patients) that mainly used consensus criteria, such as those of the EWGSOP and AWGS, found that patients with sarcopenia were associated with higher mortality as compared to those without (HR 1.87, 95% CI 1.35–2.59, I^2: 40%) [137]. At the same time, an investigation of the association of sarcopenia with hospitalization or ESKD progression in patients with CKD was conducted, although no definitive conclusions could be made due to the limited number of reports available.

6. Points of Attention for Nutritional Management

6.1. Amino Acids

Amino acids (AAs) form proteins that are necessary for structure, function including enzymatic activity, and fuel reserve throughout the body, with appropriate quantity and quality required to maintain skeletal muscle mass and function. However, a considerable loss of AAs into dialysate occurs during a hemodialysis session, resulting in a decreased concentration in plasma [138]. Furthermore, hemodiafiltration and hemofiltration can cause additional loss of AAs due to ultrafiltration [139,140]. In patients with three times of weekly hemodialysis session, the annual loss of AAs is estimated to be greater than 800 g/year, resulting in considerable loss of muscle mass [141]. In another study, 20 g of oral protein intake during the hemodialysis session could not compensate for the decline in plasma [138], thus AA supplementation is considered to be essential. Among AAs, leucine is not only a precursor of muscle protein but also a potent stimulator of muscle protein synthesis [142]. Interestingly, a recent meta-analysis showed a significant relationship between leucine supplementation and muscle mass, although there was no clear association of essential AAs with muscle mass, muscle strength, or physical performance found [143]. A balanced and tailored supplementation of AAs, possibly together with exercise as described below, is expected to improve nutritional disorders in affected dialysis patients.

6.2. Exercise

Skeletal muscle is dynamic and distinct from other organs, in which contraction plays a critical role for maintaining homeostasis [11,144]. In addition, physical exercise performed with those muscles has beneficial effects throughout the whole body, including the nervous system, hormones, and cytokines.

Aging is an inevitable risk factor for loss of skeletal muscle mass and function, known as sarcopenia. Elderly patients undergoing dialysis who suffer from both PEW and geriatric syndromes may often suffer from the vicious cycle between low physical activity and sarcopenia, thus intentional physical exercise is highly recommended. In general, aerobic exercise does not have a large effect on muscle hypertrophy. On the other hand, it may improve insulin resistance, a common component of both aging and PEW, resulting in maintenance of skeletal muscle. As compared to the anabolic action of insulin on glucose and lipid metabolism, it is unclear whether insulin has effects on protein synthesis. A recently published study clearly showed that insulin-stimulated protein synthesis in human skeletal muscle [145] in elderly subjects was found to be lower as compared to younger subjects [146]. Interestingly, aerobic exercise improved age-related protein synthesis caused by insulin resistance in the elderly group [147]. Further studies are needed to determine whether aerobic exercise can improve PEW-induced insulin resistance, resulting in protein synthesis in skeletal muscle.

As compared to aerobic exercise, resistance training is recognized to induce muscle hypertrophy and muscle strength. Using CKD model mice, the effects of aerobic as well as resistance exercise on muscle wasting were examined [148]. Although both types of exercise counteracted CKD-induced protein degradation in skeletal muscle, only resistance training improved protein synthesis, suggesting different actions associated with each type. In 23 patients receiving hemodialysis treatments, intervention by resistance training led to muscle hypertrophy, which was comparable in nine healthy subjects [149], although some of the findings reported were inconsistent [150].

In the context of nutritional management for patients undergoing dialysis, the combination of nutritional supplementation and exercise is likely the approach most expected to be used. However, this combined intervention during hemodialysis was found to not always have synergistic effects in hemodialysis patients [15,16,151,152]. A possible explanation for this unexpected observation may be due to inadequate intensity, duration, and/or timing of the performed exercise. In consideration of AA loss during a hemodialysis session, adequate replenishment of AAs is theoretically necessary. In elderly subjects, ingestion of leucin after resistance training resulted in prolonged protein synthesis in skeletal muscle [153]. Future studies should be conducted to establish an appropriate combination of nutritional supplementation and resistance exercise for elderly dialysis patients.

7. Topics of Interest Related to Nutritional Status and Infection

7.1. Infection-Related Outcomes and Medical Costs

Infection is a common cause of death in patients undergoing dialysis, apart from the recent COVID-19 pandemic. In Japan, infectious diseases were shown to be the second leading cause of death in 2018 at 21.3% [154]. Infection-related deaths have been increasing since 1993 and this is expected to be the most common cause of mortality in the near future.

From an economic perspective, hospitalization is a greater problem than death. In the US, the rate of hospitalization for patients undergoing hemodialysis is two times higher and 37% of those patients are re-hospitalized within 30 days of discharge [155], with hospitalization especially common for elderly incidental patients [156]. Among individuals receiving support from Medicare, the US federal health insurance program for those who are aged 65 years or older, younger with disabilities, or with ESKD, patients receiving hemodialysis treatment comprise only 1%, although they account for 9% of Medicare expenditures. Therefore, hospitalization drives up the cost for hemodialysis patients [155].

Among the various causes, infection is a major factor related to hospitalization [157] and infection-related hospitalizations have dramatically increased among patients receiving hemodialysis treatment [158]. The latter report noted that 28% of patients undergoing in-center hemodialysis (Medicare beneficiaries) experienced at least one infection-related hospitalization [158]. Risk factors for hospitalization were found to be higher age, lower serum albumin level, inability to ambulate or transfer, cancer, chronic obstructive pulmonary disease, drug dependence, residence in a care facility, and treatment for other than a fistula.

7.2. Hospitalization for Infection and Resultant Short-Term Outcomes in Patients Undergoing Hemodialysis

Infection is a common cause of hospitalization, thus it is important to understand the consequences of infection-related hospitalization from the viewpoint of both clinical practice and medical economics. Surprisingly, limited data are available regarding the outcomes of these cases. The HEMO study examined whether a higher dialysis dose or use of a high-flux dialyzer membrane resulted in reduced mortality, and examined infection-related hospitalization as a secondary outcome [159]. In this study, 783 (42.4%) of 1846 hemodialysis patients had at least one hospitalization for infection [160]. Among those who were hospitalized, 57.7% had a severe outcome, with 28.6% in the hospital for longer than 7 days and 15.3% treated in the intensive care unit (ICU), while 13.8% died. Older age and lower albumin were shown to be associated with worse outcome. Another study focused on 30-day outcomes after discharge following infection-related hospitalization using the US Renal Data System [161]. Of 140,665 patients, 60,270 (42.8%) experienced at least one hospitalization for infection. Furthermore, of 54,996 who survived the initial hospitalization and were available for a 30-day follow-up examination, 27% were readmitted and survived for 30 days, while 3% were readmitted and then died within 30 days of discharge, and 4% died without hospital readmission. In this study, lower albumin, lower BMI, physical inability, absence of nephrology care prior to dialysis, and non-Hispanic ethnicity were associated with readmission or death without readmission. On the other hand, older age, white race, comorbid conditions, and institutionalization were found to independently contribute to death without readmission. These results indicate a profound link to advance care planning and conservative kidney management, although these topics are beyond the scope of the present report.

7.3. Chronic Critical Illness (CCI)

As emphasized at the beginning of this study, obesity and its related complications including acute myocardial infarction (AMI) have been shown to be severe problems in the US. However, recent medical advances have changed trends in regard to those accompanied by aging. A retrospective study using Medicare data from 1996 to 2008 showed that numbers of hospitalizations for AMI showed a gradual decease, whereas those for sepsis were dramatically increased (2.7 times higher) [162]. As a result, the overall costs of acute hospitalization for AMI and sepsis were USD 3.16 and 15.73 billion, respectively, during that time period. In addition, recent treatment in an ICU has been shown to enable patients with severe illness to survive. Although saving lives is desirable, this situation has also led to the new nebulous term 'chronic critical illness (CCI)' [163,164]. Patients with CCI who tend to have recurrent infections, organ dysfunction, weakness, and/or delirium, frequently require long-term care and remain institutionalized. These reports noted that the annual cost is estimated to more than USD 20 billion.

7.4. Nutritional Disorders and Infection

It is generally accepted that a strong association exists between PEW and infection. Furthermore, a correlation between nutritional resilience and infection-related events in patients undergoing hemodialysis has been described [155]. As noted previously, short-term outcomes after infection-related hospitalization have been found to be poor [160,161]. Some factors noted in the present review were shown to be related to worse outcome, such as older age, lower albumin, and lower BMI. However, long-term outcomes in this population, which are more relevant to clinical and economical countermeasures, are largely unknown.

7.5. Nutritional Disorders and Long-Term Mortality after Hospitalization for Infection

To bridge the gap related to the association of nutritional status and infection-related long-term outcomes, we examined findings of a prospective cohort of 518 patients undergoing hemodialysis to determine whether the GNRI used as a nutritional screening tool could provide results predictive of infection-related hospitalization and subsequent death [165]. Previous reports have noted that lower GNRI was associated with higher all-cause mortality [111] as well as infection-related mortality [110] (Figure 1A). Although no data regarding a direct association between GNRI and short-term mortality after hospitalization for infection are available, lower albumin together with older age or lower BMI has been speculated to be correlated to short-term mortality [160,161] (Figure 1B).

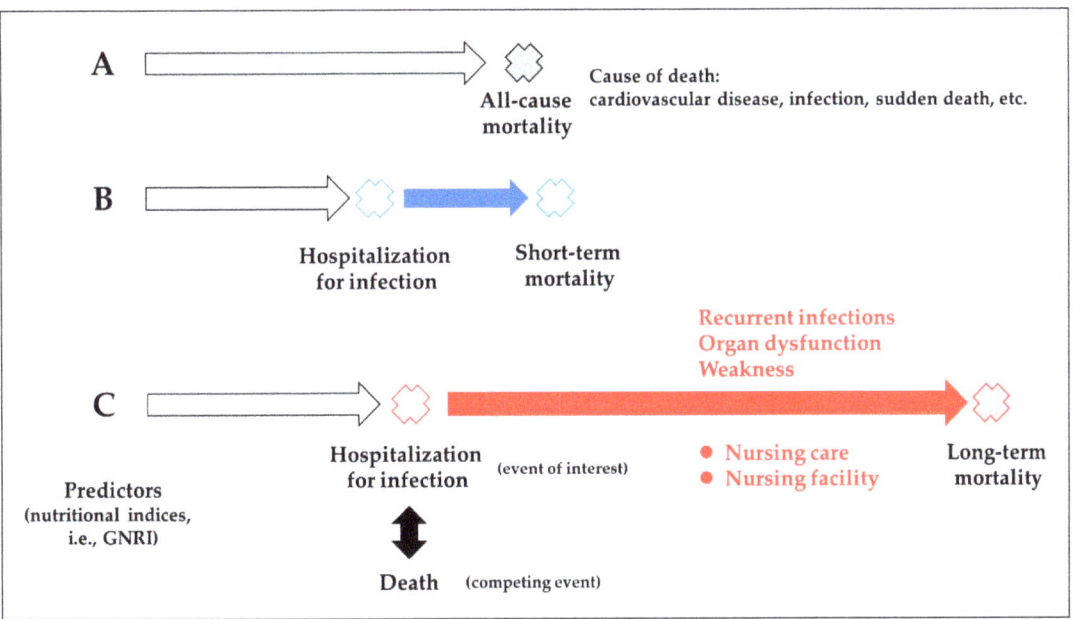

Figure 1. Short- and long-term outcomes after hospitalization for infection.

Our study was the first to show an inverse association of GNRI and all-cause mortality with reproducibility [111]. Therefore, we focused on the association of GNRI with hospitalization for infection. Patients who died are no longer at risk of hospitalization for infection, thus analysis of the multivariable-adjusted association of GNRI with hospitalization for infection was conducted with a Fine-Gray model but not a Cox model, with death as a competing risk factor (Figure 1C) [166,167]. Our prior investigation found that the GNRI was unable to predict hospitalization for infection [165], thus we examined death after hospitalization for infection. On the other hand, it is interesting to note that the GNRI could be used to predict death after hospitalization for infection during the subsequent 2.5-year follow-up period [165], suggesting that baseline GNRI findings can be used for prediction of not only mortality but also long-term death in patients who have been hospitalized for infection.

8. Missing Link among PEW, Immunodeficiency, and Infection

The presence of CKD/ESKD is profoundly associated with a type of immunodeficiency referred to as secondary immunodeficiency related to kidney disease (SIDKD) [168], with aging and malnutrition known to be involved. It is plausible that PEW in elderly patients receiving hemodialysis treatment leads to immunodeficiency, resulting in infection. However, the mechanisms are largely unknown. As described previously, patients with CCI who survive an acute illness often suffer from subsequent recurrent infections. The hallmark traits of CCI are persistent inflammation, immunosuppression, and catabolism syndrome (PICS) [169–172]. Although the trigger for CCI/PICS is critical illness, such as sepsis, common to PEW are subsequent protein catabolism/cachexia, persistent inflammation, and possibly immune suppression. Recent studies have presented findings that suggest involvement of myeloid-derived suppressor cells (MDSCs) as one of the pathogenic factors related to CCI/PICS [169–171]. Furthermore, another recent report showed that increased levels of MDSCs in patients with ESKD were positively associated with infectious events [173]. Additional studies are necessary to better reveal the associations among PEW, immunodeficiency, and infection.

9. Conclusions

Methods for early detection of nutritional disorders will be useful for developing comprehensive intervention strategies for elderly patients undergoing dialysis with the goal of preserving health. An appropriate nutritional status can result in maintaining regular physical activity, which leads to a sense of well-being that can protect from PEW, sarcopenia, and frailty. Additionally, measures against infection are a priority requirement for this population. Elucidation of the underlying mechanisms related to undernutrition, immunodeficiency, and infection should assist in the development of better treatments, resulting in improved prognosis for affected individuals.

Funding: This research was supported in part by a Grant-in-Aid for Scientific Research (C) (No. 22K08334) from the Japan Society for the Promotion of Science (to K.M.).

Institutional Review Board Statement: Not applicable.

Informed Consent Statement: Not applicable.

Data Availability Statement: Not applicable.

Conflicts of Interest: The authors declare no conflict of interest.

References

1. Popkin, B.M.; Corvalan, C.; Grummer-Strawn, L.M. Dynamics of the double burden of malnutrition and the changing nutrition reality. *Lancet* **2020**, *395*, 65–74. [CrossRef] [PubMed]
2. Sarma, S.; Sockalingam, S.; Dash, S. Obesity as a multisystem disease: Trends in obesity rates and obesity-related complications. *Diabetes Obes. Metab.* **2021**, *23* (Suppl. S1), 3–16. [CrossRef] [PubMed]
3. Mathers, C.D.; Stevens, G.A.; Boerma, T.; White, R.A.; Tobias, M.I. Causes of international increases in older age life expectancy. *Lancet* **2015**, *385*, 540–548. [CrossRef] [PubMed]
4. Fried, L.P.; Tangen, C.M.; Walston, J.; Newman, A.B.; Hirsch, C.; Gottdiener, J.; Seeman, T.; Tracy, R.; Kop, W.J.; Burke, G.; et al. Frailty in older adults: Evidence for a phenotype. *J. Gerontol. A Biol. Sci. Med. Sci.* **2001**, *56*, M146–M156. [CrossRef]
5. Rosenberg, I.H. Sarcopenia: Origins and clinical relevance. *J. Nutr.* **1997**, *127*, 990S–991S. [CrossRef] [PubMed]
6. Wang, X.; Vrtiska, T.J.; Avula, R.T.; Walters, L.R.; Chakkera, H.A.; Kremers, W.K.; Lerman, L.O.; Rule, A.D. Age, kidney function, and risk factors associate differently with cortical and medullary volumes of the kidney. *Kidney Int.* **2014**, *85*, 677–685. [CrossRef] [PubMed]
7. Denic, A.; Glassock, R.J.; Rule, A.D. Structural and Functional Changes with the Aging Kidney. *Adv. Chronic Kidney Dis.* **2016**, *23*, 19–28. [CrossRef]
8. Imai, E.; Horio, M.; Watanabe, T.; Iseki, K.; Yamagata, K.; Hara, S.; Ura, N.; Kiyohara, Y.; Moriyama, T.; Ando, Y.; et al. Prevalence of chronic kidney disease in the Japanese general population. *Clin. Exp. Nephrol.* **2009**, *13*, 621–630. [CrossRef]
9. Nitta, K.; Masakane, I.; Hanafusa, N.; Taniguchi, M.; Hasegawa, T.; Nakai, S.; Goto, S.; Wada, A.; Hamano, T.; Hoshino, J. Annual dialysis data report 2017, JSDT renal data registry. *Ren. Replace. Ther.* **2019**, *5*, 53. [CrossRef]
10. Mori, K.; Nishide, K.; Okuno, S.; Shoji, T.; Emoto, M.; Tsuda, A.; Nakatani, S.; Imanishi, Y.; Ishimura, E.; Yamakawa, T.; et al. Impact of diabetes on sarcopenia and mortality in patients undergoing hemodialysis. *BMC Nephrol.* **2019**, *20*, 105. [CrossRef]
11. Mori, K. Maintenance of Skeletal Muscle to Counteract Sarcopenia in Patients with Advanced Chronic Kidney Disease and Especially Those Undergoing Hemodialysis. *Nutrients* **2021**, *13*, 1538. [CrossRef]
12. Inaba, M.; Mori, K. Extension of Healthy Life Span of Dialysis Patients in the Era of a 100-Year Life. *Nutrients* **2021**, *13*, 2693. [CrossRef] [PubMed]
13. Isaka, Y. Optimal Protein Intake in Pre-Dialysis Chronic Kidney Disease Patients with Sarcopenia: An Overview. *Nutrients* **2021**, *13*, 1205. [CrossRef]
14. Fouque, D.; Kalantar-Zadeh, K.; Kopple, J.; Cano, N.; Chauveau, P.; Cuppari, L.; Franch, H.; Guarnieri, G.; Ikizler, T.A.; Kaysen, G.; et al. A proposed nomenclature and diagnostic criteria for protein-energy wasting in acute and chronic kidney disease. *Kidney Int.* **2008**, *73*, 391–398. [CrossRef] [PubMed]
15. Oliveira, E.A.; Zheng, R.; Carter, C.E.; Mak, R.H. Cachexia/Protein energy wasting syndrome in CKD: Causation and treatment. *Semin. Dial.* **2019**, *32*, 493–499. [CrossRef] [PubMed]
16. Ikizler, T.A. Optimal nutrition in hemodialysis patients. *Adv. Chronic Kidney Dis.* **2013**, *20*, 181–189. [CrossRef]
17. Hanna, R.M.; Ghobry, L.; Wassef, O.; Rhee, C.M.; Kalantar-Zadeh, K. A Practical Approach to Nutrition, Protein-Energy Wasting, Sarcopenia, and Cachexia in Patients with Chronic Kidney Disease. *Blood Purif.* **2020**, *49*, 202–211. [CrossRef] [PubMed]
18. Herselman, M.; Moosa, M.R.; Kotze, T.J.; Kritzinger, M.; Wuister, S.; Mostert, D. Protein-energy malnutrition as a risk factor for increased morbidity in long-term hemodialysis patients. *J. Ren. Nutr.* **2000**, *10*, 7–15. [CrossRef] [PubMed]
19. Kalantar-Zadeh, K.; Ikizler, T.A.; Block, G.; Avram, M.M.; Kopple, J.D. Malnutrition-inflammation complex syndrome in dialysis patients: Causes and consequences. *Am. J. Kidney Dis.* **2003**, *42*, 864–881. [CrossRef]

20. Pupim, L.B.; Caglar, K.; Hakim, R.M.; Shyr, Y.; Ikizler, T.A. Uremic malnutrition is a predictor of death independent of inflammatory status. *Kidney Int.* **2004**, *66*, 2054–2060. [CrossRef]
21. Mak, R.H.; Cheung, W.; Cone, R.D.; Marks, D.L. Mechanisms of disease: Cytokine and adipokine signaling in uremic cachexia. *Nat. Clin. Pract. Nephrol.* **2006**, *2*, 527–534. [CrossRef]
22. Ikizler, T.A.; Cano, N.J.; Franch, H.; Fouque, D.; Himmelfarb, J.; Kalantar-Zadeh, K.; Kuhlmann, M.K.; Stenvinkel, P.; TerWee, P.; Teta, D.; et al. Prevention and treatment of protein energy wasting in chronic kidney disease patients: A consensus statement by the International Society of Renal Nutrition and Metabolism. *Kidney Int.* **2013**, *84*, 1096–1107. [CrossRef]
23. Kanda, E.; Kato, A.; Masakane, I.; Kanno, Y. A new nutritional risk index for predicting mortality in hemodialysis patients: Nationwide cohort study. *PLoS ONE* **2019**, *14*, e0214524. [CrossRef]
24. Woodhouse, K.W.; Wynne, H.; Baillie, S.; James, O.F.; Rawlins, M.D. Who are the frail elderly? *Q. J. Med.* **1988**, *68*, 505–506.
25. Buchner, D.M.; Wagner, E.H. Preventing frail health. *Clin. Geriatr. Med.* **1992**, *8*, 1–18. [CrossRef]
26. Rockwood, K.; Mitnitski, A. Frailty in relation to the accumulation of deficits. *J. Gerontol. A Biol. Sci. Med. Sci.* **2007**, *62*, 722–727. [CrossRef] [PubMed]
27. Sabatino, A.; Cuppari, L.; Stenvinkel, P.; Lindholm, B.; Avesani, C.M. Sarcopenia in chronic kidney disease: What have we learned so far? *J. Nephrol.* **2021**, *34*, 1347–1372. [CrossRef] [PubMed]
28. Cruz-Jentoft, A.J.; Baeyens, J.P.; Bauer, J.M.; Boirie, Y.; Cederholm, T.; Landi, F.; Martin, F.C.; Michel, J.P.; Rolland, Y.; Schneider, S.M.; et al. Sarcopenia: European consensus on definition and diagnosis: Report of the European Working Group on Sarcopenia in Older People. *Age Ageing* **2010**, *39*, 412–423. [CrossRef] [PubMed]
29. Chen, L.K.; Liu, L.K.; Woo, J.; Assantachai, P.; Auyeung, T.W.; Bahyah, K.S.; Chou, M.Y.; Chen, L.Y.; Hsu, P.S.; Krairit, O.; et al. Sarcopenia in Asia: Consensus report of the Asian Working Group for Sarcopenia. *J. Am. Med. Dir. Assoc.* **2014**, *15*, 95–101. [CrossRef] [PubMed]
30. Cruz-Jentoft, A.J.; Bahat, G.; Bauer, J.; Boirie, Y.; Bruyere, O.; Cederholm, T.; Cooper, C.; Landi, F.; Rolland, Y.; Sayer, A.A.; et al. Sarcopenia: Revised European consensus on definition and diagnosis. *Age Ageing* **2019**, *48*, 601. [CrossRef] [PubMed]
31. Chen, L.K.; Woo, J.; Assantachai, P.; Auyeung, T.W.; Chou, M.Y.; Iijima, K.; Jang, H.C.; Kang, L.; Kim, M.; Kim, S.; et al. Asian Working Group for Sarcopenia: 2019 Consensus Update on Sarcopenia Diagnosis and Treatment. *J. Am. Med. Dir. Assoc.* **2020**, *21*, 300–307.e302. [CrossRef]
32. Correia, M. Nutrition Screening vs Nutrition Assessment: What's the Difference? *Nutr. Clin. Pract.* **2018**, *33*, 62–72. [CrossRef] [PubMed]
33. Correia, M. Response to Comment on 'Nutrition Screening vs Nutrition Assessment: What's the Difference?'. *Nutr Clin Pract.* **2018**, *33*, 307–308. [CrossRef]
34. Kalantar-Zadeh, K.; Kopple, J.D.; Block, G.; Humphreys, M.H. A malnutrition-inflammation score is correlated with morbidity and mortality in maintenance hemodialysis patients. *Am. J. Kidney Dis.* **2001**, *38*, 1251–1263. [CrossRef] [PubMed]
35. Park, J.; Ahmadi, S.F.; Streja, E.; Molnar, M.Z.; Flegal, K.M.; Gillen, D.; Kovesdy, C.P.; Kalantar-Zadeh, K. Obesity paradox in end-stage kidney disease patients. *Prog. Cardiovasc. Dis.* **2014**, *56*, 415–425. [CrossRef] [PubMed]
36. Kalantar-Zadeh, K.; Block, G.; Humphreys, M.H.; Kopple, J.D. Reverse epidemiology of cardiovascular risk factors in maintenance dialysis patients. *Kidney Int.* **2003**, *63*, 793–808. [CrossRef] [PubMed]
37. Yen, T.H.; Lin, J.L.; Lin-Tan, D.T.; Hsu, C.W. Association between body mass and mortality in maintenance hemodialysis patients. *Apher. Dial.* **2010**, *14*, 400–408. [CrossRef]
38. Park, J.; Jin, D.C.; Molnar, M.Z.; Dukkipati, R.; Kim, Y.L.; Jing, J.; Levin, N.W.; Nissenson, A.R.; Lee, J.S.; Kalantar-Zadeh, K. Mortality predictability of body size and muscle mass surrogates in Asian vs white and African American hemodialysis patients. *Mayo Clin. Proc.* **2013**, *88*, 479–486. [CrossRef]
39. Kalantar-Zadeh, K.; Regidor, D.L.; Kovesdy, C.P.; Van Wyck, D.; Bunnapradist, S.; Horwich, T.B.; Fonarow, G.C. Fluid retention is associated with cardiovascular mortality in patients undergoing long-term hemodialysis. *Circulation* **2009**, *119*, 671–679. [CrossRef]
40. Okuno, S. Significance of Adipose Tissue Maintenance in Patients Undergoing Hemodialysis. *Nutrients* **2021**, *13*, 1895. [CrossRef] [PubMed]
41. Postorino, M.; Marino, C.; Tripepi, G.; Zoccali, C.; Group, C.W. Abdominal obesity and all-cause and cardiovascular mortality in end-stage renal disease. *J. Am. Coll. Cardiol.* **2009**, *53*, 1265–1272. [CrossRef] [PubMed]
42. Kalantar-Zadeh, K.; Rhee, C.M.; Chou, J.; Ahmadi, S.F.; Park, J.; Chen, J.L.; Amin, A.N. The Obesity Paradox in Kidney Disease: How to Reconcile it with Obesity Management. *Kidney Int. Rep.* **2017**, *2*, 271–281. [CrossRef] [PubMed]
43. Hoogeveen, E.K.; Halbesma, N.; Rothman, K.J.; Stijnen, T.; van Dijk, S.; Dekker, F.W.; Boeschoten, E.W.; de Mutsert, R.; Netherlands Cooperative Study on the Adequacy of Dialysis-2 Study, G. Obesity and mortality risk among younger dialysis patients. *Clin. J. Am. Soc. Nephrol.* **2012**, *7*, 280–288. [CrossRef]
44. Sakao, Y.; Ojima, T.; Yasuda, H.; Hashimoto, S.; Hasegawa, T.; Iseki, K.; Tsubakihara, Y.; Kato, A. Serum Creatinine Modifies Associations between Body Mass Index and Mortality and Morbidity in Prevalent Hemodialysis Patients. *PLoS ONE* **2016**, *11*, e0150003. [CrossRef]
45. Chumlea, W.C. Anthropometric and body composition assessment in dialysis patients. *Semin. Dial.* **2004**, *17*, 466–470. [CrossRef] [PubMed]

46. Chumlea, W.C.; Dwyer, J.; Bergen, C.; Burkart, J.; Paranandi, L.; Frydrych, A.; Cockram, D.B.; Kusek, J.W.; McLeroy, S.; Hemodialysis Study, G. Nutritional status assessed from anthropometric measures in the HEMO study. *J. Ren. Nutr.* **2003**, *13*, 31–38. [CrossRef]
47. Alberti, K.G.; Zimmet, P.; Shaw, J. Metabolic syndrome—A new world-wide definition. A Consensus Statement from the International Diabetes Federation. *Diabet. Med.* **2006**, *23*, 469–480. [CrossRef]
48. Kakita, D.; Matsuzawa, R.; Yamamoto, S.; Suzuki, Y.; Harada, M.; Imamura, K.; Yoshikoshi, S.; Imai, H.; Osada, S.; Shimokado, K.; et al. Simplified discriminant parameters for sarcopenia among patients undergoing haemodialysis. *J. Cachexia Sarcopenia Muscle* **2022**, *13*, 2898–2907. [CrossRef]
49. Su, C.T.; Yabes, J.; Pike, F.; Weiner, D.E.; Beddhu, S.; Burrowes, J.D.; Rocco, M.V.; Unruh, M.L. Changes in anthropometry and mortality in maintenance hemodialysis patients in the HEMO Study. *Am. J. Kidney Dis.* **2013**, *62*, 1141–1150. [CrossRef]
50. Stosovic, M.; Stanojevic, M.; Simic-Ogrizovic, S.; Jovanovic, D.; Djukanovic, L. The predictive value of anthropometric parameters on mortality in haemodialysis patients. *Nephrol. Dial. Transpl.* **2011**, *26*, 1367–1374. [CrossRef]
51. Ohkawa, S.; Odamaki, M.; Yoneyama, T.; Hibi, I.; Miyaji, K.; Kumagai, H. Standardized thigh muscle area measured by computed axial tomography as an alternate muscle mass index for nutritional assessment of hemodialysis patients. *Am. J. Clin. Nutr.* **2000**, *71*, 485–490. [CrossRef] [PubMed]
52. Noori, N.; Kopple, J.D.; Kovesdy, C.P.; Feroze, U.; Sim, J.J.; Murali, S.B.; Luna, A.; Gomez, M.; Luna, C.; Bross, R.; et al. Mid-arm muscle circumference and quality of life and survival in maintenance hemodialysis patients. *Clin. J. Am. Soc. Nephrol.* **2010**, *5*, 2258–2268. [CrossRef] [PubMed]
53. Barazzoni, R.; Jensen, G.L.; Correia, M.; Gonzalez, M.C.; Higashiguchi, T.; Shi, H.P.; Bischoff, S.C.; Boirie, Y.; Carrasco, F.; Cruz-Jentoft, A.; et al. Guidance for assessment of the muscle mass phenotypic criterion for the Global Leadership Initiative on Malnutrition (GLIM) diagnosis of malnutrition. *Clin. Nutr.* **2022**, *41*, 1425–1433. [CrossRef] [PubMed]
54. Kaizu, Y.; Ohkawa, S.; Kumagai, H. Muscle mass index in haemodialysis patients: A comparison of indices obtained by routine clinical examinations. *Nephrol. Dial. Transpl.* **2002**, *17*, 442–448. [CrossRef] [PubMed]
55. Lowrie, E.G.; Lew, N.L. Death risk in hemodialysis patients: The predictive value of commonly measured variables and an evaluation of death rate differences between facilities. *Am. J. Kidney Dis.* **1990**, *15*, 458–482. [CrossRef]
56. Mazairac, A.H.; de Wit, G.A.; Grooteman, M.P.; Penne, E.L.; van der Weerd, N.C.; van den Dorpel, M.A.; Nube, M.J.; Levesque, R.; Ter Wee, P.M.; Bots, M.L.; et al. A composite score of protein-energy nutritional status predicts mortality in haemodialysis patients no better than its individual components. *Nephrol. Dial. Transpl.* **2011**, *26*, 1962–1967. [CrossRef]
57. Kittiskulnam, P.; Chuengsaman, P.; Kanjanabuch, T.; Katesomboon, S.; Tungsanga, S.; Tiskajornsiri, K.; Praditpornsilpa, K.; Eiam-Ong, S. Protein-Energy Wasting and Mortality Risk Prediction Among Peritoneal Dialysis Patients. *J. Ren. Nutr.* **2021**, *31*, 679–686. [CrossRef]
58. de Roij van Zuijdewijn, C.L.; ter Wee, P.M.; Chapdelaine, I.; Bots, M.L.; Blankestijn, P.J.; van den Dorpel, M.A.; Nube, M.J.; Grooteman, M.P. A Comparison of 8 Nutrition-Related Tests to Predict Mortality in Hemodialysis Patients. *J. Ren. Nutr.* **2015**, *25*, 412–419. [CrossRef]
59. Kaysen, G.A.; Dubin, J.A.; Muller, H.G.; Mitch, W.E.; Rosales, L.M.; Levin, N.W. Relationships among inflammation nutrition and physiologic mechanisms establishing albumin levels in hemodialysis patients. *Kidney Int.* **2002**, *61*, 2240–2249. [CrossRef]
60. Don, B.R.; Kaysen, G. Serum albumin: Relationship to inflammation and nutrition. *Semin. Dial.* **2004**, *17*, 432–437. [CrossRef]
61. de Mutsert, R.; Grootendorst, D.C.; Indemans, F.; Boeschoten, E.W.; Krediet, R.T.; Dekker, F.W.; Netherlands Cooperative Study on the Adequacy of Dialysis, I.I.S.G. Association between serum albumin and mortality in dialysis patients is partly explained by inflammation, and not by malnutrition. *J. Ren. Nutr.* **2009**, *19*, 127–135. [CrossRef] [PubMed]
62. Suzuki, Y.; Harada, M.; Matsuzawa, R.; Hoshi, K.; Koh, Y.M.; Aoyama, N.; Uemura, K.; Yamamoto, S.; Imamura, K.; Yoshikoshi, S.; et al. Trajectory of Serum Albumin Prior to Death in Patients Receiving Hemodialysis. *J. Ren. Nutr.* **2022**. [CrossRef] [PubMed]
63. Kalantar-Zadeh, K.; Kilpatrick, R.D.; Kuwae, N.; McAllister, C.J.; Alcorn, H., Jr.; Kopple, J.D.; Greenland, S. Revisiting mortality predictability of serum albumin in the dialysis population: Time dependency, longitudinal changes and population-attributable fraction. *Nephrol. Dial. Transpl.* **2005**, *20*, 1880–1888. [CrossRef] [PubMed]
64. Eriguchi, R.; Obi, Y.; Streja, E.; Tortorici, A.R.; Rhee, C.M.; Soohoo, M.; Kim, T.; Kovesdy, C.P.; Kalantar-Zadeh, K. Longitudinal Associations among Renal Urea Clearance-Corrected Normalized Protein Catabolic Rate, Serum Albumin, and Mortality in Patients on Hemodialysis. *Clin. J. Am. Soc. Nephrol.* **2017**, *12*, 1109–1117. [CrossRef]
65. Kim, H.W.; Jhee, J.H.; Joo, Y.S.; Yang, K.H.; Jung, J.J.; Shin, J.H.; Han, S.H.; Yoo, T.H.; Kang, S.W.; Park, J.T. Clinical significance of hemodialysis quality of care indicators in very elderly patients with end stage kidney disease. *J. Nephrol.* **2022**, *35*, 2351–2361. [CrossRef]
66. Kanno, Y.; Kanda, E. Comparison of accuracy between pre-hemodialysis and post-hemodialysis levels of nutritional factors for prediction of mortality in hemodialysis patients. *Clin. Nutr.* **2019**, *38*, 383–388. [CrossRef]
67. Spiekerman, A.M. Proteins used in nutritional assessment. *Clin. Lab. Med.* **1993**, *13*, 353–369. [CrossRef]
68. Chertow, G.M.; Ackert, K.; Lew, N.L.; Lazarus, J.M.; Lowrie, E.G. Prealbumin is as important as albumin in the nutritional assessment of hemodialysis patients. *Kidney Int.* **2000**, *58*, 2512–2517. [CrossRef]
69. Chertow, G.M.; Goldstein-Fuchs, D.J.; Lazarus, J.M.; Kaysen, G.A. Prealbumin, mortality, and cause-specific hospitalization in hemodialysis patients. *Kidney Int.* **2005**, *68*, 2794–2800. [CrossRef]

70. Rambod, M.; Kovesdy, C.P.; Bross, R.; Kopple, J.D.; Kalantar-Zadeh, K. Association of serum prealbumin and its changes over time with clinical outcomes and survival in patients receiving hemodialysis. *Am. J. Clin. Nutr.* **2008**, *88*, 1485–1494. [CrossRef]
71. Caglar, K.; Fedje, L.; Dimmitt, R.; Hakim, R.M.; Shyr, Y.; Ikizler, T.A. Therapeutic effects of oral nutritional supplementation during hemodialysis. *Kidney Int.* **2002**, *62*, 1054–1059. [CrossRef] [PubMed]
72. Gkouvatsos, K.; Papanikolaou, G.; Pantopoulos, K. Regulation of iron transport and the role of transferrin. *Biochim. Biophys. Acta* **2012**, *1820*, 188–202. [CrossRef] [PubMed]
73. Schmaier, A.H. Transferrin: A blood coagulation modifier. *Cell Res.* **2020**, *30*, 101–102. [CrossRef] [PubMed]
74. Kalantar-Zadeh, K.; Kleiner, M.; Dunne, E.; Ahern, K.; Nelson, M.; Koslowe, R.; Luft, F.C. Total iron-binding capacity-estimated transferrin correlates with the nutritional subjective global assessment in hemodialysis patients. *Am. J. Kidney Dis.* **1998**, *31*, 263–272. [CrossRef] [PubMed]
75. Bross, R.; Zitterkoph, J.; Pithia, J.; Benner, D.; Rambod, M.; Kovesdy, C.P.; Kopple, J.D.; Kalantar-Zadeh, K. Association of serum total iron-binding capacity and its changes over time with nutritional and clinical outcomes in hemodialysis patients. *Am. J. Nephrol.* **2009**, *29*, 571–581. [CrossRef]
76. Patel, S.S.; Molnar, M.Z.; Tayek, J.A.; Ix, J.H.; Noori, N.; Benner, D.; Heymsfield, S.; Kopple, J.D.; Kovesdy, C.P.; Kalantar-Zadeh, K. Serum creatinine as a marker of muscle mass in chronic kidney disease: Results of a cross-sectional study and review of literature. *J. Cachexia Sarcopenia Muscle* **2013**, *4*, 19–29. [CrossRef]
77. Inaba, M.; Kurajoh, M.; Okuno, S.; Imanishi, Y.; Yamada, S.; Mori, K.; Ishimura, E.; Yamakawa, T.; Nishizawa, Y. Poor muscle quality rather than reduced lean body mass is responsible for the lower serum creatinine level in hemodialysis patients with diabetes mellitus. *Clin. Nephrol.* **2010**, *74*, 266–272.
78. Gracia-Iguacel, C.; Gonzalez-Parra, E.; Mahillo, I.; Ortiz, A. Criteria for classification of protein-energy wasting in dialysis patients: Impact on prevalence. *Br. J. Nutr.* **2019**, *121*, 1271–1278. [CrossRef]
79. Rhee, C.M. Low-T3 Syndrome in Peritoneal Dialysis: Metabolic Adaptation, Marker of Illness, or Mortality Mediator? *Clin. J. Am. Soc. Nephrol.* **2015**, *10*, 917–919. [CrossRef]
80. Chang, T.I.; Nam, J.Y.; Shin, S.K.; Kang, E.W. Low Triiodothyronine Syndrome and Long-Term Cardiovascular Outcome in Incident Peritoneal Dialysis Patients. *Clin. J. Am. Soc. Nephrol.* **2015**, *10*, 975–982. [CrossRef]
81. Inaba, M.; Mori, K.; Tsujimoto, Y.; Yamada, S.; Yamazaki, Y.; Emoto, M.; Shoji, T. Association of Reduced Free T3 to Free T4 Ratio with Lower Serum Creatinine in Japanese Hemodialysis Patients. *Nutrients* **2021**, *13*, 4537. [CrossRef] [PubMed]
82. Klag, M.J.; Ford, D.E.; Mead, L.A.; He, J.; Whelton, P.K.; Liang, K.Y.; Levine, D.M. Serum cholesterol in young men and subsequent cardiovascular disease. *N. Engl. J. Med.* **1993**, *328*, 313–318. [CrossRef] [PubMed]
83. Kalantar-Zadeh, K.; Block, G.; Horwich, T.; Fonarow, G.C. Reverse epidemiology of conventional cardiovascular risk factors in patients with chronic heart failure. *J. Am. Coll. Cardiol.* **2004**, *43*, 1439–1444. [CrossRef] [PubMed]
84. Iseki, K.; Yamazato, M.; Tozawa, M.; Takishita, S. Hypocholesterolemia is a significant predictor of death in a cohort of chronic hemodialysis patients. *Kidney Int.* **2002**, *61*, 1887–1893. [CrossRef] [PubMed]
85. Shoji, T.; Masakane, I.; Watanabe, Y.; Iseki, K.; Tsubakihara, Y.; Committee of Renal Data Registry, J.S.f.D.T. Elevated non-high-density lipoprotein cholesterol (non-HDL-C) predicts atherosclerotic cardiovascular events in hemodialysis patients. *Clin. J. Am. Soc. Nephrol.* **2011**, *6*, 1112–1120. [CrossRef]
86. Losappio, V.; Franzin, R.; Infante, B.; Godeas, G.; Gesualdo, L.; Fersini, A.; Castellano, G.; Stallone, G. Molecular Mechanisms of Premature Aging in Hemodialysis: The Complex Interplay Between Innate and Adaptive Immune Dysfunction. *Int. J. Mol. Sci.* **2020**, *21*, 3422. [CrossRef]
87. Turkmen, K.; Guney, I.; Yerlikaya, F.H.; Tonbul, H.Z. The relationship between neutrophil-to-lymphocyte ratio and inflammation in end-stage renal disease patients. *Ren. Fail.* **2012**, *34*, 155–159. [CrossRef]
88. Neuen, B.L.; Leather, N.; Greenwood, A.M.; Gunnarsson, R.; Cho, Y.; Mantha, M.L. Neutrophil-lymphocyte ratio predicts cardiovascular and all-cause mortality in hemodialysis patients. *Ren. Fail.* **2016**, *38*, 70–76. [CrossRef]
89. Catabay, C.; Obi, Y.; Streja, E.; Soohoo, M.; Park, C.; Rhee, C.M.; Kovesdy, C.P.; Hamano, T.; Kalantar-Zadeh, K. Lymphocyte Cell Ratios and Mortality among Incident Hemodialysis Patients. *Am. J. Nephrol.* **2017**, *46*, 408–416. [CrossRef]
90. Bross, R.; Noori, N.; Kovesdy, C.P.; Murali, S.B.; Benner, D.; Block, G.; Kopple, J.D.; Kalantar-Zadeh, K. Dietary assessment of individuals with chronic kidney disease. *Semin. Dial.* **2010**, *23*, 359–364. [CrossRef]
91. Conway, J.M.; Ingwersen, L.A.; Vinyard, B.T.; Moshfegh, A.J. Effectiveness of the US Department of Agriculture 5-step multiple-pass method in assessing food intake in obese and nonobese women. *Am. J. Clin. Nutr.* **2003**, *77*, 1171–1178. [CrossRef] [PubMed]
92. He, Y.; Lu, Y.; Yang, S.; Li, Y.; Yang, Y.; Chen, J.; Huang, Y.; Lin, Z.; Li, Y.; Kong, Y.; et al. Dietary Plant Protein and Mortality Among Patients Receiving Maintenance Hemodialysis: A Cohort Study. *Am. J. Kidney. Dis.* **2021**, *78*, 649–657.e641. [CrossRef] [PubMed]
93. Kalantar-Zadeh, K.; Supasyndh, O.; Lehn, R.S.; McAllister, C.J.; Kopple, J.D. Normalized protein nitrogen appearance is correlated with hospitalization and mortality in hemodialysis patients with Kt/V greater than 1.20. *J. Ren. Nutr.* **2003**, *13*, 15–25. [CrossRef] [PubMed]
94. Kalantar-Zadeh, K.; Kovesdy, C.P.; Bross, R.; Benner, D.; Noori, N.; Murali, S.B.; Block, T.; Norris, J.; Kopple, J.D.; Block, G. Design and development of a dialysis food frequency questionnaire. *J. Ren. Nutr.* **2011**, *21*, 257–262. [CrossRef]

95. Norman, K.; Stobaus, N.; Pirlich, M.; Bosy-Westphal, A. Bioelectrical phase angle and impedance vector analysis—Clinical relevance and applicability of impedance parameters. *Clin. Nutr.* **2012**, *31*, 854–861. [CrossRef]
96. Khalil, S.F.; Mohktar, M.S.; Ibrahim, F. The theory and fundamentals of bioimpedance analysis in clinical status monitoring and diagnosis of diseases. *Sensors* **2014**, *14*, 10895–10928. [CrossRef]
97. Campa, F.; Colognesi, L.A.; Moro, T.; Paoli, A.; Casolo, A.; Santos, L.; Correia, R.R.; Lemes, I.R.; Milanez, V.F.; Christofaro, D.D.; et al. Effect of resistance training on bioelectrical phase angle in older adults: A systematic review with Meta-analysis of randomized controlled trials. *Rev. Endocr. Metab. Disord.* **2022**, 1–11. [CrossRef]
98. Sabatino, A.; D'Alessandro, C.; Regolisti, G.; di Mario, F.; Guglielmi, G.; Bazzocchi, A.; Fiaccadori, E. Muscle mass assessment in renal disease: The role of imaging techniques. *Quant. Imaging Med. Surg.* **2020**, *10*, 1672–1686. [CrossRef]
99. Chumlea, W.C.; Guo, S.S.; Zeller, C.M.; Reo, N.V.; Siervogel, R.M. Total body water data for white adults 18 to 64 years of age: The Fels Longitudinal Study. *Kidney Int.* **1999**, *56*, 244–252. [CrossRef]
100. Beberashvili, I.; Azar, A.; Sinuani, I.; Kadoshi, H.; Shapiro, G.; Feldman, L.; Sandbank, J.; Averbukh, Z. Longitudinal changes in bioimpedance phase angle reflect inverse changes in serum IL-6 levels in maintenance hemodialysis patients. *Nutrition* **2014**, *30*, 297–304. [CrossRef]
101. Shin, J.H.; Kim, C.R.; Park, K.H.; Hwang, J.H.; Kim, S.H. Predicting clinical outcomes using phase angle as assessed by bioelectrical impedance analysis in maintenance hemodialysis patients. *Nutrition* **2017**, *41*, 7–13. [CrossRef]
102. Correia, M.I.; Caiaffa, W.T.; da Silva, A.L.; Waitzberg, D.L. Risk factors for malnutrition in patients undergoing gastroenterological and hernia surgery: An analysis of 374 patients. *Nutr. Hosp.* **2001**, *16*, 59–64. [PubMed]
103. Fontes, D.; Generoso Sde, V.; Toulson Davisson Correia, M.I. Subjective global assessment: A reliable nutritional assessment tool to predict outcomes in critically ill patients. *Clin. Nutr.* **2014**, *33*, 291–295. [CrossRef] [PubMed]
104. Rambod, M.; Bross, R.; Zitterkoph, J.; Benner, D.; Pithia, J.; Colman, S.; Kovesdy, C.P.; Kopple, J.D.; Kalantar-Zadeh, K. Association of Malnutrition-Inflammation Score with quality of life and mortality in hemodialysis patients: A 5-year prospective cohort study. *Am. J. Kidney Dis.* **2009**, *53*, 298–309. [CrossRef]
105. Borges, M.C.; Vogt, B.P.; Martin, L.C.; Caramori, J.C. Malnutrition Inflammation Score cut-off predicting mortality in maintenance hemodialysis patients. *Clin. Nutr. ESPEN* **2017**, *17*, 63–67. [CrossRef] [PubMed]
106. Bouillanne, O.; Morineau, G.; Dupont, C.; Coulombel, I.; Vincent, J.P.; Nicolis, I.; Benazeth, S.; Cynober, L.; Aussel, C. Geriatric Nutritional Risk Index: A new index for evaluating at-risk elderly medical patients. *Am. J. Clin. Nutr.* **2005**, *82*, 777–783. [CrossRef]
107. Yamada, K.; Furuya, R.; Takita, T.; Maruyama, Y.; Yamaguchi, Y.; Ohkawa, S.; Kumagai, H. Simplified nutritional screening tools for patients on maintenance hemodialysis. *Am. J. Clin. Nutr.* **2008**, *87*, 106–113. [CrossRef]
108. Kobayashi, I.; Ishimura, E.; Kato, Y.; Okuno, S.; Yamamoto, T.; Yamakawa, T.; Mori, K.; Inaba, M.; Nishizawa, Y. Geriatric Nutritional Risk Index, a simplified nutritional screening index, is a significant predictor of mortality in chronic dialysis patients. *Nephrol. Dial. Transpl.* **2010**, *25*, 3361–3365. [CrossRef]
109. Takahashi, H.; Ito, Y.; Ishii, H.; Aoyama, T.; Kamoi, D.; Kasuga, H.; Yasuda, K.; Maruyama, S.; Matsuo, S.; Murohara, T.; et al. Geriatric nutritional risk index accurately predicts cardiovascular mortality in incident hemodialysis patients. *J. Cardiol.* **2014**, *64*, 32–36. [CrossRef]
110. Matsukuma, Y.; Tanaka, S.; Taniguchi, M.; Nakano, T.; Masutani, K.; Hirakata, H.; Kitazono, T.; Tsuruya, K. Association of geriatric nutritional risk index with infection-related mortality in patients undergoing hemodialysis: The Q-Cohort Study. *Clin. Nutr.* **2019**, *38*, 279–287. [CrossRef]
111. Xiong, J.; Wang, M.; Zhang, Y.; Nie, L.; He, T.; Wang, Y.; Huang, Y.; Feng, B.; Zhang, J.; Zhao, J. Association of Geriatric Nutritional Risk Index with Mortality in Hemodialysis Patients: A Meta-Analysis of Cohort Studies. *Kidney Blood Press. Res.* **2018**, *43*, 1878–1889. [CrossRef]
112. Cederholm, T.; Jensen, G.L.; Correia, M.; Gonzalez, M.C.; Fukushima, R.; Higashiguchi, T.; Baptista, G.; Barazzoni, R.; Blaauw, R.; Coats, A.; et al. GLIM criteria for the diagnosis of malnutrition—A consensus report from the global clinical nutrition community. *Clin. Nutr.* **2019**, *38*, 1–9. [CrossRef] [PubMed]
113. Avesani, C.M.; Sabatino, A.; Guerra, A.; Rodrigues, J.; Carrero, J.J.; Rossi, G.M.; Garibotto, G.; Stenvinkel, P.; Fiaccadori, E.; Lindholm, B. A Comparative Analysis of Nutritional Assessment Using Global Leadership Initiative on Malnutrition Versus Subjective Global Assessment and Malnutrition Inflammation Score in Maintenance Hemodialysis Patients. *J. Ren. Nutr.* **2022**, *32*, 476–482. [CrossRef] [PubMed]
114. Kanno, Y.; Kanda, E.; Kato, A. Methods and Nutritional Interventions to Improve the Nutritional Status of Dialysis Patients in JAPAN-A Narrative Review. *Nutrients* **2021**, *13*, 1390. [CrossRef] [PubMed]
115. Shimamoto, S.; Yamada, S.; Hiyamuta, H.; Arase, H.; Taniguchi, M.; Tsuruya, K.; Nakano, T.; Kitazono, T. Association of the nutritional risk index for Japanese hemodialysis patients with long-term mortality: The Q-Cohort Study. *Clin. Exp. Nephrol.* **2022**, *26*, 59–67. [CrossRef] [PubMed]
116. Goodpaster, B.H.; Park, S.W.; Harris, T.B.; Kritchevsky, S.B.; Nevitt, M.; Schwartz, A.V.; Simonsick, E.M.; Tylavsky, F.A.; Visser, M.; Newman, A.B. The loss of skeletal muscle strength, mass, and quality in older adults: The health, aging and body composition study. *J. Gerontol. A Biol. Sci. Med. Sci.* **2006**, *61*, 1059–1064. [CrossRef]

117. Delmonico, M.J.; Harris, T.B.; Visser, M.; Park, S.W.; Conroy, M.B.; Velasquez-Mieyer, P.; Boudreau, R.; Manini, T.M.; Nevitt, M.; Newman, A.B.; et al. Longitudinal study of muscle strength, quality, and adipose tissue infiltration. *Am. J. Clin. Nutr.* **2009**, *90*, 1579–1585. [CrossRef]
118. Sousa-Santos, A.R.; Amaral, T.F. Differences in handgrip strength protocols to identify sarcopenia and frailty—A systematic review. *BMC Geriatr.* **2017**, *17*, 238. [CrossRef]
119. Matos, C.M.; Silva, L.F.; Santana, L.D.; Santos, L.S.; Protasio, B.M.; Rocha, M.T.; Ferreira, V.L.; Azevedo, M.F.; Martins, M.T.; Lopes, G.B.; et al. Handgrip strength at baseline and mortality risk in a cohort of women and men on hemodialysis: A 4-year study. *J. Ren. Nutr.* **2014**, *24*, 157–162. [CrossRef]
120. Vogt, B.P.; Borges, M.C.C.; Goes, C.R.; Caramori, J.C.T. Handgrip strength is an independent predictor of all-cause mortality in maintenance dialysis patients. *Clin. Nutr.* **2016**, *35*, 1429–1433. [CrossRef]
121. Kittiskulnam, P.; Chertow, G.M.; Carrero, J.J.; Delgado, C.; Kaysen, G.A.; Johansen, K.L. Sarcopenia and its individual criteria are associated, in part, with mortality among patients on hemodialysis. *Kidney Int.* **2017**, *92*, 238–247. [CrossRef]
122. Isoyama, N.; Qureshi, A.R.; Avesani, C.M.; Lindholm, B.; Barany, P.; Heimburger, O.; Cederholm, T.; Stenvinkel, P.; Carrero, J.J. Comparative associations of muscle mass and muscle strength with mortality in dialysis patients. *Clin. J. Am. Soc. Nephrol.* **2014**, *9*, 1720–1728. [CrossRef] [PubMed]
123. Yang, L.; He, Y.; Li, X. Physical function and all-cause mortality in patients with chronic kidney disease and end-stage renal disease: A systematic review and meta-analysis. *Int. Urol. Nephrol.* **2022**, 1–10. [CrossRef]
124. Kutsuna, T.; Matsunaga, A.; Matsumoto, T.; Ishii, A.; Yamamoto, K.; Hotta, K.; Aiba, N.; Takagi, Y.; Yoshida, A.; Takahira, N.; et al. Physical activity is necessary to prevent deterioration of the walking ability of patients undergoing maintenance hemodialysis. *Apher. Dial.* **2010**, *14*, 193–200. [CrossRef] [PubMed]
125. Matsuzawa, R.; Matsunaga, A.; Wang, G.; Yamamoto, S.; Kutsuna, T.; Ishii, A.; Abe, Y.; Yoneki, K.; Yoshida, A.; Takahira, N. Relationship between lower extremity muscle strength and all-cause mortality in Japanese patients undergoing dialysis. *Phys. Ther.* **2014**, *94*, 947–956. [CrossRef] [PubMed]
126. Carrero, J.J.; Thomas, F.; Nagy, K.; Arogundade, F.; Avesani, C.M.; Chan, M.; Chmielewski, M.; Cordeiro, A.C.; Espinosa-Cuevas, A.; Fiaccadori, E.; et al. Global Prevalence of Protein-Energy Wasting in Kidney Disease: A Meta-analysis of Contemporary Observational Studies from the International Society of Renal Nutrition and Metabolism. *J. Ren. Nutr.* **2018**, *28*, 380–392. [CrossRef]
127. Kim, J.C.; Kalantar-Zadeh, K.; Kopple, J.D. Frailty and protein-energy wasting in elderly patients with end stage kidney disease. *J. Am. Soc. Nephrol.* **2013**, *24*, 337–351. [CrossRef]
128. Johansen, K.L.; Dalrymple, L.S.; Delgado, C.; Kaysen, G.A.; Kornak, J.; Grimes, B.; Chertow, G.M. Association between body composition and frailty among prevalent hemodialysis patients: A US Renal Data System special study. *J. Am. Soc. Nephrol.* **2014**, *25*, 381–389. [CrossRef]
129. Lee, H.J.; Son, Y.J. Prevalence and Associated Factors of Frailty and Mortality in Patients with End-Stage Renal Disease Undergoing Hemodialysis: A Systematic Review and Meta-Analysis. *Int. J. Environ. Res. Public Health* **2021**, *18*, 3471. [CrossRef]
130. Shu, X.; Lin, T.; Wang, H.; Zhao, Y.; Jiang, T.; Peng, X.; Yue, J. Diagnosis, prevalence, and mortality of sarcopenia in dialysis patients: A systematic review and meta-analysis. *J. Cachexia Sarcopenia Muscle* **2022**, *13*, 145–158. [CrossRef]
131. Giglio, J.; Kamimura, M.A.; Lamarca, F.; Rodrigues, J.; Santin, F.; Avesani, C.M. Association of Sarcopenia with Nutritional Parameters, Quality of Life, Hospitalization, and Mortality Rates of Elderly Patients on Hemodialysis. *J. Ren. Nutr.* **2018**, *28*, 197–207. [CrossRef] [PubMed]
132. Reis, J.M.S.; Alves, L.S.; Vogt, B.P. According to Revised EWGSOP Sarcopenia Consensus Cut-Off Points, Low Physical Function Is Associated with Nutritional Status and Quality of Life in Maintenance Hemodialysis Patients. *J. Ren. Nutr.* **2022**, *32*, 469–475. [CrossRef] [PubMed]
133. Lin, Y.L.; Liou, H.H.; Lai, Y.H.; Wang, C.H.; Kuo, C.H.; Chen, S.Y.; Hsu, B.G. Decreased serum fatty acid binding protein 4 concentrations are associated with sarcopenia in chronic hemodialysis patients. *Clin. Chim. Acta* **2018**, *485*, 113–118. [CrossRef] [PubMed]
134. Ren, H.; Gong, D.; Jia, F.; Xu, B.; Liu, Z. Sarcopenia in patients undergoing maintenance hemodialysis: Incidence rate, risk factors and its effect on survival risk. *Ren. Fail.* **2016**, *38*, 364–371. [CrossRef] [PubMed]
135. Kurajoh, M.; Mori, K.; Miyabe, M.; Matsufuji, S.; Ichii, M.; Morioka, T.; Kizu, A.; Tsujimoto, Y.; Emoto, M. Nutritional Status Association with Sarcopenia in Patients Undergoing Maintenance Hemodialysis Assessed by Nutritional Risk Index. *Front Nutr.* **2022**, *9*, 896427. [CrossRef]
136. Sy, J.; Johansen, K.L. The impact of frailty on outcomes in dialysis. *Curr. Opin. Nephrol. Hypertens.* **2017**, *26*, 537–542. [CrossRef]
137. Ribeiro, H.S.; Neri, S.G.R.; Oliveira, J.S.; Bennett, P.N.; Viana, J.L.; Lima, R.M. Association between sarcopenia and clinical outcomes in chronic kidney disease patients: A systematic review and meta-analysis. *Clin. Nutr.* **2022**, *41*, 1131–1140. [CrossRef]
138. Hendriks, F.K.; Smeets, J.S.J.; Broers, N.J.H.; van Kranenburg, J.M.X.; van der Sande, F.M.; Kooman, J.P.; van Loon, L.J.C. End-Stage Renal Disease Patients Lose a Substantial Amount of Amino Acids during Hemodialysis. *J. Nutr.* **2020**, *150*, 1160–1166. [CrossRef]
139. Murtas, S.; Aquilani, R.; Deiana, M.L.; Iadarola, P.; Secci, R.; Cadeddu, M.; Salis, S.; Serpi, D.; Bolasco, P. Differences in Amino Acid Loss Between High-Efficiency Hemodialysis and Postdilution and Predilution Hemodiafiltration Using High Convection Volume Exchange-A New Metabolic Scenario? A Pilot Study. *J. Ren. Nutr.* **2019**, *29*, 126–135. [CrossRef]

140. Murtas, S.; Aquilani, R.; Iadarola, P.; Deiana, M.L.; Secci, R.; Cadeddu, M.; Bolasco, P. Differences and Effects of Metabolic Fate of Individual Amino Acid Loss in High-Efficiency Hemodialysis and Hemodiafiltration. *J. Ren. Nutr.* **2020**, *30*, 440–451. [CrossRef]
141. Bolasco, P. Hemodialysis-Nutritional Flaws in Diagnosis and Prescriptions. Could Amino Acid Losses be the Sharpest "Sword of Damocles"? *Nutrients* **2020**, *12*, 1773. [CrossRef] [PubMed]
142. Wolfson, R.L.; Chantranupong, L.; Saxton, R.A.; Shen, K.; Scaria, S.M.; Cantor, J.R.; Sabatini, D.M. Sestrin2 is a leucine sensor for the mTORC1 pathway. *Science* **2016**, *351*, 43–48. [CrossRef] [PubMed]
143. Gielen, E.; Beckwee, D.; Delaere, A.; De Breucker, S.; Vandewoude, M.; Bautmans, I.; Sarcopenia Guidelines Development Group of the Belgian Society of Gerontology and Geriatrics. Nutritional interventions to improve muscle mass, muscle strength, and physical performance in older people: An umbrella review of systematic reviews and meta-analyses. *Nutr. Rev.* **2021**, *79*, 121–147. [CrossRef]
144. Hoshino, J. Renal Rehabilitation: Exercise Intervention and Nutritional Support in Dialysis Patients. *Nutrients* **2021**, *13*, 1444. [CrossRef] [PubMed]
145. Fujita, S.; Rasmussen, B.B.; Cadenas, J.G.; Grady, J.J.; Volpi, E. Effect of insulin on human skeletal muscle protein synthesis is modulated by insulin-induced changes in muscle blood flow and amino acid availability. *Am. J. Physiol. Endocrinol. Metab.* **2006**, *291*, E745–E754. [CrossRef] [PubMed]
146. Rasmussen, B.B.; Fujita, S.; Wolfe, R.R.; Mittendorfer, B.; Roy, M.; Rowe, V.L.; Volpi, E. Insulin resistance of muscle protein metabolism in aging. *FASEB J.* **2006**, *20*, 768–769. [CrossRef] [PubMed]
147. Fujita, S.; Rasmussen, B.B.; Cadenas, J.G.; Drummond, M.J.; Glynn, E.L.; Sattler, F.R.; Volpi, E. Aerobic exercise overcomes the age-related insulin resistance of muscle protein metabolism by improving endothelial function and Akt/mammalian target of rapamycin signaling. *Diabetes* **2007**, *56*, 1615–1622. [CrossRef]
148. Wang, X.H.; Du, J.; Klein, J.D.; Bailey, J.L.; Mitch, W.E. Exercise ameliorates chronic kidney disease-induced defects in muscle protein metabolism and progenitor cell function. *Kidney Int.* **2009**, *76*, 751–759. [CrossRef]
149. Kirkman, D.L.; Mullins, P.; Junglee, N.A.; Kumwenda, M.; Jibani, M.M.; Macdonald, J.H. Anabolic exercise in haemodialysis patients: A randomised controlled pilot study. *J. Cachexia Sarcopenia Muscle* **2014**, *5*, 199–207. [CrossRef]
150. Johansen, K.L.; Painter, P.L.; Sakkas, G.K.; Gordon, P.; Doyle, J.; Shubert, T. Effects of resistance exercise training and nandrolone decanoate on body composition and muscle function among patients who receive hemodialysis: A randomized, controlled trial. *J. Am. Soc. Nephrol.* **2006**, *17*, 2307–2314. [CrossRef]
151. Dong, J.; Sundell, M.B.; Pupim, L.B.; Wu, P.; Shintani, A.; Ikizler, T.A. The effect of resistance exercise to augment long-term benefits of intradialytic oral nutritional supplementation in chronic hemodialysis patients. *J. Ren. Nutr.* **2011**, *21*, 149–159. [CrossRef]
152. Hendriks, F.K.; Kooman, J.P.; van Loon, L.J.C. Dietary protein interventions to improve nutritional status in end-stage renal disease patients undergoing hemodialysis. *Curr. Opin. Clin. Nutr. Metab. Care* **2021**, *24*, 79–87. [CrossRef] [PubMed]
153. Dickinson, J.M.; Gundermann, D.M.; Walker, D.K.; Reidy, P.T.; Borack, M.S.; Drummond, M.J.; Arora, M.; Volpi, E.; Rasmussen, B.B. Leucine-enriched amino acid ingestion after resistance exercise prolongs myofibrillar protein synthesis and amino acid transporter expression in older men. *J. Nutr.* **2014**, *144*, 1694–1702. [CrossRef]
154. Nitta, K.; Goto, S.; Masakane, I.; Hanafusa, N.; Taniguchi, M.; Hasegawa, T.; Nakai, S.; Wada, A.; Hamano, T.; Hoshino, J. Annual dialysis data report for 2018, JSDT Renal Data Registry: Survey methods, facility data, incidence, prevalence, and mortality. *Ren. Replace. Ther.* **2020**, *6*, 41. [CrossRef]
155. Golestaneh, L. Decreasing hospitalizations in patients on hemodialysis: Time for a paradigm shift. *Semin. Dial.* **2018**, *31*, 278–288. [CrossRef] [PubMed]
156. Schoonover, K.L.; Hickson, L.J.; Norby, S.M.; Hogan, M.C.; Chaudhary, S.; Albright, R.C., Jr.; Dillon, J.J.; McCarthy, J.T.; Williams, A.W. Risk factors for hospitalization among older, incident haemodialysis patients. *Nephrology* **2013**, *18*, 712–717. [CrossRef] [PubMed]
157. Chavers, B.M.; Solid, C.A.; Gilbertson, D.T.; Collins, A.J. Infection-related hospitalization rates in pediatric versus adult patients with end-stage renal disease in the United States. *J. Am. Soc. Nephrol.* **2007**, *18*, 952–959. [CrossRef]
158. Dalrymple, L.S.; Mu, Y.; Nguyen, D.V.; Romano, P.S.; Chertow, G.M.; Grimes, B.; Kaysen, G.A.; Johansen, K.L. Risk Factors for Infection-Related Hospitalization in In-Center Hemodialysis. *Clin. J. Am. Soc. Nephrol.* **2015**, *10*, 2170–2180. [CrossRef]
159. Eknoyan, G.; Beck, G.J.; Cheung, A.K.; Daugirdas, J.T.; Greene, T.; Kusek, J.W.; Allon, M.; Bailey, J.; Delmez, J.A.; Depner, T.A.; et al. Effect of dialysis dose and membrane flux in maintenance hemodialysis. *N. Engl. J. Med.* **2002**, *347*, 2010–2019. [CrossRef]
160. Allon, M.; Radeva, M.; Bailey, J.; Beddhu, S.; Butterly, D.; Coyne, D.W.; Depner, T.A.; Gassman, J.J.; Kaufman, A.M.; Kaysen, G.A.; et al. The spectrum of infection-related morbidity in hospitalized haemodialysis patients. *Nephrol. Dial. Transpl.* **2005**, *20*, 1180–1186. [CrossRef]
161. Dalrymple, L.S.; Mu, Y.; Romano, P.S.; Nguyen, D.V.; Chertow, G.M.; Delgado, C.; Grimes, B.; Kaysen, G.A.; Johansen, K.L. Outcomes of infection-related hospitalization in Medicare beneficiaries receiving in-center hemodialysis. *Am. J. Kidney Dis.* **2015**, *65*, 754–762. [CrossRef] [PubMed]
162. Iwashyna, T.J.; Cooke, C.R.; Wunsch, H.; Kahn, J.M. Population burden of long-term survivorship after severe sepsis in older Americans. *J. Am. Geriatr. Soc.* **2012**, *60*, 1070–1077. [CrossRef] [PubMed]
163. Nelson, J.E.; Cox, C.E.; Hope, A.A.; Carson, S.S. Chronic critical illness. *Am. J. Respir. Crit. Care Med.* **2010**, *182*, 446–454. [CrossRef] [PubMed]

164. Lamas, D. Chronic critical illness. *N. Engl. J. Med.* **2014**, *370*, 175–177. [CrossRef] [PubMed]
165. Machiba, Y.; Mori, K.; Shoji, T.; Nagata, Y.; Uedono, H.; Nakatani, S.; Ochi, A.; Tsuda, A.; Morioka, T.; Yoshida, H.; et al. Nutritional Disorder Evaluated by the Geriatric Nutritional Risk Index Predicts Death After Hospitalization for Infection in Patients Undergoing Maintenance Hemodialysis. *J. Ren. Nutr.* **2022**, *32*, 751–757. [CrossRef]
166. Noordzij, M.; Leffondre, K.; van Stralen, K.J.; Zoccali, C.; Dekker, F.W.; Jager, K.J. When do we need competing risks methods for survival analysis in nephrology? *Nephrol. Dial. Transpl.* **2013**, *28*, 2670–2677. [CrossRef]
167. Hsu, J.Y.; Roy, J.A.; Xie, D.; Yang, W.; Shou, H.; Anderson, A.H.; Landis, J.R.; Jepson, C.; Wolf, M.; Isakova, T.; et al. Statistical Methods for Cohort Studies of CKD: Survival Analysis in the Setting of Competing Risks. *Clin. J. Am. Soc. Nephrol.* **2017**, *12*, 1181–1189. [CrossRef]
168. Steiger, S.; Rossaint, J.; Zarbock, A.; Anders, H.J. Secondary Immunodeficiency Related to Kidney Disease (SIDKD)-Definition, Unmet Need, and Mechanisms. *J. Am. Soc. Nephrol.* **2022**, *33*, 259–278. [CrossRef]
169. Gentile, L.F.; Cuenca, A.G.; Efron, P.A.; Ang, D.; Bihorac, A.; McKinley, B.A.; Moldawer, L.L.; Moore, F.A. Persistent inflammation and immunosuppression: A common syndrome and new horizon for surgical intensive care. *J. Trauma Acute Care Surg.* **2012**, *72*, 1491–1501. [CrossRef]
170. Mira, J.C.; Gentile, L.F.; Mathias, B.J.; Efron, P.A.; Brakenridge, S.C.; Mohr, A.M.; Moore, F.A.; Moldawer, L.L. Sepsis Pathophysiology, Chronic Critical Illness, and Persistent Inflammation-Immunosuppression and Catabolism Syndrome. *Crit. Care Med.* **2017**, *45*, 253–262. [CrossRef]
171. Darden, D.B.; Kelly, L.S.; Fenner, B.P.; Moldawer, L.L.; Mohr, A.M.; Efron, P.A. Dysregulated Immunity and Immunotherapy after Sepsis. *J. Clin. Med.* **2021**, *10*, 1742. [CrossRef] [PubMed]
172. Rosenthal, M.D.; Vanzant, E.L.; Moore, F.A. Chronic Critical Illness and PICS Nutritional Strategies. *J. Clin. Med.* **2021**, *10*, 2294. [CrossRef] [PubMed]
173. Xing, Y.F.; Cai, R.M.; Lin, Q.; Ye, Q.J.; Ren, J.H.; Yin, L.H.; Li, X. Expansion of polymorphonuclear myeloid-derived suppressor cells in patients with end-stage renal disease may lead to infectious complications. *Kidney Int.* **2017**, *91*, 1236–1242. [CrossRef] [PubMed]

Disclaimer/Publisher's Note: The statements, opinions and data contained in all publications are solely those of the individual author(s) and contributor(s) and not of MDPI and/or the editor(s). MDPI and/or the editor(s) disclaim responsibility for any injury to people or property resulting from any ideas, methods, instructions or products referred to in the content.

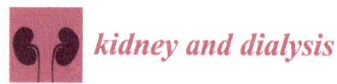 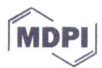

Review

Renal Rehabilitation—Its Theory and Clinical Application to Patients Undergoing Daily Dialysis Therapy

Ryota Matsuzawa [1,*] and Daisuke Kakita [2]

[1] Department of Physical Therapy, School of Rehabilitation, Hyogo Medical University, Kobe 650-8530, Japan
[2] Course of Health Science, Hyogo Medical University Graduate School of Health Science, Kobe 650-8530, Japan
* Correspondence: ryota122560@gmail.com; Tel.: +81-78-304-3181; Fax: +81-78-304-2811

Abstract: An aging population and the prevalence of lifestyle-related ailments have led to a worldwide increase in the rate of chronic kidney disease requiring renal replacement therapy. The mean age of people requiring dialysis has been rising, and Japanese patients are aging more rapidly than those in the United States and Europe. Compared to people with normal kidney function, those undergoing hemodialysis are at increased risk of sarcopenia or frailty and serious health problems that limit access to kidney transplantation and lead to adverse health outcomes such as functional dependence, hospitalization, and death in patients on dialysis treatment. The Japanese Society of Renal Rehabilitation, established in 2011, published a clinical practice guideline for renal rehabilitation in 2019. Although the concept has become widely known among kidney health providers in recent years, efforts have still not focused on routine clinical care for patients with chronic kidney disease. In this review, the theory and clinical application of renal rehabilitation for patients undergoing daily hemodialysis were investigated.

Keywords: sarcopenia; frailty; exercise; CKD; dialysis

1. Introduction

As the world's population ages, the rate of chronic kidney disease requiring renal replacement therapy is increasing [1], along with the mean age of patients undergoing dialysis. Significant increases in the age of these patients is the result of improved survival and reduced transplant availability, which has been observed in almost all 12 nations in the international cohort "Dialysis Outcomes and Practice Patterns Study (DOPPS)" [2]. With previously reported data, Japanese patients on dialysis are aging more rapidly than those in the United States or Europe [3]. The rate of patients aged 65 years and older in the United States rose to 38.4% from 21.1% between 1980 and 2015, meanwhile, the rate in Japan rose to 59.8% from 12.2%. According to the nationwide data of the Japanese Society for Dialysis Therapy, the mean age of the Japanese dialysis population was 68.8 years at the end of 2018, a 14.22-year increase since the end of 1990. Furthermore, patients aged 60 years or older represented 79.1% of those who started dialysis therapy in 2018 and 78.1% of the entire dialysis population [4].

The health management of older hemodialysis patients poses serious issues that are not only clinical but also social. In 2016, the advisory board of European Renal Best Practice published guidelines on the management of older patients with chronic kidney disease [5]. In 2019, the Japanese Society of Renal Rehabilitation, which was established in 2011, also published a clinical practice guide for renal rehabilitation, targeting patients who were and were not dependent on dialysis and had a renal transplant [6]. In recent years, the concept of renal rehabilitation has gradually become widely known among kidney health providers, but it is currently still not included in routine clinical care for patients undergoing dialysis because of the lack of medical staff who can evaluate physical functions and provide exercise guidance adequately. This review focused on the theory of renal rehabilitation and its clinical application for patients on daily dialysis.

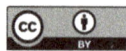

2. Functional Status and Physical Frailty

The mortality rate for patients on hemodialysis was approximately 10% in 2018 [4] and is still high despite continued improvements in dialysis technology. One of the potential contributors to poor survival might be a high burden of functional dependence [7], which is an individual's inability to perform day-to-day tasks associated with personal care and maintaining a household. A previous study that included almost all 12 nations demonstrated a high level of disability in daily activities in most patients undergoing hemodialysis, and a dose–response association was noted between poor functional status and adverse clinical outcomes [8]. Furthermore, the association between a yearly change in functional status and all-cause mortality among 817 Japanese individuals requiring hemodialysis therapy was examined [9]. Among the patients free of disability at the baseline, 19.9% experienced a functional decline during the one-year observation, which was strongly associated with a higher mortality risk. Importantly, even after adjusting for baseline characteristics including functional status, the reduction still had a negative effect on survival in patients with end-stage renal disease. We underscore the importance of regular monitoring of a patient's functional status and interventions to prevent deterioration. Impaired mobility, poor physical functioning, and muscle weakness, the main components of physical frailty, contribute to an increased likelihood of disabilities not only in community-dwelling older adults [10,11] but also in patients on hemodialysis [12].

Frailty is generally considered to be an age-related fragile state characterized by physiological vulnerability to stress, associated with an increased risk of adverse health outcomes [13,14]. The frailty phenotype was first defined by Fried and colleagues based on the following five criteria: shrinking, weakness, poor endurance and energy, slowness, and a low level of physical activity [13]. Frailty is identified by the presence of three or more of the above criteria, and an intermediate frailty phenotype is commonly defined as having one or two. Satake et al. proposed a revised Japanese version of the Cardiovascular Health Study (J-CHS) criteria (Table 1) [15], which was constructed by simplifying the original CHS criteria to suit older Japanese people.

Table 1. The revised Japanese version of the Cardiovascular Health Study (J-CHS) criteria, created based on a reference from Satake et al. [15].

Component	Questions and Measurements	Answer
Shrinking	Have you unintentionally lost 2 or more kg in the past 6 months?	Yes = 1 No = 0
Weakness	Grip strength <28 kg in men or 18 kg in women	Yes = 1 No = 0
Exhaustion	In the past 2 weeks, have you felt tired without reason?	Yes = 1 No = 0
Slowness	Gait speed <1.0 m/s	Yes = 1 No = 0
Low activity	Do you engage in a moderate level of physical exercise or sports? Do you engage in a low level of physical exercise aimed at health?	No to both questions = 1 Other = 0

Frailty, prefrailty, and robustness were defined as 3–5, 1–2, and 0 points, respectively.

Frailty is highly prevalent in patients with chronic kidney disease who require hemodialysis. The prevalence of frailty in this population was 36.8% based on a previously performed meta-analysis [16] compared with 7.4% of community-dwelling older adults [17]. Many factors were mutually connected and could be unified theoretically into a cycle of frailty, which we have reported elsewhere (Figure 1) [18]. Patients with kidney diseases also have an increased risk of sarcopenia, which is defined as a state with low muscle mass and low muscle strength or low physical performance, and it is thought that sarcopenia occurs due to a comorbidity burden, long-standing malnutrition, chronic inflammation, metabolic acidosis, anabolic resistance, hormonal changes, physical inactivity, and amino acid loss via dialysis [19–22]. Sarcopenia and physical frailty decrease access to kidney transplantation [23] and lead to adverse health outcomes including hospitalization [24] and death [25] in patients on hemodialysis. Thus, early identification and treatment are especially needed for these populations.

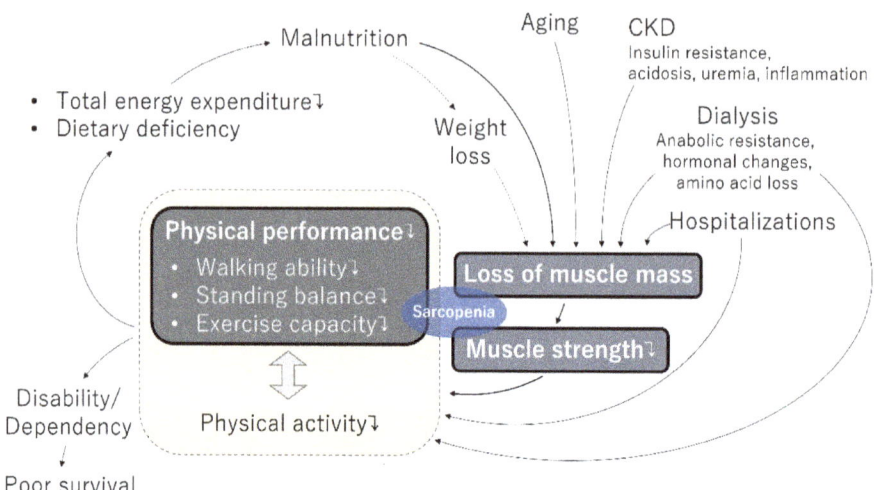

Figure 1. Cycle of frailty in patients with chronic kidney disease (CKD), adapted from Matsuzawa et al. [18].

3. Sarcopenia in the Cycle of Frailty

Sarcopenia has been described as a geriatric syndrome characterized by the loss of skeletal muscle mass and decreased muscle function and is at the center of the cycle of frailty. Patients with end-stage renal disease are at an increased risk of developing sarcopenia due to various factors [19–21,26]. Sarcopenia is diagnosed when patients have low muscle mass and low muscle strength or low physical performance according to the criteria of the Asian Working Group for Sarcopenia 2019 (AWGS2) [27]. The diagnostic criteria proposed by different working groups are summarized in Table 2 [27–30]. According to a recently performed meta-analysis, the prevalence of sarcopenia in patients on dialysis treatment was 28.5% [31], which is extremely high compared to rates ranging from 10.0 to 14.1% in the general population [32,33]. We examined the proportion of patients with sarcopenia according to the AWGS2 criteria among older Japanese patients on hemodialysis from three dialysis facilities and found that approximately 40% had been diagnosed with sarcopenia, and one in two aged 65 years and older had sarcopenia (Figure 2) [34]. Troublingly, sarcopenia ranges from asymptomatic to life-threatening, [35] and silent sarcopenia needs to be identified early via objective assessments. A diagnosis is essential for clinical management and therapeutic decision-making; however, it is not feasible in routine clinical practice for populations undergoing hemodialysis because it is time-consuming and resources are limited. Therefore, a convenient, objective, and rapid screening tool that can be used in clinical practice for hemodialysis patients whose physical conditions are dramatically altered, even for a short period, is needed. We recently conducted a study aimed to evaluate the ability of simplified tools to detect sarcopenia among patients on hemodialysis [34]. Our findings demonstrate that calf circumference and the creatinine-derived index could be considered as alternative means of discriminating sarcopenia in hemodialysis patients (Figure 3) [34]. The calf circumference was measured using a non-elastic tape at the point of the largest circumference. Both legs were measured, and the maximum value of both calves was used [34]. The creatinine-derived index, a disease-specific measure identifying low muscle mass and poor physical function [36,37], was calculated using the following formula:

Table 2. Diagnostic criteria of sarcopenia proposed by different working groups.

Working Group	(A) Low Muscle Mass	(B) Low Muscle Strength	(C) Low Physical Performance	Diagnosis
IWGS (2011) [28]	ASM/height^2 (DXA): men ≤7.23 kg/m^2, women ≤5.67 kg/m^2	-	Gait speed: <1.0 m/s	• Sarcopenia: (C) and (A)
EWGSOP2 (2019) [29]	ASM (BIA or DXA): men <20 kg, women <15 kg or ASM/height^2 (BIA or DXA): men <7.0 kg/m^2, women <6.0 kg/m^2	Handgrip strength: men <27 kg, women <16 kg or five-time chair stand time: >15 s	Gait speed: ≤0.8 m/s or SPPB: ≤8 points or timed up and go test: ≥20 s or 400 m walk test: non-completion or ≥6 min for completion	• Sarcopenia probable: (B) • Sarcopenia: (B) and (A) • Sarcopenia severe: (B), (A) and (C)
AWGS (2020) [27]	ASM/height^2 (BIA): men <7.0 kg/m^2, women <5.7 kg/m^2 or ASM/height^2 (DXA): men <7.0 kg/m^2, women <5.4 kg/m^2	Handgrip strength: men <28 kg, women <18 kg	Gait speed: <1.0 m/s or SPPB: ≤9 points or five-time chair stand time: ≥12 s	• Sarcopenia: (A) and (B) or (A) and (C) • Sarcopenia severe: (A), (B) and (C)
ISPRM (2021) [30]	STAR (ultrasound): men <1.4, women <1.0	Handgrip strength: men <32 kg, women <19 kg or five-time chair stand time: ≥12 s	Rise from a chair: inability or gait speed: ≤0.8 m/s	• Sarcopenia: (B) and (A) • Sarcopenia severe: (B), (A) and (C)

IWGS: the International Working Group on Sarcopenia; EWGSOP: the European Working Group on Sarcopenia in Older People; AWGS: the Asian Working Group for Sarcopenia; ISPRM: the International Society of Physical and Rehabilitation Medicine; ASM: appendicular skeletal muscle mass; DXA: dual-energy X-ray absorptiometry; BIA: bioimpedance; STAR: sonographic anterior thigh ratio; SPPB:, short physical performance battery.

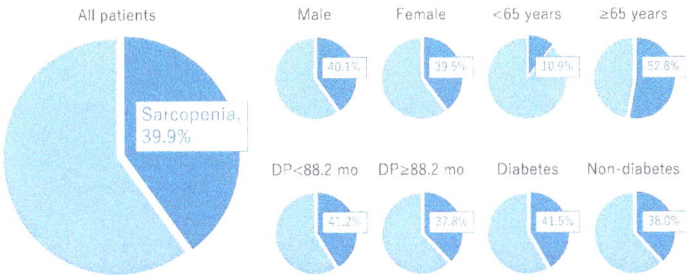

Figure 2. Prevalence rate of sarcopenia in patients undergoing hemodialysis, created based on a reference from Kakita et al. [34]. DP: dialysis period.

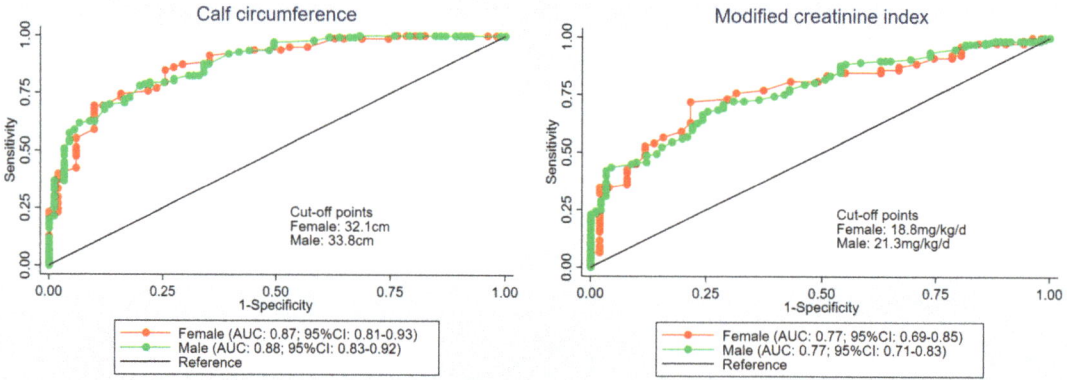

Figure 3. ROC curves of the simplified discriminant parameters against sarcopenia, created based on a reference from Kakita et al. [34].

Modified creatinine index (mg/kg/d) = 16.21 + 1.12 × (1 for men; 0 for women) − 0.06 × age (year) − 0.08 × single-pool Kt/V urea + 0.009 × serum creatinine level before dialysis (mmol/L) [36].

These are objective indicators that are easy to apply in clinical practice. Adding these assessments into routine clinical care will be valuable, not only for diagnosing sarcopenia, but also for improving prognostic stratification in patients on hemodialysis.

4. Management of Physical Frailty

In 2016, the European Renal Best Practice guideline development group underscored the importance of managing older patients with chronic kidney disease, especially with a routine assessment of physical function and activity [5]. An early identification of poor physical function and activity is essential for establishing a comprehensive management plan for patients on hemodialysis. We recommended a clinical physical frailty management algorithm for patients who require hemodialysis (Figure 4) [38], a modified version of Roshanravan's algorithm [39] tailored to Japanese populations. It consists of understanding a patient's physical function and activity level and exercise interventions. For low-functioning or sedentary patients who had been screened by routine evaluation, we encouraged participation in a supervised or home-based exercise program. We had previously evaluated the effects of a management program for physical frailty that consisted of the routine assessment of physical function and activity with feedback on the results of all-cause mortality and cardiovascular events for hemodialysis patients [40]. As a result, a lower proportion of program attendance was strongly associated with increased risks of mortality and cardiovascular events compared to those who attended the program more regularly. These results emphasize the importance of managing physical function and activity as part of routine clinical care.

Poor physical functioning, especially leg muscle strength, is common among hemodialysis patients and is strongly associated with decreased walking ability and lower basic and instrumental daily activity [41]. We previously evaluated thee lower extremity muscle strength using a handheld dynamometer in 190 clinically stable hemodialysis patients who did not require walking assistance. Approximately half of them had muscle strength below the cutoff value [42], which is used to determine whether patients can walk independently. This finding indicated that decreased muscle strength was already present. Given that lower extremity muscle strength correlated strongly and positively with gait speed and standing balance function [42], maintaining leg muscle strength seems to be a critical factor for preventing falls, fall-related fractures, and bedridden status. Fortunately, hemodialysis patients can improve poor muscle strength by resistance training. Low-intensity training with ankle weights during dialysis sessions was shown to improve leg muscle strength and functional status in older patients [12].

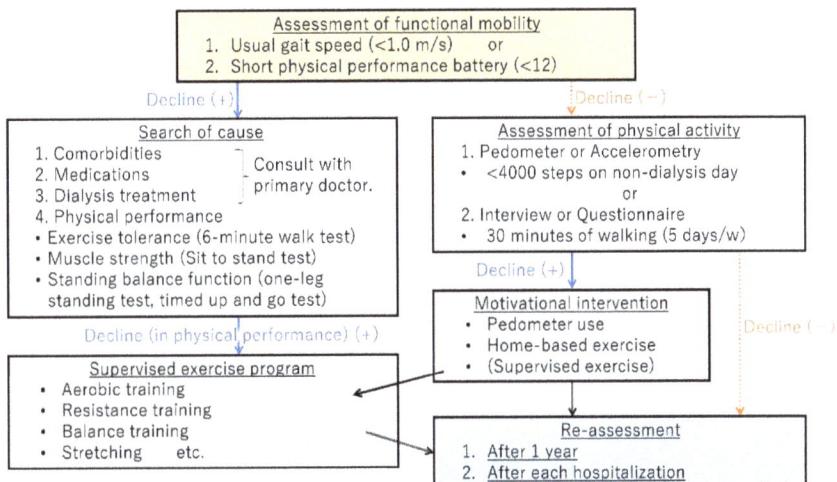

Figure 4. Clinical algorithm for the management of physical frailty in patients on hemodialysis, adapted from Matsuzawa et al. [18].

A systematic review and meta-analysis were previously conducted to evaluate the physical activity levels in patients with chronic kidney disease at different stages. The daily step counts in pre-dialysis patients, patients on peritoneal dialysis, patients on hemodialysis, and kidney transplant recipients were 5638 steps/day, 4264 steps/day, 4112 steps/day, and 8690 steps/day, respectively [43]. Patients on hemodialysis remained substantially less active as with patients on peritoneal dialysis and decreased physical activity assessed by questionnaire [44–48] or accelerometer-based methods [49,50] was strongly associated with higher mortality among patients on maintenance hemodialysis therapy. Goal setting is well-known to be a key motivational factor for increasing physical activity and is essential for successful intervention. We proposed walking 4000 steps per non-dialysis day as an initial minimum requirement for patients who require no assistance in walking [50]. This is a realistic goal for older adults that is consistent with the recommendations of the American College of Sports Medicine [51]. In addition, a decline in physical activity of >30% over the previous year was observed in almost one-quarter of patients undergoing hemodialysis and was associated with an elevated mortality risk independent of patient characteristics and baseline activity level [52]. On the other hand, we recently revealed that a lower physical activity level on "dialysis days" was also associated with higher risks of cardiovascular events and all-cause mortality independent to that on non-dialysis days [53]. Physical activity on dialysis days was restricted due to large fluctuations in vital signs during treatment or symptoms such as fatigue [54], so it is necessary to investigate the cause of decreased physical activity on dialysis days and to consider whether intradialytic exercise could be safely performed to cover the shortfall.

5. Frailty and Renal Transplantation

A previous prospective cohort study revealed that kidney transplant candidates with frailty were 38% less likely to be listed for kidney transplantation, had a 1.7-fold higher risk of waitlist mortality, and were 32% less likely to undergo kidney transplantation compared with non-frail individuals, even after adjusting for baseline characteristics including age, body mass index, and cause of end-stage renal disease [23]. Although the number of preemptive kidney transplants (PEKT) in Japan has increased recently, 60% of living kidney transplant recipients and 85% of cadaveric kidney transplant recipients still experience dialysis therapy before transplantation and the average durations of dialysis were 2.6 years and 13.9 years, respectively. Therefore, for successful renal transplantation in older people, routine management of physical frailty in patients undergoing dialysis is essential. Additionally, exercise interventions against physical frailty need to be considered after kidney transplantation because that alone does not improve poor walking ability, low muscle function, or muscle loss.

6. Exercise Intervention after Kidney Transplantation

A recent meta-analysis showed that exercise therapy for patients with kidney transplant improved physical performance and quality of life [55], but most of this evidence targeted chronic, stable patients after a certain period of time had passed since transplantation. There have been few studies that have investigated exercise therapy in the early post-kidney transplantation period.

We started an early-phase exercise program for renal transplant patients, and after discharge from hospital, we reported its effect on physical performance and activity, quality of life, and kidney function [56]. Our program consisted of supervised aerobic training by physical therapists and physical activity in the ward and at home (Figure 5). Patients started the program on day 6 after transplantation. Supervised aerobic training was conducted during hospitalization and was performed for 3–4 weeks until discharge. Participants attended one or two sessions of supervised structured aerobic training per day at a rehabilitation center in the hospital 5 days/week. Aerobic training consisted of a 35–45 min/session on a treadmill walking or cycle ergometer exercise including a warmup and cool-down [56]. Exercise intensity was prescribed for patients at a 13–15 rating of perceived exertion on the Borg scale. Exercise therapy was stopped or the intensity was changed according to the criteria in Table 3. Physical activity instruction was provided for up to two months after kidney transplantation. On day 6 after transplantation, participants were instructed to wear a pedometer while performing a walking exercise. The following progressive target values were a guide: 3000 steps/day in the first week, 5000 in the second, and 5000 plus stair climbing movement in the third. The number of steps was confirmed by a physiotherapist during supervised aerobic training, and the target step count was corrected as necessary. As a result, exercise capacity and lower extremity muscle strength at 2 months after kidney transplantation were significantly higher in the exercise group than in the control. Regarding kidney function, in both the control and exercise groups, all patients succeeded in withdrawing from, or avoiding dialysis therapy, and there was no significant difference in the recovery curve of kidney function.

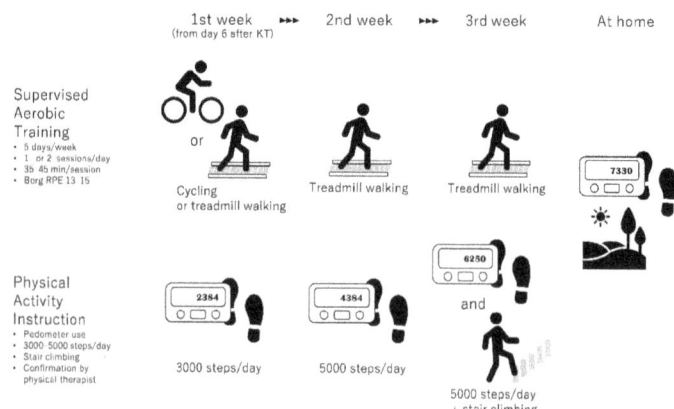

Figure 5. Protocol exercise intervention for patients after kidney transplantation, created based on a reference from Yamamoto et al. [56]. KT: kidney transplantation; RPE: rating of perceived exertion.

Table 3. Key points to note for safe implementation of exercise interventions among patients after kidney transplantation, created based on a reference from Yamamoto S. et al. [56].

In the following cases, exercise therapy should be stopped or exercise intensity should be changed:
(1) Temperature higher than 38 °C.   (2) Surgical wound pain higher than 7/10 on the visual analog scale.   (3) Increase in the serum creatinine value for more than two days.   (4) Increase in the serum creatinine value by 30% or more compared with the previous day.   (5) Severe anemia (serum hemoglobin <7.0 g/dL).   (6) Abstinence from eating.   (7) Patients judged unsuitable for exercise therapy by the responsible nurses or the primary doctor for reasons other than the ones above.

7. Summary

The mortality rates among patients on hemodialysis remain high, and one of the potential contributors might be the high burden of functional dependence, caused by impaired mobility, poor physical functioning, and muscle weakness—the main components of physical frailty. As recent evidence has revealed, physical frailty can constitute a limiting factor for successful transplantation in patients with end-stage renal disease with or without hemodialysis. In addition, frailty among patients after transplantation has been identified as a risk factor for poor health outcomes. Therefore, initiating an exercise program to reduce or prevent physical frailty during the post-transplantation phase could be necessary. Although the concept of renal rehabilitation has become widely known among kidney health providers in recent years, kidney health professionals should make serious efforts to manage sarcopenia and physical frailty based on the evaluations of physical function and activity as well as exercise therapy.

Author Contributions: Conceptualization, R.M.; Formal analysis, R.M. and D.K.; Writing—original draft preparation, R.M.; Writing—review and editing, D.K.; Visualization, D.K. All authors have read and agreed to the published version of the manuscript.

Funding: This work was supported by research funding from Hyogo Medical University, Japan (R.M.) and the JSPS KAKENHI: 20K19332, Japan (R.M.).

Institutional Review Board Statement: No ethical approval was required because this study did not include confidential personal data and did not involve patient intervention.

Informed Consent Statement: Not applicable.

Data Availability Statement: Not applicable.

Conflicts of Interest: The authors declare no conflict of interest.

References

1. Hamer, R.A.; El Nahas, A.M. The burden of chronic kidney disease. *BMJ* **2006**, *332*, 563–564. [CrossRef] [PubMed]
2. Canaud, B.; Tong, L.; Tentori, F.; Akiba, T.; Karaboyas, A.; Gillespie, B.; Akizawa, T.; Pisoni, R.L.; Bommer, J.; Port, F.K. Clinical Practices and Outcomes in Elderly Hemodialysis Patients: Results from the Dialysis Outcomes and Practice Patterns Study (DOPPS). *Clin. J. Am. Soc. Nephrol.* **2011**, *6*, 1651–1662. [CrossRef]
3. Kimata, N.; Tsuchiya, K.; Akiba, T.; Nitta, K. Differences in the Characteristics of Dialysis Patients in Japan Compared with Those in Other Countries. *Blood Purif.* **2015**, *40*, 275–279. [CrossRef] [PubMed]
4. Nitta, K.; Goto, S.; Masakane, I.; Hanafusa, N.; Taniguchi, M.; Hasegawa, T.; Nakai, S.; Wada, A.; Hamano, T.; Hoshino, J.; et al. Annual dialysis data report for 2018, JSDT Renal Data Registry: Survey methods, facility data, incidence, prevalence, and mortality. *Ren. Replace. Ther.* **2020**, *6*, 41. [CrossRef]
5. Farrington, K.; Covic, A.; Aucella, F.; Clyne, N.; De Vos, L.; Findlay, A.; Fouque, D.; Grodzicki, T.; Iyasere, O.; Jager, K.J.; et al. Clinical Practice Guideline on management of older patients with chronic kidney disease stage 3b or higher (eGFR < 45 mL/min/1.73 m^2). *Nephrol. Dial. Transpl.* **2016**, *31*, 1–66. [CrossRef]

6. Yamagata, K.; Hoshino, J.; Sugiyama, H.; Hanafusa, N.; Shibagaki, Y.; Komatsu, Y.; Konta, T.; Fujii, N.; Kanda, E.; Sofue, T.; et al. Clinical practice guideline for renal rehabilitation: Systematic reviews and recommendations of exercise therapies in patients with kidney diseases. *Ren. Replace. Ther.* **2019**, *5*, 1–19. [CrossRef]
7. Tamura, M.K.; Covinsky, K.E.; Chertow, G.M.; Yaffe, K.; Landefeld, C.S.; McCulloch, C.E. Faculty Opinions recommendation of Functional status of elderly adults before and after initiation of dialysis. *N. Engl. J. Med.* **2009**, *361*, 1539–1547. [CrossRef]
8. Jassal, S.V.; Karaboyas, A.; Comment, L.A.; Bieber, B.; Morgenstern, H.; Sen, A.; Gillespie, B.W.; De Sequera, P.; Marshall, M.R.; Fukuhara, S.; et al. Functional Dependence and Mortality in the International Dialysis Outcomes and Practice Patterns Study (DOPPS). *Am. J. Kidney Dis.* **2016**, *67*, 283–292. [CrossRef]
9. Matsuzawa, R.; Kamitani, T.; Roshanravan, B.; Fukuma, S.; Joki, N.; Fukagawa, M. Decline in the Functional Status and Mortality in Patients on Hemodialysis: Results from the Japan Dialysis Outcome and Practice Patterns Study. *J. Ren. Nutr.* **2019**, *29*, 504–510. [CrossRef]
10. Heiland, E.G.; Welmer, A.-K.; Wang, R.; Santoni, G.; Angleman, S.; Fratiglioni, L.; Qiu, C. Association of mobility limitations with incident disability among older adults: A population-based study. *Age Ageing* **2016**, *45*, 812–819. [CrossRef]
11. Goto, R.; Watanabe, H.; Haruta, J.; Tsutsumi, M.; Yokoya, S.; Maeno, T. Identification of prognostic factors for activities of daily living in elderly patients after hospitalization for acute infectious disease in Japan: A 6-month follow-up study. *Geriatr. Gerontol. Int.* **2017**, *18*, 615–622. [CrossRef] [PubMed]
12. Chen, J.L.; Godfrey, S.; Ng, T.T.; Moorthi, R.; Liangos, O.; Ruthazer, R.; Jaber, B.L.; Levey, A.S.; Castaneda-Sceppa, C. Effect of intra-dialytic, low-intensity strength training on functional capacity in adult haemodialysis patients: A randomized pilot trial. *Nephrol. Dial. Transpl.* **2010**, *25*, 1936–1943. [CrossRef] [PubMed]
13. Fried, L.P.; Tangen, C.M.; Walston, J.; Newman, A.B.; Hirsch, C.; Gottdiener, J.; Seeman, T.; Tracy, R.; Kop, W.J.; Burke, G.; et al. Cardiovascular Health Study Collaborative Research G. Frailty in older adults: Evidence for a phenotype. *J. Gerontol. A Biol. Sci. Med. Sci.* **2001**, *56*, 146–156. [CrossRef] [PubMed]
14. Walston, J.; Hadley, E.C.; Ferrucci, L.; Guralnik, J.M.; Newman, A.B.; Studenski, S.A.; Ershler, W.B.; Harris, T.; Fried, L.P. Research Agenda for Frailty in Older Adults: Toward a Better Understanding of Physiology and Etiology: Summary from the American Geriatrics Society/National Institute on Aging Research Conference on Frailty in Older Adults. *J. Am. Geriatr. Soc.* **2006**, *54*, 991–1001. [CrossRef] [PubMed]
15. Satake, S.; Arai, H. The revised Japanese version of the Cardiovascular Health Study criteria (revised J-CHS criteria). *Geriatr. Gerontol. Int.* **2020**, *20*, 992–993. [CrossRef] [PubMed]
16. Kojima, G. Prevalence of frailty in end-stage renal disease: A systematic review and meta-analysis. *Int. Urol. Nephrol.* **2017**, *49*, 1989–1997. [CrossRef]
17. Kojima, G.; Iliffe, S.; Taniguchi, Y.; Shimada, H.; Rakugi, H.; Walters, K. Prevalence of frailty in Japan: A systematic review and meta-analysis. *J. Epidemiol.* **2017**, *27*, 347–353. [CrossRef]
18. Matsuzawa, R. Renal rehabilitation as a management strategy for physical frailty in CKD. *Ren. Replace. Ther.* **2022**, *8*, 1–9. [CrossRef]
19. Hendriks, F.K.; Smeets, J.S.; van der Sande, F.M.; Kooman, J.P.; van Loon, L.J. Dietary Protein and Physical Activity Interventions to Support Muscle Maintenance in End-Stage Renal Disease Patients on Hemodialysis. *Nutrients* **2019**, *11*, 2972. [CrossRef]
20. Vettoretti, S.; Caldiroli, L.; Armelloni, S.; Ferrari, C.; Cesari, M.; Messa, P. Sarcopenia is Associated with Malnutrition but Not with Systemic Inflammation in Older Persons with Advanced CKD. *Nutrients* **2019**, *11*, 1378. [CrossRef]
21. Kim, J.K.; Choi, S.R.; Choi, M.J.; Kim, S.G.; Lee, Y.K.; Noh, J.W.; Kim, H.J.; Song, Y.R. Prevalence of and factors associated with sarcopenia in elderly patients with end-stage renal disease. *Clin. Nutr.* **2014**, *33*, 64–68. [CrossRef] [PubMed]
22. Gungor, O.; Ulu, S.; Hasbal, N.B.; Anker, S.D.; Kalantar-Zadeh, K. Effects of hormonal changes on sarcopenia in chronic kidney disease: Where are we now and what can we do? *J. Cachexia Sarcopenia Muscle* **2021**, *12*, 1380–1392. [CrossRef] [PubMed]
23. Haugen, C.E.; Chu, N.; Ying, H.; Warsame, F.; Holscher, C.M.; Desai, N.M.; Jones, M.R.; Norman, S.P.; Brennan, D.C.; Garonzik-Wang, J.; et al. Frailty and Access to Kidney Transplantation. *Clin. J. Am. Soc. Nephrol.* **2019**, *14*, 576–582. [CrossRef] [PubMed]
24. McAdams-DeMarco, M.A.; Law, A.; Salter, M.L.; Boyarsky, B.; Gimenez, L.F.; Jaar, B.; Walston, J.D.; Segev, D.L. Frailty as a Novel Predictor of Mortality and Hospitalization in Individuals of All Ages Undergoing Hemodialysis. *J. Am. Geriatr. Soc.* **2013**, *61*, 896–901. [CrossRef]
25. Alfaadhel, T.A.; Soroka, S.D.; Kiberd, B.A.; Landry, D.; Moorhouse, P.; Tennankore, K.K. Frailty and Mortality in Dialysis: Evaluation of a Clinical Frailty Scale. *Clin. J. Am. Soc. Nephrol.* **2015**, *10*, 832–840. [CrossRef]
26. Kim, J.C.; Shapiro, B.B.; Zhang, M.; Li, Y.; Porszasz, J.; Bross, R.; Feroze, U.; Upreti, R.; Kalantar-Zadeh, K.; Kopple, J.D. Daily physical activity and physical function in adult maintenance hemodialysis patients. *J. Cachex Sarcopenia Muscle* **2014**, *5*, 209–220. [CrossRef]
27. Chen, L.-K.; Woo, J.; Assantachai, P.; Auyeung, T.-W.; Chou, M.-Y.; Iijima, K.; Jang, H.C.; Kang, L.; Kim, M.; Kim, S.; et al. Asian Working Group for Sarcopenia: 2019 Consensus Update on Sarcopenia Diagnosis and Treatment. *J. Am. Med. Dir. Assoc.* **2020**, *21*, 300–307. [CrossRef]
28. Fielding, R.A.; Vellas, B.; Evans, W.J.; Bhasin, S.; Morley, J.E.; Newman, A.B.; van Kan, G.A.; Andrieu, S.; Bauer, J.; Breuille, D.; et al. Sarcopenia: An Undiagnosed Condition in Older Adults. Current Consensus Definition: Prevalence, Etiology, and Consequences. International Working Group on Sarcopenia. *J. Am. Med. Dir. Assoc.* **2011**, *12*, 249–256. [CrossRef]

29. Cruz-Jentoft, A.J.; Bahat, G.; Bauer, J.; Boirie, Y.; Bruyere, O.; Cederholm, T.; Cooper, C.; Landi, F.; Rolland, Y.; Sayer, A.A.; et al. Sarcopenia: Revised European consensus on definition and diagnosis. *Age Ageing* **2019**, *48*, 16–31. [CrossRef]
30. Kara, M.; Kaymak, B.; Frontera, W.; Ata, A.M.; Ricci, V.; Ekiz, T.; Chang, K.V.; Han, D.S.; Michail, X.; Quittan, M.; et al. Diagnosing sarcopenia: Functional perspectives and a new algorithm from the ISarcoPRM. *J. Rehabil. Med.* **2021**, *53*, jrm00209. [CrossRef]
31. Shu, X.; Lin, T.; Wang, H.; Zhao, Y.; Jiang, T.; Peng, X.; Yue, J. Diagnosis, prevalence, and mortality of sarcopenia in dialysis patients: A systematic review and meta-analysis. *J. Cachexia Sarcopenia Muscle* **2022**, *13*, 145–158. [CrossRef] [PubMed]
32. Shafiee, G.; Keshtkar, A.; Soltani, A.; Ahadi, Z.; Larijani, B.; Heshmat, R. Prevalence of sarcopenia in the world: A systematic review and meta- analysis of general population studies. *J. Diabetes Metab. Disord.* **2017**, *16*, 21. [CrossRef]
33. Kitamura, A.; Seino, S.; Abe, T.; Nofuji, Y.; Yokoyama, Y.; Amano, H.; Nishi, M.; Taniguchi, Y.; Narita, M.; Fujiwara, Y.; et al. Sarcopenia: Prevalence, associated factors, and the risk of mortality and disability in Japanese older adults. *J. Cachex Sarcopenia Muscle* **2020**, *12*, 30–38. [CrossRef] [PubMed]
34. Kakita, D.; Matsuzawa, R.; Yamamoto, S.; Suzuki, Y.; Harada, M.; Imamura, K.; Yoshikoshi, S.; Imai, H.; Osada, S.; Shimokado, K.; et al. Simplified discriminant parameters for sarcopenia among patients undergoing hemodialysis. *J. Cachexia Sarcopenia Muscle* 2022, in press.
35. Imamura, K.; Yamamoto, S.; Suzuki, Y.; Matsuzawa, R.; Harada, M.; Yoshikoshi, S.; Yoshida, A.; Matsunaga, A. Limitations of SARC-F as a Screening Tool for Sarcopenia in Patients on Hemodialysis. *Nephron Exp. Nephrol.* **2021**, *146*, 32–39. [CrossRef]
36. Canaud, B.; Ye, X.; Usvyat, L.; Kooman, J.; van der Sande, F.; Raimann, J.; Wang, Y.; Kotanko, P. Clinical and predictive value of simplified creatinine index used as muscle mass surrogate in end-stage kidney disease haemodialysis patients—Results from the international MONitoring Dialysis Outcome initiative. *Nephrol. Dial. Transplant.* **2020**, *35*, 2161–2171. [CrossRef]
37. Yamamoto, S.; Matsuzawa, R.; Hoshi, K.; Suzuki, Y.; Harada, M.; Watanabe, T.; Isobe, Y.; Imamura, K.; Osada, S.; Yoshida, A.; et al. Modified Creatinine Index and Clinical Outcomes of Hemodialysis Patients: An Indicator of Sarcopenia? *J. Ren. Nutr.* **2021**, *31*, 370–379. [CrossRef]
38. Matsuzawa, R.; Roshanravan, B. Management of Physical Frailty in Patients Requiring Hemodialysis Therapy. *Contrib. Nephrol.* **2018**, *196*, 101–109. [CrossRef]
39. Roshanravan, B.; Gamboa, J.; Wilund, K. Exercise and CKD: Skeletal Muscle Dysfunction and Practical Application of Exercise to Prevent and Treat Physical Impairments in CKD. *Am. J. Kidney Dis.* **2017**, *69*, 837–852. [CrossRef]
40. Yamamoto, S.; Matsuzawa, R.; Abe, Y.; Hoshi, K.; Yoneki, K.; Harada, M.; Watanabe, T.; Shimoda, T.; Suzuki, Y.; Matsunaga, Y.; et al. Utility of Regular Management of Physical Activity and Physical Function in Hemodialysis Patients. *Kidney Blood Press. Res.* **2018**, *43*, 1505–1515. [CrossRef]
41. Kojima, G. Quick and Simple FRAIL Scale Predicts Incident Activities of Daily Living (ADL) and Instrumental ADL (IADL) Disabilities: A Systematic Review and Meta-analysis. *J. Am. Med. Dir. Assoc.* **2018**, *19*, 1063–1068. [CrossRef] [PubMed]
42. Matsuzawa, R.; Matsunaga, A.; Wang, G.; Yamamoto, S.; Kutsuna, T.; Ishii, A.; Abe, Y.; Yoneki, K.; Yoshida, A.; Takahira, N. Relationship Between Lower Extremity Muscle Strength and All-Cause Mortality in Japanese Patients Undergoing Dialysis. *Phys. Ther.* **2014**, *94*, 947–956. [CrossRef] [PubMed]
43. Zhang, F.; Ren, Y.; Wang, H.; Bai, Y.; Huang, L. Daily Step Counts in Patients with Chronic Kidney Disease: A Systematic Review and Meta-Analysis of Observational Studies. *Front. Med.* **2022**, *17*, 842423. [CrossRef] [PubMed]
44. Johansen, K.L.; Kaysen, G.A.; Dalrymple, L.S.; Grimes, B.A.; Glidden, D.; Anand, S.; Chertow, G.M. Association of Physical Activity with Survival among Ambulatory Patients on Dialysis: The Comprehensive Dialysis Study. *Clin. J. Am. Soc. Nephrol.* **2012**, *8*, 248–253. [CrossRef]
45. Lopes, A.A.; Lantz, B.; Morgenstern, H.; Wang, M.; Bieber, B.; Gillespie, B.W.; Li, Y.; Painter, P.; Jacobson, S.H.; Rayner, H.C.; et al. Associations of Self-Reported Physical Activity Types and Levels with Quality of Life, Depression Symptoms, and Mortality in Hemodialysis Patients: The DOPPS. *Clin. J. Am. Soc. Nephrol.* **2014**, *9*, 1702–1712. [CrossRef]
46. O'Hare, A.M.; Tawney, K.; Bacchetti, P.; Johansen, K.L. Decreased survival among sedentary patients undergoing dialysis: Results from the dialysis morbidity and mortality study wave 2. *Am. J. Kidney Dis.* **2003**, *41*, 447–454. [CrossRef]
47. Stack, A.G.; Molony, D.A.; Rives, T.; Tyson, J.; Murthy, B.V. Association of physical activity with mortality in the US dialysis population. *Am. J. Kidney Dis.* **2005**, *45*, 690–701. [CrossRef]
48. Tentori, F.; Elder, S.J.; Thumma, J.; Pisoni, R.L.; Bommer, J.; Fissell, R.B.; Fukuhara, S.; Jadoul, M.; Keen, M.L.; Saran, R.; et al. Physical exercise among participants in the Dialysis Outcomes and Practice Patterns Study (DOPPS): Correlates and associated outcomes. *Nephrol. Dial. Transpl.* **2010**, *25*, 3050–3062. [CrossRef]
49. Matsuzawa, R.; Matsunaga, A.; Wang, G.; Kutsuna, T.; Ishii, A.; Abe, Y.; Takagi, Y.; Yoshida, A.; Takahira, N. Habitual Physical Activity Measured by Accelerometer and Survival in Maintenance Hemodialysis Patients. *Clin. J. Am. Soc. Nephrol.* **2012**, *7*, 2010–2016. [CrossRef]
50. Matsuzawa, R.; Roshanravan, B.; Shimoda, T.; Mamorita, N.; Yoneki, K.; Harada, M.; Watanabe, T.; Yoshida, A.; Takeuchi, Y.; Matsunaga, A. Physical Activity Dose for Hemodialysis Patients: Where to Begin? Results from a Prospective Cohort Study. *J. Ren. Nutr.* **2018**, *28*, 45–53. [CrossRef]
51. Chodzko-Zajko, W. ; American College of Sports Medicine. *ACSM's Exercise for Older Adults*, 1st ed.; Lippincott Williams & Wilkins: New York, NY, USA, 2014.

52. Shimoda, T.; Matsuzawa, R.; Yoneki, K.; Harada, M.; Watanabe, T.; Matsumoto, M.; Yoshida, A.; Takeuchi, Y.; Matsunaga, A. Changes in physical activity and risk of all-cause mortality in patients on maintenance hemodialysis: A retrospective cohort study. *BMC Nephrol.* **2017**, *18*, 154. [CrossRef]
53. Yamamoto, S.; Matsuzawa, R.; Hoshi, K.; Harada, M.; Watanabe, T.; Suzuki, Y.; Isobe, Y.; Imamura, K.; Osada, S.; Yoshida, A.; et al. Impact of Physical Activity on Dialysis and Nondialysis Days and Clinical Outcomes Among Patients on Hemodialysis. *J. Ren. Nutr.* **2021**, *31*, 380–388. [CrossRef] [PubMed]
54. Debnath, S.; Rueda, R.; Bansal, S.; Kasinath, B.S.; Sharma, K.; Lorenzo, C. Fatigue characteristics on dialysis and non-dialysis days in patients with chronic kidney failure on maintenance hemodialysis. *BMC Nephrol.* **2021**, *22*, 1–9. [CrossRef] [PubMed]
55. Oguchi, H.; Tsujita, M.; Yazawa, M.; Kawaguchi, T.; Hoshino, J.; Kohzuki, M.; Ito, O.; Yamagata, K.; Shibagaki, Y.; Sofue, T. The efficacy of exercise training in kidney transplant recipients: A meta-analysis and systematic review. *Clin. Exp. Nephrol.* **2018**, *23*, 275–284. [CrossRef] [PubMed]
56. Yamamoto, S.; Matsuzawa, R.; Kamitani, T.; Hoshi, K.; Ishii, D.; Noguchi, F.; Hamazaki, N.; Nozaki, K.; Ichikawa, T.; Maekawa, E.; et al. Efficacy of Exercise Therapy Initiated in the Early Phase After Kidney Transplantation: A Pilot Study. *J. Ren. Nutr.* **2020**, *30*, 518–525. [CrossRef]

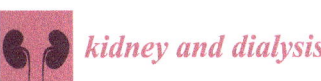

Review

Toward Revision of the 'Best Practice for Diabetic Patients on Hemodialysis 2012'

Masanori Abe *, Tomomi Matsuoka, Shunsuke Kawamoto, Kota Miyasato and Hiroki Kobayashi

Division of Nephrology, Hypertension and Endocrinology, Department of Medicine, Nihon University School of Medicine, Tokyo 173-8610, Japan
* Correspondence: abe.masanori@nihon-u.ac.jp; Tel.: +81-3-3972-8111

Abstract: Diabetic nephropathy is the leading cause of dialysis therapy worldwide. The number of diabetes patients on dialysis in clinical settings has been increasing in Japan. In 2013, the Japanese Society for Dialysis Therapy (JSDT) published the "Best Practice for Diabetic Patients on Hemodialysis 2012". While glycated hemoglobin (HbA1c) is used mainly as a glycemic control index for dialysis patients overseas, Japan is the first country in the world to use glycated albumin (GA) for assessment. According to a survey conducted by the JSDT in 2018, the number of facilities measuring only HbA1c has decreased compared with 2013, while the number of facilities measuring GA or both has significantly increased. Ten years have passed since the publication of the first edition of the guidelines, and several clinical studies regarding the GA value and mortality of dialysis patients have been reported. In addition, novel antidiabetic agents have appeared, and continuous glucose monitoring of dialysis patients has been adopted. On the other hand, Japanese dialysis patients are rapidly aging, and the proportion of patients with malnutrition is increasing. Therefore, there is great variation among diabetes patients on dialysis with respect to their backgrounds and characteristics. This review covers the indices and targets of glycemic control, the treatment of hyperglycemia, and diet recommendations for dialysis patients with diabetes.

Keywords: antidiabetic agents; burnt-out diabetes; continuous glucose monitoring; diabetes mellitus; dialysis; glycated albumin; glycated hemoglobin; glycemic control

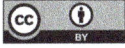

1. Introduction

Diabetes is, globally, the leading cause of end-stage kidney disease (ESKD) for patients on dialysis. In Japan, diabetic nephropathy has been the most common cause of ESKD since 1998, accounting for 42.3% of the incidence of dialysis patients in 2018 [1]. Furthermore, the rate of diabetic nephropathy was 39.0% in all dialysis patients in 2018 [1]. Although many dialysis patients have diabetes, there are no guidelines for the management of diabetes patients on dialysis. Therefore, the Japanese Society for Dialysis Therapy (JSDT) published the "Best Practice for Diabetic Patients on Hemodialysis 2012" [2]. Glycated hemoglobin (HbA1c) is commonly used worldwide as an index of glycemic control for dialysis patients. However, it has been demonstrated that it does not provide accurate glycemic control in patients on hemodialysis (HD) [3–5]. In addition to the shortened red-blood-cell lifespan (approximately 60 days), patients experience blood loss and hemorrhage due to HD therapy, and the administration of erythropoiesis-stimulating agents (ESAs) for the treatment of renal anemia increases the proportion of immature erythrocytes. Therefore, in HD patients, the HbA1c levels tend to be lower. On the other hand, it was reported that glycated albumin (GA) is a useful control index instead of HbA1c because it is not affected by the lifespan of red blood cells or ESA treatment [3–5]. Therefore, the "Best Practice for Diabetic Patients on Hemodialysis 2012" of JSDT first recommended GA as an indicator of glycemic control for HD patients with diabetes. The guidelines describe the management required for diabetes HD patients: (1) indices of glycemic control and its frequency of measurement; (2) glucose concentrations in dialysate; (3) approach of hyperglycemia and hypoglycemia during HD; (4) treatment by oral antidiabetic agents and insulin; (5) diet therapy; and (6) management of complications such as diabetic retinopathy, orthostatic hypotension, arteriosclerosis, and bone diseases [2]. However, in the ten years that have passed since the publication of the first edition, the background of diabetes patients on dialysis has changed and novel treatments have emerged; hence, revision is required. This review covers the indices and targets of glycemic control, the treatment of hyperglycemia, and diet recommendations for dialysis patients with diabetes.

2. Which Glycemic Index, GA or HbA1c, Demonstrates Better Performance in Dialysis Patients?

In HD patients, GA is a better indicator of glycemic control than HbA1c, which is known to underestimate and not accurately reflect mean blood-glucose levels [3–5]. HbA1c in HD patients is influenced by various factors, such as shortened erythrocyte lifespan, ESA for the treatment of renal anemia, the administration of iron preparations, uremia, and blood transfusion, thus potentially resulting in inaccurate measurements. ESA administration or iron supplementation can rapidly reduce HbA1c levels without improving glycemic control. The stimulation of erythropoiesis increases the proportion of young erythrocytes compared to old erythrocytes and leads to a decrease in HbA1c levels. GA is more strongly correlated with plasma glucose levels than HbA1c and is unaffected by red-blood-cell lifespan or ESA administration, making it a more reliable indicator of glycemic control in HD patients [6].

3. Target GA Levels in Hemodialysis Patients from Observational Studies and Meta-analyses

An association between GA levels and outcomes in HD patients with diabetes has been reported in multiple observational studies conducted in Japan. It has been reported that the incidence of cardiovascular complications is higher in HD patients with diabetes with GA levels $\geq 23\%$ [7], and poor glycemic control in patients with GA levels $\geq 29\%$ at the time of dialysis initiation is associated with increased cardiovascular morbidity and shortened survival [8]. It was reported that the prognosis appeared better in a group of patients with GA <20% without a history of cardiovascular events upon the start of the observation compared with higher GA groups (20.0–24.5% and >24.5%) [9]. There are also some studies from the United States that report associations between GA level, the onset of cardiovascular events [10], prognosis [10,11], admission rate [11], and duration of hospitalization in dialysis patients with diabetes [12]. Based on these results, the "Best Practice for Diabetic Patients on Hemodialysis 2012" recommends GA levels <20.0% as the tentative target values for glycemic control in HD patients with diabetes. However, in patients with cardiovascular disease or who have a tendency toward hypoglycemia, GA levels < 24.0% are recommended [2]. More recently, it was reported in Taiwan that higher GA levels might be predictors of mortality not only for patients with diabetes on HD but also those without diabetes [13].

In 2018, the JSDT Renal Data Registry Committee (JRDR) reported an association between a glycemic control indicator and prognosis based on an investigation on 22,441 HD patients with diabetes [14]. The patients were stratified by deciles of the baseline GA level and HbA1c level and analyzed for the potential association with one-year mortality, a prognostic indicator for HD patients with diabetes. As a result, the groups with GA levels $\geq 22.9\%$ had significantly higher adjusted hazard ratio (HR) values than the reference, with GA levels of 17.1 to <18.2% (Figure 1). Meanwhile, the groups with HbA1c of <5.3% and $\geq 7.6\%$ had a significantly higher adjusted HR than the reference, with HbA1c levels of 6.0% to <6.3%, demonstrating a U-shaped trend for the HR (Figure 1) [14]. The JRDR also reported the association between three-year mortality and GA levels in 40,417 HD patients with diabetes [15]. In that report, three-year mortality showed a linear association with GA levels $\geq 18\%$, whereas this association was not observed between lower GA levels and three-year mortality. In malnourished patients treated with oral antidiabetic agents, increased mortality was associated with GA levels $\geq 24\%$. These results suggest a need to set the target GA value for glycemic control based on consideration of such factors as the use of antidiabetic agents, nutritional status, and patient background, such as cancer development status.

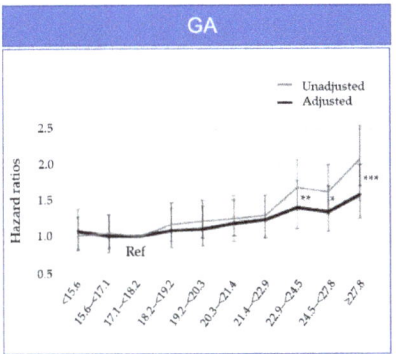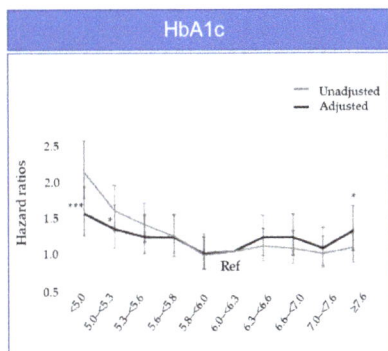

Figure 1. Hazard ratios of all-cause mortality divided by deciles of GA levels and HbA1c levels in 22,441 hemodialysis patients. Adjusted variables include age, sex, vintage, modality, body mass index, smoking, type of diabetes, antihypertensive agents use, type of hypoglycemic agent use, hemoglobin, albumin, C-reactive protein, parathyroid hormone, calcium, phosphate, high-density lipoprotein, Kt/V, normalized protein catabolic rate, history of cardiovascular disease, and type of dialysis center. * $p < 0.05$, ** $p < 0.01$, *** $p < 0.001$ vs. Ref. (Adjusted).

Furthermore, based on the multicenter prospective observational study of 841 chronic dialysis patients with diabetes for a mean study period of 3.1 years, GA levels could be a prognostic factor in predicting atherosclerotic cardiovascular disease (ASCVD)-related mortality [16]. Overall, it was suggested that GA might be a more suitable parameter than HbA1c for accurately predicting the prognosis of dialysis patients with diabetes.

In 2018, the results of a meta-analysis were reported. The relationship between average blood glucose levels and HbA1c and GA levels was investigated [17]. The meta-analysis included 24 studies with 3928 patients, and it was concluded that GA was superior to HbA1c in assessing glycemic status in diabetes patients with advanced chronic kidney disease (CKD), including CKD stages 4 and 5 and dialysis. Furthermore, the results of another meta-analysis, including 12 studies with 25,932 dialysis patients, demonstrated that GA can be an effective indicator for predicting the prognosis of dialysis patients with diabetes [18].

4. Current Glycemic Status in Diabetes Patients on Dialysis

Although JSDT presented the "Best Practice for Diabetic Patients on Hemodialysis 2012" in Japan in 2013, the annual dialysis data report for 2013 by JRDR found that 53.5% of dialysis patients with diabetes had been assessed based on GA measurement, whereas 46.5% of the patients had been assessed solely on the basis of HbA1c at the end of 2013 [19]. The 2013 survey examined HbA1c and GA levels, while the 2018 survey also examined casual plasma glucose levels in addition to HbA1c and GA. The proportion of patients who were assessed according to GA was 75.9%, whereas the proportion for HbA1c only was 24.1%. Thus, the popularity of GA measurements has increased in Japan [20]. In addition, glycemic indices were investigated in two treatment groups, which were the hemodialysis, including HD and HDF patients, and the peritoneal dialysis (PD) groups.

Casual plasma glucose levels were measured in 111,005 patients of 160,021 diabetes patients on dialysis. The casual plasma glucose levels in the HD and HDF groups were 151.5 ± 56.1 and 150.8 ± 55.4 mg/dL, respectively, while those in the PD group were 140.3 ± 53.4 mg/dL, lower than those in HD and HDF patients. The mean casual plasma glucose levels were equivalent between the HD and HDF patients. In total, 84.4% of the diabetes patients on HD and HDF achieved the target casual plasma glucose levels of below 200 mg/dL (Figure 2). On the other hand, 89.1% of the PD patients achieved casual plasma glucose levels of <200 mg/dL, and this rate was higher than that of the hemodialysis patients. Casual plasma glucose levels < 50 mg/dL, a finding suggestive of severe hypoglycemia, was observed in 237 hemodialysis patients (0.2%), but only 1 PD patient.

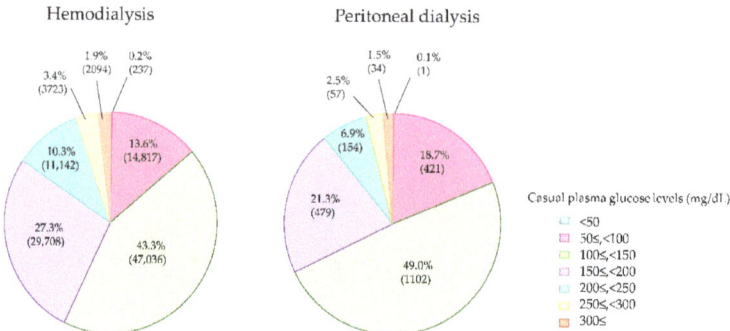

Figure 2. Casual plasma glucose levels of diabetes patients on hemodialysis and peritoneal dialysis in 2018.

The GA levels were 16.9% ± 4.4% for the PD group and 20.9% ± 5.1% for the HD group. The levels were clearly lowered in the PD group irrespective of whether the plasma glucose levels were equivalent between the two groups (Figure 3). This finding suggests that the half-life of serum albumin is shortened in PD patients due to the loss of albumin into PD fluid. The target GA level of less than 20.0%, which is recommended in the "Best Practice for Diabetic Patients on Hemodialysis 2012", was achieved in 51.4% in 2018, which is more than the 46.6% in the 2013 survey. In total, 80.4% of the patients achieved the target GA level of <24.0%, which is the target for patients with a history of cardiovascular diseases or who are prone to hypoglycemia.

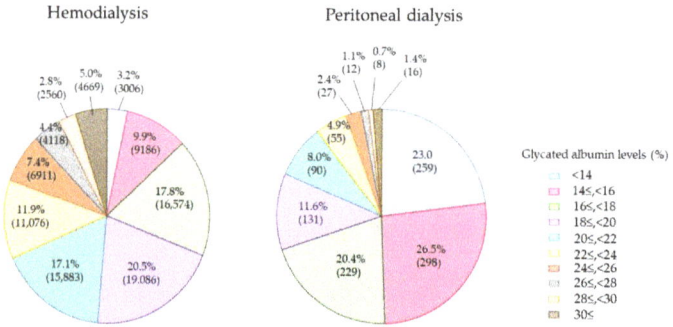

Figure 3. Glycated albumin (GA) levels of diabetes patients on hemodialysis and peritoneal dialysis in 2018.

According to the 2018 survey, the average HbA1c values were almost equivalent between the three groups of PD, HD, and HDF, at 6.14% ± 1.11%, 6.17% ± 1.16%, and 6.23% ± 1.19%, respectively. These values are similar to the value of 6.19% ± 1.16% in the 2013 survey. As shown in Figure 4, when the patients were divided into groups according to HbA1c levels and the distribution ratios compared, there was no difference in the ratios between the two groups. This finding suggests that the HbA1c levels were apparently lowered in all of the dialysis patients because both the HD and the PD patients had renal anemia and were treated with ESAs.

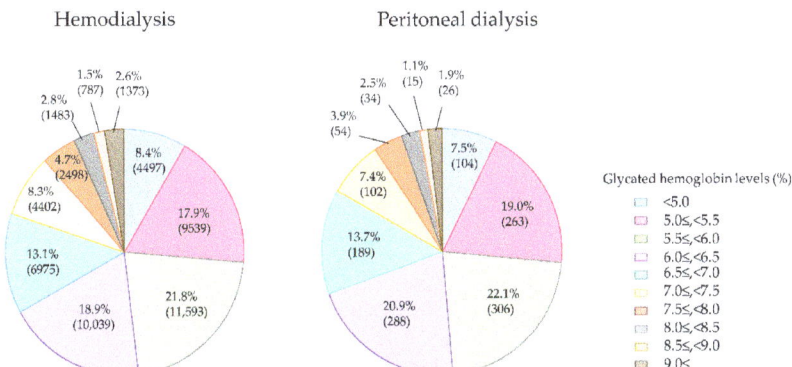

Figure 4. Glycated hemoglobin (HbA1c) levels of diabetes patients on hemodialysis and peritoneal dialysis in 2018.

5. Association between GA Levels and Mortality in PD Patients

There are few reports examining the relationship between GA values and mortality in PD patients. It was reported that the GA levels are 4.5% lower in PD than in HD patients [21]. Nevertheless, there are reports that, compared with HbA1c, GA more accurately reflects glycemic control in PD patients and is associated with prognosis. In addition, JRDR reported the results of analysis of the relationship between HbA1c and GA as indicators of glycemic control and 2-year mortality in PD patients [22]. Although no association was found between HbA1c and mortality, the hazard ratio of death significantly increased when the GA value was 20.0% or higher. However, there are few studies that have examined the relationship between GA levels and mortality in PD patients. Therefore, further evidence is needed to substantiate this relationship.

6. Limitations of GA

GA levels are affected not only by plasma glucose levels but also by albumin metabolism. In patients with a prolonged albumin half-life, such as those with liver cirrhosis or untreated hypothyroidism, GA levels are increased [23,24]. Decreased GA levels may be found in patients with untreated hyperthyroidism or nephrotic syndrome [23,25]. Patients with proteinuria are known to have lower GA levels due to a shortened albumin half-life. In particular, proteinuria with nephrotic range, i.e., over 3.5 g/day, has been reported to decrease GA levels regardless of glycemic status [25]. Furthermore, GA can be falsely lowered in PD patients because the lifespan of albumin is shortened due to albumin loss into PD fluid [25,26].

7. 'Burnt-Out Diabetes' Phenomenon in Patients on Dialysis

Diabetes patients undergoing dialysis due to diabetic nephropathy experience naturally improved glycemic control and normal-to-low HbA1c levels with the worsening of kidney function and decline in residual kidney function after starting renal replacement therapy, with or without antidiabetic agents. This phenomenon is called 'burnt-out diabetes' [27–29].

In a 2-year cohort study of 23,618 diabetes patients on HD in the United States, 33% of the patients had HbA1c < 6.0% [30]. When the HbA1c level of 5.0–5.9% was used as a reference, the survival rate was significantly lower both for the group with HbA1c of 7.0% or higher and with HbA1c < 5.0%. In a 6-year cohort study of 54,757 diabetes patients on dialysis in the United States, 40% of the patients had HbA1c of <6.0% [31]. When HbA1c levels of 7.0–7.9% were used as a reference, the hazard ratio (HR) for all-cause mortality increased with increasing HbA1c levels: 8.0–8.9% (HR 1.11), 9.0–9.9% (HR 1.36), and 10% or more (HR 1.59). Furthermore, the HR for all-cause mortality increased with decreasing HbA1c levels; 6.0–6.9% (1.05), 5.0–5.9% (HR 1.08), and <5.0% (HR 1.35). In the

Dialysis Outcomes and Practice Patterns Study (DOPPS), the survival was significantly lower in the HbA1c of ≥9.0%, <5.0%, 5–5.9%, and 6–6.9% groups when the HbA1c 7–7.9% group was used as a reference [32]. However, when analyzed according to the presence or absence of malnutrition, which was defined as BMI < 19 kg/m², serum albumin concentrations < 3.0 g/dL, or cachexia, the survival was significantly worse in patients with HbA1c < 5% and malnutrition. Therefore, it was suggested that the patients with lower HbA1c levels due to malnutrition might have poorer prognoses among patients with 'burnt-out diabetes'. As shown in Figure 5, there are several factors that induce 'burnt-out diabetes'.

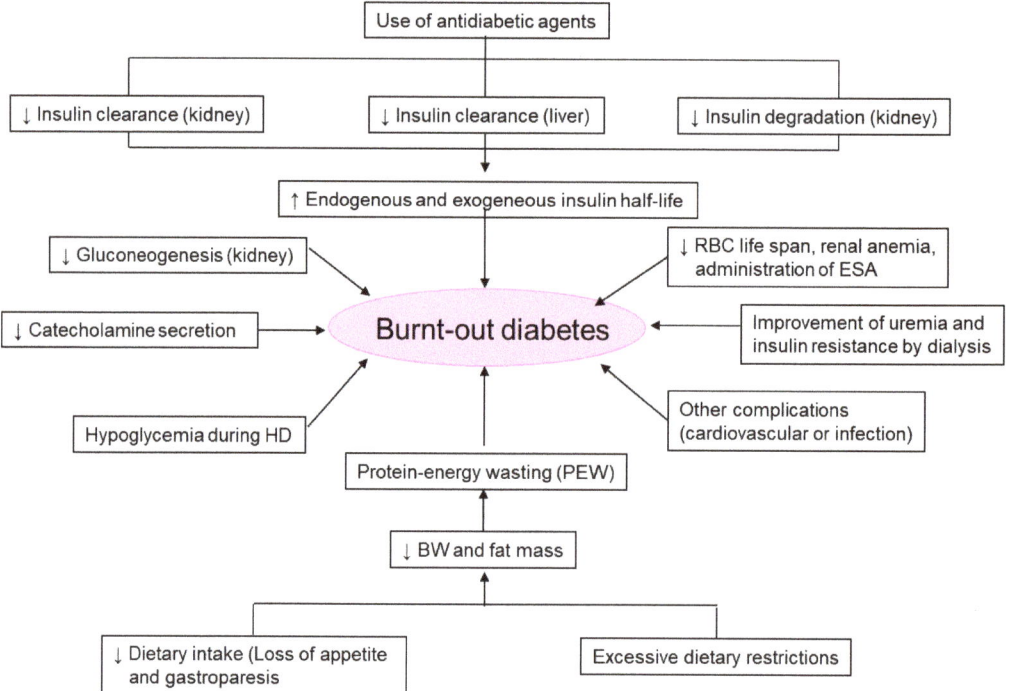

Figure 5. Leading factors of 'burnt-out diabetes'. BW, body weight; ESA, erythropoiesis stimulating agent; HD, hemodialysis; RBC, red blood cell.

In dialysis patients who have renal anemia and are treated with ESAs, HbA1c levels can be falsely lowered and, therefore, hyperglycemia overlooked. The two abovementioned cohort studies conducted in the United States measured only the HbA1c levels; GA and the use or non-use of antidiabetic agents were not investigated. Therefore, we conducted an investigation in order to confirm the 'true burnt-out diabetes' based on HbA1c, GA levels, and the use or non-use of antidiabetic agents according to the JRDR in 2013 [33]. When 'burnt-out diabetes' was defined as those who had HbA1c < 6.0% and were not treated with antidiabetic agents, it was found in 20.7% of HD patients. However, if we defined 'burnt-out diabetes' as HbA1c < 6.0%, GA < 16.0% (which was the normal value), and without antidiabetic medications, it was diagnosed in 5.4% of the patients. Therefore, the prognosis for patients with 'true burnt-out diabetes' must be confirmed in the future.

8. Continuous Glucose Monitoring in Patients on Dialysis

Continuous glucose monitoring (CGM) measures interstitial fluid glucose-levels, indirectly estimates plasma glucose concentrations, and provides estimates of average sensor glucose values, glucose excursions, and time in range [34–38]. Previous studies have suggested that high mean glucose levels and glycemic abnormalities such as glucose fluctuation and hypoglycemia accelerate the progression of atherosclerosis in patients with type 2 diabetes [39,40]. GA or HbA1c indicate only average plasma glucose levels and not fluctuations in plasma glucose levels or hypoglycemia, both of which may play an important role in the development of cardiovascular disease (CVD). However, CGM provides a subtle picture of daily blood-glucose fluctuations over 24 h. Therefore, evaluating various aspects of glycemic status may help identify patients with a high probability of developing CVD, and may lead to improving patients' outcomes. CGM is now frequently used to monitor glycemic control and contributes to improvements in glycemic control in patients with type 1 and type 2 diabetes who are not on dialysis [41–43].

Not all CGM devices are approved for use in dialysis patients, because their efficacy in dialysis patients has not yet been investigated (Table 1) [44–50]. However, many studies have reported that CGM is adaptable for glucose monitoring in patients on dialysis [51–53]. Nevertheless, whether the glycemic control of patients on dialysis can be improved by the use of CGM remains to be determined. Two reports suggested that CGM is useful for dialysis patients. The use of CGM to adjust the insulin dose significantly decreased sensor glucose levels at the 3-month follow-up [54]. Furthermore, a comparative study of blood-glucose monitoring by finger prick and CGM was performed on dialysis patients. Antidiabetic treatment was adjusted by the results of the blood-glucose monitoring by finger prick and CGM. The adjustment of diabetes medications together with use of CGM was associated with improvements in glycemic control but not in blood-glucose monitoring by finger prick [55]. It has been reported that plasma glucose concentrations in dialysis patients tend to be underestimated when inferred from HbA1c levels rather than CGM, GA, or fructosamine [56–58]. Furthermore, the results of the meta-analysis revealed that there was a significant correlation between CGM and the self-monitoring of blood-glucose levels [59]. Furthermore, CGM had similar correlations with HbA1c and GA values [59]. Although the question of whether CGM variables can predict late-onset diabetic complications remains to be established, CGM could play a useful role in modifying glycemic control in dialysis populations. The efficiency of CGM, which can optimize glucose levels by detecting and preventing hypoglycemia, is also worth investigating for patients on dialysis.

Table 1. Overview of CGM models.

	Eversense XL	Dexcom G6	Dexcom G6 Pro	FreeStyle Libre	FreeStyle Libre Pro	Freestyle Libre 2	Medtronic Guardian Connect
Approved for CKD (not on dialysis)	Yes	Yes	Yes	Yes	Yes	Yes	Yes
Approved for hemodialysis	Yes	No	No	Yes	Yes	No	Yes
Approved for peritoneal dialysis	Yes	No	No	Yes	Yes	No	Yes

CGM, continuous glucose monitoring; CKD, chronic kidney disease.

An international consensus report in 2019 provided the targets of 'time in range' for the general diabetes populations, such as those with type 1 and type 2 diabetes, and for high-risk populations, including the elderly [34]. Dialysis patients are included in this high-risk population. The guidelines recommend that dialysis patients should be within the target range (70–180 mg/dL) at least 50% of the time and below the range (<70 mg/dL) less than 1% of the time. However, this has not yet been fully evaluated in dialysis patients. The CGM goals for the high-risk group are focused on reducing the time spent below the target range even though they spend less time within the target range. Therefore, the average plasma glucose level is allowed to rise, and this guideline emphasizes the avoidance of hypoglycemia. However, it is unclear whether CGM can provide adequate glycemic control to prevent late-onset diabetic complications in dialysis patients. KDIGO highlights the unreliability of HbA1c in the dialysis population and recommends the use of CGM, especially for those treated with antidiabetic agents who are at high risk of hypoglycemia [60].

CGM may be an effective tool for detecting hypoglycemia, lowering overall blood glucose levels, and reducing daily fluctuation even in patients on dialysis. However, the effects of long-term CGM use in dialysis patients have not been fully evaluated, and further evaluations are required.

9. Peculiarities of Glycemic Control in Dialysis Patients

The disruption of blood glucose homeostasis occurs due to decreased renal function in dialysis patients. Dialysis patients have increased insulin resistance due to uremia, renal anemia, metabolic acidosis, and secondary hyperparathyroidism, and plasma glucose levels tend to increase. On the other hand, the kidney produces a large amount of gluconeogenesis secondary to the liver. Additionally, it also plays a role as an insulin clearance organ as well as the liver. Therefore, hypoglycemia is likely to occur due to reduced gluconeogenesis and insulin clearance in patients with impaired kidney function. Therefore, while dialysis patients have impaired glucose tolerance, they are simultaneously susceptible to hypoglycemia [61].

In addition, HD itself has a significant effect on plasma glucose levels. HD therapy often starts when plasma glucose levels rise after a meal. In Japan, many facilities use dialysate with a glucose concentration of 100 mg/dL, and plasma glucose is removed by diffusion via a dialyzer after the start of HD. In particular, a rapid drop in plasma glucose levels occurs in patients with higher plasma glucose levels before the start of HD. Therefore, when plasma glucose levels exceed 100 mg/dL during a HD session, plasma glucose is diffused from the plasma to the dialysate following the concentration gradient. Contrary to theory, the countercurrent transit of plasma through the dialyzer reduces glucose levels to less than 100 mg/dL at the post-dialyzer site in many patients [62]. This mechanism assumes that the plasma glucose is diffused into erythrocytes. Plasma glucose may be consumed within erythrocytes as a result of accelerated anaerobic metabolism, because the erythrocyte cytosolic pH changes during HD [63]. This phenomenon is thus called 'hemodialysis-induced hypoglycemia'.

On the other hand, insulin is adsorbed and removed by the dialyzer; therefore, the concentration of plasma insulin is decreased after HD [63–66]. A rapid drop in plasma glucose levels due to HD leads to stimulated secretion of counterregulatory hormones, such as glucagon, growth hormone, and adrenocorticotropic hormone. These factors lead to increased plasma glucose levels after HD. This phenomenon is called 'hemodialysis-associated hyperglycemia' [61,67–69]. It is difficult to estimate the changes in plasma glucose levels in HD patients, as the effect of factors vary depending on the individual case.

10. Medications for Glycemic Control in Diabetes Patients on Dialysis

Antidiabetic agents exert their pharmacological action and then disappear as they are metabolized and excreted. However, the metabolism and excretion of antidiabetic agents is impaired by deteriorated kidney function. In particular, agents whose active metabolites are excreted by the kidney have a significant effect, requiring dose reduction, careful administration, or are contraindicated. The "Best Practice for Diabetic Patients on Hemodialysis 2012" states that sulfonylureas (SU), biguanides, and thiazolidinediones are contraindicated in patients on dialysis [2]. The oral antidiabetic agents that can be administered to dialysis patients are α-glucosidase inhibitors (α-GI), dipeptidyl peptidase-4 (DPP-4) inhibitors, mitiglinide, and repaglinide (rapid-acting insulin secretagogues) [2,70]. The dose recommendations for antidiabetic agents other than insulin are shown in Table 2.

Table 2. Dose recommendation in diabetes patients on dialysis.

Classification	Drug	Regular Dose (mg/Day)	Optimal Dose for Dialysis Patients (mg/Day)
Sulfonylureas	Tolbutamide	250–2000	Contraindication
	Acetohexamide	250–1000	Contraindication
	Chlorpropamide	100–500	Contraindication
	Glyclopyramide	250–500	Contraindication
	Glibenclamide	1.25–10	Contraindication
	Glipizide [*1]	2.5–20	Regular dose
	Gliclazide	40–160	Regular dose [*2]
	Glimepiride	0.5–6	Contraindication
	Gliquidone [*1]	15–60	Regular dose
Fast-acting insulin secretagogues	Nateglinide	270–360	Contraindication
	Mitiglinide	15–30	Careful administration
	Repaglinide	0.75–3	Careful administration
Biguanides	Metformin	500–2250	Contraindication
	Buformin	50–150	Contraindication
Thiazolidinediones	Pioglitazone	15–45	Regular dose [*2]
α-Glucosidase inhibitors	Acarbose	150–300	Regular dose [*3]
	Voglibose	0.6–0.9	Regular dose
	Miglitol	150–225	Careful administration
DPP-4 inhibitors	Sitagliptin	50–100	12.5–25
	Vildagliptin	50–100	Careful administration
	Alogliptin	25	6.25
	Linagliptin	5	Regular dose
	Teneligliptin [*4]	20–40	Regular dose
	Anagliptin [*4]	200–400	100
	Saxagliptin	5	2.5
	Trelagliptin [*4]	100 mg once a week	25 mg once a week
	Omarigliptin [*4]	25 mg once a week	12.5 mg once a week
GLP-1 receptor agonist	Liraglutide	0.3–0.9	Careful administration
	Exenatide	10–20 μg	Contraindication
	Exenatide	2 mg once a week	Contraindication
	Lixisenatide	10–20 μg	Careful administration
	Dulaglutide	0.75 mg once a week	Regular dose
	Semaglutide	0.25–1.0 mg once a week	Regular dose
	Semaglutide (oral)	3–14 mg	Regular dose
SGLT2 inhibitor	Ipragliflozin [*4]	50–100	Avoid; not effective
	Dapagliflozin	5–10	Avoid; not effective
	Luseogliflozin [*4]	2.5–5	Avoid; not effective
	Tofogliflozin [*4]	20	Avoid; not effective
	Canagliflozin	100	Avoid; not effective
	Empagliflozin	10–25	Avoid; not effective

[*1] Not available in Japan. [*2] Not recommended in Japan for patients on dialysis. [*3] Not recommended in KDOQI guidelines for patients on dialysis. [*4] Not available in the United States.

10.1. SUs

It is not possible to remove all SUs by HD because of their high protein-binding rate. Although the key metabolic pathway is the liver, SU readily induces hypoglycemia, because active metabolites have hypoglycemic effects and accumulate in dialysis patients. Therefore, they are contraindicated in patients on dialysis in Japan. However, gliclazide is metabolized in the liver, and more than 99% of its metabolites are excreted via the kidneys and feces, approximately 70% and 20%, respectively. Furthermore, their metabolites have very low activity. Therefore, the Kidney Disease Outcomes Quality Initiative (KDOQI) guidelines state that gliclazide can be used even in patients on dialysis [71]. In addition, glipizide and gliquidone, which are not marketed in Japan, can be administered at regular doses to patients on dialysis, according to the European Best Practice Guidelines (ERBP) [72].

10.2. Biguanide

Biguanides are not metabolized and are primarily excreted unchanged by the kidneys, and they accumulate in patients with renal impairment. It is well known that the administration of biguanide to patients with renal dysfunction is likely to induce lactic acidosis. Therefore, biguanides are contraindicated in patients with severe renal impairment as well as dialysis patients [70,73].

10.3. Fast-Acting Insulin Secretagogues

Fast-acting insulin secretagogues stimulate insulin secretion via a mechanism similar to that for SUs. However, those effects have a faster onset of action than SUs, resulting in a rapid increase in plasma insulin levels and a shorter duration of hypoglycemic effects. The risk of hypoglycemia with fast-acting insulin secretagogues is less than that with SUs. Although there are three types of fast-acting insulin secretagogues, nateglinide, mitiglinide, and repaglinide, only nateglinide cannot be used for patients on dialysis. Because its metabolites have the effect of lowering plasma glucose levels and are excreted by the kidneys, the use of nateglinide in dialysis patients increases the risk of hypoglycemia [70]. Repaglinide is characterized by an excretion route via bile, and its metabolites have no effect on lowering plasma glucose levels. Therefore, repaglinide can be safely used even in patients on dialysis, but it is recommended that it be initiated at a low dose.

10.4. α-Glucosidase Inhibitors (α-GIs)

The use of α-GIs is rarely associated with hypoglycemia, and these agents are carefully administered to dialysis patients without dose adjustment in Japan [2,73]. However, the plasma concentrations of acarbose and miglitol may rise in patients with kidney dysfunction, and the accumulation of these agents may lead to liver failure. Therefore, the KDOQI guidelines recommend the avoidance of acarbose and miglitol in dialysis patients [71]. Moreover, caution is required with αGI administration because gastrointestinal symptoms such as flatulence, abdominal bloating, constipation, and diarrhea may occur.

10.5. Thiazolidinedione

In Japan, thiazolidinedione is contraindicated in diabetes patients with a history of cardiac failure and severe renal impairment [2,73]. Thiazolidinedione has an adverse effect on fluid retention and may induce edema, anemia, and cardiac failure. Therefore, it is also contraindicated in patients on dialysis in Japan. By contrast, thiazolidinediones are completely metabolized by the liver, and no dose adjustments are needed for patients on dialysis in other countries [71,72].

10.6. DPP-4 Inhibitors

DPP-4 inhibitors have a lower risk of hypoglycemia when administered alone, and because they are oral agents, the prescription rate has risen rapidly and had a great impact on diabetic treatment in recent years. Many investigations have reported on the efficacy and safety of DPP-4 inhibitors in patients on dialysis [73–75]. All currently marketed DPP-4 inhibitors are available for dialysis patients. However, dose adjustments must be made for the use of sitagliptin, saxagliptin, alogliptin, and anagliptin according to kidney function. On the other hand, linagliptin and teneligliptin can be administered without dose adjustment, even in patients on dialysis. Furthermore, the once-weekly DPP-4 inhibitors, omarigliptin and trelagliptin, are also available with dose adjustment for patients on dialysis [76,77]. However, further studies are needed to clarify the efficacy and safety of these agents, since few reports have investigated the efficacy and safety of once-weekly DPP-4 inhibitors for dialysis patients.

10.7. SGLT2 Inhibitors

Several large-scale clinical trials have demonstrated not only the hypoglycemic effect of SGLT2 inhibitors but also their effect in suppressing the progression of CKD and heart failure [78–83]. Therefore, it is now possible to administer them to CKD and heart-failure patients. However, they cannot be administered to dialysis patients because they cannot exert their hypoglycemic effect.

10.8. GLP-1 Receptor Agonists

Glucagon-like peptide-1 (GLP-1) receptor agonists are the same class as incretin-related drugs such as DPP-4 inhibitors but stronger hypoglycemic effects in addition to extra-pancreatic effects. The once-weekly agents, duraglutide and semaglutide, can be administered at their regular dose to dialysis patients [84,85]. On the other hand, liraglutide and lixisenatide can be used with careful administration [86–88]. Exenatide is contraindicated in patients on dialysis. The injection of once-weekly GLP-1 receptor agonists at a dialysis facility by medical staff is one of the therapeutic options.

10.9. Insulin Therapy

Although intensive insulin therapy helps achieve target glycemic control, it increases the risk of severe hypoglycemia in diabetes patients with normal kidney function. The dose of insulin is reduced as the kidney function declines [59,87–89]. The dose of insulin can be reduced by 25% relative to normal kidney function when GFR decreases to <50 mL/min/1.73 m^2. Furthermore, when GFR falls to <10 mL/min/1.73 m^2, the dose is reduced by 50% relative to normal kidney function [61,89–91]. The initiation of dialysis may improve peripheral insulin resistance, further reducing insulin requirements. Basal-supported oral therapy, which involves long-acting insulin with oral antidiabetic agents, may also be possible. Long-acting insulin can also be administered by medical staff on the day of HD for patients who have difficulty injecting themselves with insulin [92].

The advantage of insulin therapy is that it has no adverse effects, other than hypoglycemia, compared with oral antidiabetic agents, similar to those with normal kidney function. Furthermore, the incidence of prolonged hypoglycemia is also low. On the other hand, the disadvantage is that it is limited to patients who can self-manage and who can obtain the cooperation of family members to watch over and administer the injections on their behalf.

11. Dietary Recommendations

The nutritional management for diabetes patients on dialysis considers energy, protein, potassium, phosphate, salt, and vitamins [93,94], and there are few dietary guidelines specific to diabetes dialysis patients. Similar to the general diabetes population, the energy-intake requirements for dialysis patients vary by gender, age, and physical activity [95,96]. We must consider the ideal body mass index (BMI) of each patient. Considering the better outcomes observed for HD patients with a higher BMI, a BMI of at least >23.0 kg/m^2 should be maintained [93,94,97]. It was reported that the maintenance of BMI above the upper 50th percentile might be associated with a higher survival rate for patients on maintenance HD [98]. However, Japanese dialysis patients are aging, and the proportion of patients with protein energy wasting (PEW) and frailty is increasing. Although the mechanisms of PEW are complex and not fully understood, several studies reported that PEW is a major cause of morbidity and mortality in dialysis patients, and the prevalence of PEW was higher in diabetes patients than in non-diabetes patients on dialysis. Non-diabetes patients on dialysis [99–101]. The possible risk factors for PEW include increased nutrient loss, nutritional deficiencies, increased catabolism, and metabolic acidosis, which are shared by HD patients with and without diabetes. In dialysis patients with diabetes, increased muscle protein breakdown, increased complications, increased prevalence of gastroparesis, increased inflammatory cytokines, and impaired taste are additional risk factors that may be associated with the increased prevalence of PEW [102–106].

Some guidelines recommend a protein intake of at least 1.1 g/kg of ideal body weight (IBW) for HD patients [93–96]. In Japan, the "Best Practice for Diabetic Patients on Hemodialysis 2012" recommends a protein intake per reference body weight in the range of 0.9–1.2 g/kg/day. This target does not differentiate between diabetes and non-diabetes patients. In addition, it is recommended not to exceed 60 g/day for men and 50 g/day for women [2]. Fat intake in the range of 20–25% of total energy intake is recommended, and recommended intakes for salt, water, potassium, and phosphorus were the same as those for non-diabetes HD patients and were not differentiated [2]. The KDOQI guidelines recommend that the composition of the total energy intake should comprise 50–60% from carbohydrates, less than 30% from fat, and at least 15% from protein [94]. Therefore, protein intake in dialysis patients should correspond to 1.1 g protein/kg IBW and at least 15% of the total energy intake. However, it was suggested that the average protein intake in Japanese dialysis patients is below 0.9 g/kg/day [107]. Therefore, the assessment tool for nutritional status should be incorporated into daily clinical practice.

Previous studies did not evaluate which nutrients and nutritional products can improve plasma glucose levels and prognosis in diabetes patients on dialysis. In addition, the question of whether nutritional interventions can increase or maintain muscle mass in dialysis patients with diabetes was not investigated. Therefore, further studies are required to elucidate these points.

12. Conclusions

Levels of GA might be a better indicator of glycemic control than levels of HbA1c in patients on HD. Although a U-shaped relationship is observed between the HbA1c levels and mortality, GA is linearly associated with mortality in dialysis patients and may predict mortality in this population. Therefore, JSDT recommends GA as an alternative indicator of glycemic control to HbA1c for diabetes patients on HD. Because there have been no randomized controlled trials on dialysis patients, however, further studies are needed to clarify the target GA levels. Moreover, additional studies are warranted to clarify the superiority of periodic CGM to standard care in order to improve glycemic control, and CGMs can help to reduce hypoglycemic episodes and other diabetic complications in the dialysis population. Once-weekly DPP-4 inhibitors and some GLP-1 receptor agonists have been added as new treatment options. Additional research is required to clarify the efficacy and safety of these agents for diabetes patients on dialysis.

Funding: This research received no external funding.

Institutional Review Board Statement: Not applicable.

Informed Consent Statement: Not applicable.

Conflicts of Interest: The authors declare no conflict of interest.

References

1. Nitta, K.; Goto, S.; Masakane, I.; Hanafusa, N.; Taniguchi, M.; Hasegawa, T.; Nakai, S.; Wada, A.; Hamano, T.; Hoshino, J.; et al. Annual dialysis data report for 2018, JSDT Renal Data Registry: Survey methods, facility data, incidence, prevalence, and mortality. *Ren. Replace. Ther.* **2020**, *6*, 41. [CrossRef]
2. Nakao, T.; Inaba, M.; Abe, M.; Kaizu, K.; Shima, K.; Babazono, T.; Tomo, T.; Hirakata, H.; Akizawa, T.; Japanese Society for Dialysis Therapy. Best practice for diabetic patients on hemodialysis 2012. *Ther. Apher. Dial.* **2015**, *19* (Suppl. S1), 40–66. [CrossRef]
3. Inaba, M.; Okuno, S.; Kumeda, Y.; Yamada, S.; Imanishi, Y.; Tabata, T.; Okamura, M.; Okada, S.; Yamakawa, T.; Ishimura, E.; et al. Glycated albumin is a better glycemic indicator than glycated hemoglobin values in hemodialysis patients with diabetes: Effect of anemia and erythropoietin injection. *J. Am. Soc. Nephrol.* **2007**, *18*, 896–903. [CrossRef] [PubMed]
4. Abe, M.; Matsumoto, K. Glycated hemoglobin or glycated albumin for assessment of glycemic control in hemodialysis patients with diabetes? *Nat. Clin. Pract. Nephrol.* **2008**, *4*, 482–483. [CrossRef] [PubMed]
5. Peacock, T.P.; Shihabi, Z.K.; Bleyer, A.J.; Dolbare, E.L.; Byers, J.R.; Knovich, M.A.; Calles-Escandon, J.; Russell, G.B.; Freedman, B.I. Comparison of glycated albumin and hemoglobin A(1c) levels in diabetic subjects on hemodialysis. *Kidney Int.* **2008**, *73*, 1062–1068. [CrossRef] [PubMed]

6. Kohzuma, T.; Tao, X.; Koga, M. Glycated albumin as biomarker: Evidence and its outcomes. *J. Diabetes Complicat.* **2021**, *35*, 108040. [CrossRef] [PubMed]
7. Okada, T.; Nakao, T.; Matsumoto, H.; Shino, T.; Nagaoka, Y.; Tomaru, R.; Wada, T. Association between markers of glycemic control, cardiovascular complications and survival in type 2 diabetic patients with end-stage renal disease. *Intern. Med.* **2007**, *46*, 807–814. [CrossRef] [PubMed]
8. Fukuoka, K.; Nakao, K.; Morimoto, H.; Nakao, A.; Takatori, Y.; Arimoto, K.; Taki, M.; Wada, J.; Makino, H. Glycated albumin levels predict long-term survival in diabetic patients undergoing haemodialysis. *Nephrology* **2008**, *13*, 278–283. [CrossRef]
9. Inaba, M.; Maekawa, K.; Okuno, S.; Imanishi, Y.; Hayashino, Y.; Emoto, M.; Shoji, T.; Ishimura, E.; Yamakawa, T.; Nishizawa, Y. Impact of atherosclerosis on the relationship of glycemic control and mortality in diabetic patients on hemodialysis. *Clin. Nephrol.* **2012**, *78*, 273–280. [CrossRef]
10. Shafi, T.; Sozio, S.M.; Plantinga, L.C.; Jaar, B.G.; Kim, E.T.; Parekh, R.S.; Steffes, M.W.; Powe, N.R.; Coresh, J.; Selvin, E. Serum fructosamine and glycated albumin and risk of mortality and clinical outcomes in hemodialysis patients. *Diabetes Care* **2013**, *36*, 1522–1533. [CrossRef]
11. Freedman, B.I.; Andries, L.; Shihabi, Z.K.; Rocco, M.V.; Byers, J.R.; Cardona, C.Y.; Pickard, M.A.; Henderson, D.L.; Sadler, M.V.; Courchene, L.M.; et al. Glycated albumin and risk of death and hospitalizations in diabetic dialysis patients. *Clin. J. Am. Soc. Nephrol.* **2011**, *6*, 1635–1643. [CrossRef]
12. Murea, M.; Moran, T.; Russell, G.B.; Shihabi, Z.K.; Byers, J.R.; Andries, L.; Bleyer, A.J.; Freedman, B.I. Glycated albumin, not hemoglobin A1c, predicts cardiovascular hospitalization and length of stay in diabetic patients on dialysis. *Am. J. Nephrol.* **2012**, *36*, 488–496. [CrossRef] [PubMed]
13. Lu, C.L.; Ma, W.Y.; Lin, Y.F.; Shyu, J.F.; Wang, Y.H.; Liu, Y.M.; Wu, C.C.; Lu, K.C. Glycated Albumin Predicts Long-term Survival in Patients Undergoing Hemodialysis. *Int. J. Med. Sci.* **2016**, *13*, 395–402. [CrossRef] [PubMed]
14. Hoshino, J.; Hamano, T.; Abe, M.; Hasegawa, T.; Wada, A.; Ubara, Y.; Takaichi, K.; Inaba, M.; Nakai, S.; Masakane, I.; et al. Glycated albumin versus hemoglobin A1c and mortality in diabetic hemodialysis patients: A cohort study. *Nephrol. Dial. Transplant.* **2018**, *33*, 1150–1158. [CrossRef] [PubMed]
15. Hoshino, J.; Abe, M.; Hamano, T.; Hasegawa, T.; Wada, A.; Ubara, Y.; Takaichi, K.; Nakai, S.; Masakane, I.; Nitta, K. Glycated albumin and hemoglobin A1c levels and cause-specific mortality by patients' conditions among hemodialysis patients with diabetes: A 3-year nationwide cohort study. *BMJ Open Diabetes Res. Care* **2020**, *8*, e001642. [CrossRef]
16. Hanai, K.; Akamatsu, M.; Fujimori, A.; Higashi, H.; Horie, Y.; Itaya, Y.; Ito, M.; Kanamaru, T.; Kawaguchi, H.; Kikuchi, K.; et al. Usefulness of glycated albumin as a predictor of mortality in chronic hemodialysis patients with diabetes: A multi-center, prospective cohort study. *Ren. Replace. Ther.* **2020**, *6*, 17. [CrossRef]
17. Gan, T.; Liu, X.; Xu, G. Glycated Albumin Versus HbA1c in the Evaluation of Glycemic Control in Patients With Diabetes and CKD. *Kidney Int. Rep.* **2017**, *3*, 542–554. [CrossRef]
18. Copur, S.; Siriopol, D.; Afsar, B.; Comert, M.C.; Uzunkopru, G.; Sag, A.A.; Ortiz, A.; Covic, A.; van Raalte, D.H.; Cherney, D.Z.; et al. Serum glycated albumin predicts all-cause mortality in dialysis patients with diabetes mellitus: Meta-analysis and systematic review of a predictive biomarker. *Acta. Diabetol.* **2021**, *58*, 81–91. [CrossRef]
19. Masakane, I.; Nakai, S.; Ogata, S.; Kimata, N.; Hanafusa, N.; Hamano, T.; Wakai, K.; Wada, A.; Nitta, K. An Overview of Regular Dialysis Treatment in Japan (As of 31 December 2013). *Ther. Apher. Dial.* **2015**, *19*, 540–574. [CrossRef]
20. Nitta, K.; Abe, M.; Masakane, I.; Hanafusa, N.; Taniguchi, M.; Hasegawa, T.; Nakai, S.; Wada, A.; Hamano, T.; Hoshino, J.; et al. Annual dialysis data report 2018, JSDT Renal Data Registry: Dialysis fluid quality, hemodialysis and hemodiafiltration, peritoneal dialysis, and diabetes. *Ren. Replace. Ther.* **2020**, *6*, 51. [CrossRef]
21. Miyabe, M.; Kurajoh, M.; Mori, K.; Okuno, S.; Okada, S.; Emoto, M.; Tsujimoto, Y.; Inaba, M. Superiority of glycated albumin over glycated haemoglobin as indicator of glycaemic control and predictor of all-cause mortality in patients with type 2 diabetes mellitus receiving peritoneal dialysis. *Ann. Clin. Biochem.* **2019**, *56*, 684–691. [CrossRef] [PubMed]
22. Abe, M.; Hamano, T.; Hoshino, J.; Wada, A.; Nakai, S.; Masakane, I. Glycemic control and survival in peritoneal dialysis patients with diabetes: A 2-year nationwide cohort study. *Sci. Rep.* **2019**, *9*, 3320. [CrossRef] [PubMed]
23. Koga, M.; Murai, J.; Saito, H.; Matsumoto, S.; Kasayama, S. Effects of thyroid hormone on serum glycated albumin levels: Study on non-diabetic subjects. *Diabetes Res. Clin. Pract.* **2009**, *84*, 163–167. [CrossRef]
24. Koga, M.; Kasayama, S.; Kanehara, H.; Bando, Y. CLD (chronic liver disease)-HbA1c as a suitable indicator for estimation of mean plasma glucose in patients with chronic liver diseases. *Diabetes Res. Clin. Pract.* **2008**, *81*, 258–262. [CrossRef] [PubMed]
25. Okada, T.; Nakao, T.; Matsumoto, H.; Nagaoka, Y.; Tomaru, R.; Iwasawa, H.; Wada, T. Influence of proteinuria on glycated albumin values in diabetic patients with chronic kidney disease. *Intern. Med.* **2011**, *50*, 23–29. [CrossRef]
26. Freedman, B.I.; Shenoy, R.N.; Planer, J.A.; Clay, K.D.; Shihabi, Z.K.; Burkart, J.M.; Cardona, C.Y.; Andries, L.; Peacock, T.P.; Sabio, H.; et al. Comparison of glycated albumin and hemoglobin A1c concentrations in diabetic subjects on peritoneal and hemodialysis. *Perit. Dial. Int.* **2010**, *30*, 72–79. [CrossRef] [PubMed]
27. Kalantar-Zadeh, K.; Derose, S.F.; Nicholas, S.; Benner, D.; Sharma, K.; Kovesdy, C.P. Burnt-out diabetes: Impact of chronic kidney disease progression on the natural course of diabetes mellitus. *J. Ren. Nutr.* **2009**, *19*, 33–37. [CrossRef] [PubMed]
28. Kovesdy, C.P.; Park, J.C.; Kalantar-Zadeh, K. Glycemic control and burnt-out diabetes in ESRD. *Semin. Dial.* **2010**, *23*, 148–156. [CrossRef]

29. Park, J.; Lertdumrongluk, P.; Molnar, M.Z.; Kovesdy, C.P.; Kalantar-Zadeh, K. Glycemic control in diabetic dialysis patients and the burnt-out diabetes phenomenon. *Curr. Diab. Rep.* **2012**, *12*, 432–439. [CrossRef]
30. Kalantar-Zadeh, K.; Kopple, J.D.; Regidor, D.L.; Jing, J.; Shinaberger, C.S.; Aronovitz, J.; McAllister, C.J.; Whellan, D.; Sharma, K. A1C and survival in maintenance hemodialysis patients. *Diabetes Care* **2007**, *30*, 1049–1055. [CrossRef]
31. Rhee, C.M.; Leung, A.M.; Kovesdy, C.P.; Lynch, K.E.; Brent, G.A.; Kalantar-Zadeh, K. Updates on the management of diabetes in dialysis patients. *Semin. Dial.* **2014**, *27*, 135–145. [CrossRef]
32. Ramirez, S.P.; McCullough, K.P.; Thumma, J.R.; Nelson, R.G.; Morgenstern, H.; Gillespie, B.W.; Inaba, M.; Jacobson, S.H.; Vanholder, R.; Pisoni, R.L.; et al. Hemoglobin A(1c) levels and mortality in the diabetic hemodialysis population: Findings from the Dialysis Outcomes and Practice Patterns Study (DOPPS). *Diabetes Care* **2012**, *35*, 2527–2532. [CrossRef]
33. Abe, M.; Hamano, T.; Hoshino, J.; Wada, A.; Inaba, M.; Nakai, S.; Masakane, I. Is there a "burnt-out diabetes" phenomenon in patients on hemodialysis? *Diabetes Res. Clin. Pract.* **2017**, *130*, 211–220. [CrossRef]
34. Battelino, T.; Danne, T.; Bergenstal, R.M.; Amiel, S.A.; Beck, R.; Biester, T.; Bosi, E.; Buckingham, B.A.; Cefalu, W.T.; Close, K.L.; et al. Clinical Targets for Continuous Glucose Monitoring Data Interpretation: Recommendations From the International Consensus on Time in Range. *Diabetes Care* **2019**, *42*, 1593–1603. [CrossRef]
35. Freckmann, G.; Pleus, S.; Grady, M.; Setford, S.; Levy, B. Measures of Accuracy for Continuous Glucose Monitoring and Blood Glucose Monitoring Devices. *J. Diabetes. Sci. Technol.* **2019**, *13*, 575–583. [CrossRef] [PubMed]
36. Elbalshy, M.; Haszard, J.; Smith, H.; Kuroko, S.; Galland, B.; Oliver, N.; Shah, V.; de Bock, M.I.; Wheeler, B.J. Effect of divergent continuous glucose monitoring technologies on glycaemic control in type 1 diabetes mellitus: A systematic review and meta-analysis of randomised controlled trials. *Diabet. Med.* **2022**, *39*, e14854. [CrossRef]
37. Gordon, I.; Rutherford, C.; Makarounas-Kirchmann, K.; Kirchmann, M. Meta-analysis of average change in laboratory-measured HbA1c among people with type 1 diabetes mellitus using the 14 day flash glucose monitoring system. *Diabetes Res. Clin. Pract.* **2020**, *164*, 108158. [CrossRef]
38. Bianchi, C.; Aragona, M.; Rodia, C.; Baronti, W.; de Gennaro, G.; Bertolotto, A.; Del Prato, S. Freestyle Libre trend arrows for the management of adults with insulin-treated diabetes: A practical approach. *J. Diabetes Complicat.* **2019**, *33*, 6–12. [CrossRef]
39. Gerbaud, E.; Darier, R.; Montaudon, M.; Beauvieux, M.C.; Coffin-Boutreux, C.; Coste, P.; Douard, H.; Ouattara, A.; Catargi, B. Glycemic variability is a powerful independent predictive factor of midterm major adverse cardiac events in patients with diabetes with acute coronary syndrome. *Diabetes Care* **2019**, *42*, 674–681. [CrossRef]
40. Su, G.; Mi, S.H.; Tao, H.; Li, Z.; Yang, H.X.; Zheng, H.; Zhou, Y.; Tian, L. Impact of admission glycemic variability, glucose, and glycosylated hemoglobin on major adverse cardiac events after acute myocardial infarction. *Diabetes Care* **2013**, *36*, 1026–1032. [CrossRef]
41. Aleppo, G.; Ruedy, K.J.; Riddlesworth, T.D.; Kruger, D.F.; Peters, A.L.; Hirsch, I.; Bergenstal, R.M.; Toschi, E.; Ahmann, A.J.; Shah, V.N.; et al. REPLACE-BG: A Randomized Trial Comparing Continuous Glucose Monitoring With and Without Routine Blood Glucose Monitoring in Adults With Well-Controlled Type 1 Diabetes. *Diabetes Care* **2017**, *40*, 538–545. [CrossRef] [PubMed]
42. Martens, T.; Beck, R.W.; Bailey, R.; Ruedy, K.J.; Calhoun, P.; Peters, A.L.; Pop-Busui, R.; Philis-Tsimikas, A.; Bao, S.; Umpierrez, G.; et al. Effect of Continuous Glucose Monitoring on Glycemic Control in Patients With Type 2 Diabetes Treated With Basal Insulin: A Randomized Clinical Trial. *JAMA* **2021**, *325*, 2262–2272. [CrossRef]
43. Karter, A.J.; Parker, M.M.; Moffet, H.H.; Gilliam, L.K.; Dlott, R. Association of Real-time Continuous Glucose Monitoring With Glycemic Control and Acute Metabolic Events Among Patients With Insulin-Treated Diabetes. *JAMA* **2021**, *325*, 2273–2284. [CrossRef] [PubMed]
44. Eversense, X.L. User Guide [Internet]. Available online: https://global.eversensediabetes.com/sites/default/files/2021-11/LBL-1402-31-001_Rev_E_Eversense_User_Guide_mgdL_UK-ENG.pdf (accessed on 8 August 2022).
45. Dexcom. Dexcom G6 Continuous Glucose Monitoring System. User Guide [Internet]. Available online: https://s3-us-west-2.amazonaws.com/dexcompdf/G6-CGM-Users-Guide.pdf#page=21 (accessed on 8 August 2022).
46. Dexcom. Dexcom G6 Pro Continuous Glucose Monitoring System. User Guide [Internet]. Available online: https://www.dexcom.com/faq/what-dexcom-g6-pro-continuous-glucose-monitoring-cgm-system (accessed on 8 August 2022).
47. Abbott. FreeStyle Libre 14 Day System. Available online: https://www.freestyleprovider.abbott/us-en/freestyle-libre-14-day-system.html (accessed on 8 August 2022).
48. Abbott. FreeStyle Libre Pro Flash Glucose Monitoring System [Internet]. Available online: https://www.freestyle.abbott/in-en/products/freestyle-libre-pro.html (accessed on 8 August 2022).
49. Abbott. FreeStyle Libre 2 System IN-SERVICE GUIDE [Internet]. Available online: https://provider.myfreestyle.com/pdf/In-Service-FreeStyle-Libre-2-HCP-Sales.pdf (accessed on 8 August 2022).
50. Medtronic. Guardian Connect System. User Guide [Internet]. Available online: https://www.medtronicdiabetes.com/download-library/guardian-connect (accessed on 8 August 2022).
51. Mambelli, E.; Cristino, S.; Mosconi, G.; Göbl, C.; Tura, A. Flash Glucose Monitoring to Assess Glycemic Control and Variability in Hemodialysis Patients: The GIOTTO Study. *Front. Med.* **2021**, *8*, 617891. [CrossRef]
52. Toyoda, M.; Murata, T.; Saito, N.; Kimura, M.; Takahashi, H.; Ishida, N.; Kitamura, M.; Hida, M.; Hayashi, A.; Moriguchi, I.; et al. Assessment of the accuracy of an intermittent-scanning continuous glucose monitoring device in patients with type 2 diabetes mellitus undergoing hemodialysis (AIDT2H) study. *Ther. Apher. Dial.* **2021**, *25*, 586–594. [CrossRef] [PubMed]

53. Narasaki, Y.; Park, E.; You, A.S.; Daza, A.; Peralta, R.A.; Guerrero, Y.; Novoa, A.; Amin, A.N.; Nguyen, D.V.; Price, D.; et al. Continuous glucose monitoring in an end-stage renal disease patient with diabetes receiving hemodialysis. *Semin. Dial.* **2021**, *34*, 388–393. [CrossRef]
54. Képénékian, L.; Smagala, A.; Meyer, L.; Imhoff, O.; Alenabi, F.; Serb, L.; Fleury, D.; Dorey, F.; Krummel, T.; Le Floch, J.P.; et al. Continuous glucose monitoring in hemodialyzedpatients with type 2 diabetes: A multicenter pilot study. *Clin. Nephrol.* **2014**, *82*, 240–246. [CrossRef] [PubMed]
55. Joubert, M.; Fourmy, C.; Henri, P.; Ficheux, M.; Lobbedez, T.; Reznik, Y. Effectiveness of continuous glucose monitoring in dialysis patients with diabetes: The DIALYDIAB pilot study. *Diabetes Res. Clin. Pract.* **2015**, *107*, 348–354. [CrossRef]
56. Bomholt, T.; Kofod, D.; Nørgaard, K.; Rossing, P.; Feldt-Rasmussen, B.; Hornum, M. Can the Use of Continuous Glucose Monitoring Improve Glycemic Control in Patients with Type 1 and 2 Diabetes Receiving Dialysis? *Nephron* **2022**, *13*, 1–6. [CrossRef]
57. Hayashi, A.; Takano, K.; Masaki, T.; Yoshino, S.; Ogawa, A.; Shichiri, M. Distinct biomarker roles for HbA1c and glycated albumin in patients with type 2 diabetes on hemodialysis. *J. Diabetes Complicat.* **2016**, *30*, 1494–1499. [CrossRef]
58. Bomholt, T.; Feldt-Rasmussen, B.; Butt, R.; Borg, R.; Sarwary, M.H.; Elung-Jensen, T.; Almdal, T.; Knop, F.K.; Nørgaard, K.; Ranjan, A.G.; et al. Hemoglobin A1c and Fructosamine Evaluated in Patients with Type 2 Diabetes Receiving Peritoneal Dialysis Using Long-Term Continuous Glucose Monitoring. *Nephron* **2022**, *146*, 146–152. [CrossRef] [PubMed]
59. Wang, F.; Wang, D.; Lyu, X.L.; Sun, X.M.; Duan, B.H. Continuous glucose monitoring in diabetes patients with chronic kidney disease on dialysis: A meta-analysis. *Minerva Endocrinol.* **2022**, *47*, 325–333. [CrossRef] [PubMed]
60. Kidney Disease: Improving Global Outcomes (KDIGO) Diabetes Work Group. KDIGO 2020 Clinical Practice Guideline for Diabetes Management in Chronic Kidney Disease. *Kidney Int.* **2020**, *98*, S1–S115. [CrossRef] [PubMed]
61. Abe, M.; Kalantar-Zadeh, K. Haemodialysis-induced hypoglycaemia and glycaemic disarrays. *Nat. Rev. Nephrol.* **2015**, *11*, 302–313. [CrossRef] [PubMed]
62. Abe, M.; Kaizu, K.; Matsumoto, K. Plasma insulin is removed by hemodialysis: Evaluation of the relation between plasma insulin and glucose by using a dialysate with or without glucose. *Ther. Apher. Dial.* **2007**, *11*, 280–287. [CrossRef] [PubMed]
63. Takahashi, A.; Kubota, T.; Shibahara, N.; Terasaki, J.; Kagitani, M.; Ueda, H.; Inoue, T.; Katsuoka, Y. The mechanism of hypoglycemia caused by hemodialysis. *Clin. Nephrol.* **2004**, *62*, 362–368. [CrossRef] [PubMed]
64. Abe, M.; Kikuchi, F.; Kaizu, K.; Matsumoto, K. The influence of hemodialysis membranes on the plasma insulin level of diabetic patients on maintenance hemodialysis. *Clin. Nephrol.* **2008**, *69*, 354–360. [CrossRef] [PubMed]
65. Abe, M.; Okada, K.; Matsumoto, K. Plasma insulin and C-peptide concentrations in diabetic patients undergoing hemodialysis: Comparison with five types of high-flux dialyzer membranes. *Diabetes Res. Clin. Pract.* **2008**, *82*, e17–e19. [CrossRef] [PubMed]
66. Abe, M.; Okada, K.; Ikeda, K.; Matsumoto, S.; Soma, M.; Matsumoto, K. Characterization of insulin adsorption behavior of dialyzer membranes used in hemodialysis. *Artif. Organs.* **2011**, *35*, 398–403. [CrossRef] [PubMed]
67. Abe, M.; Kaizu, K.; Matsumoto, K. Evaluation of the hemodialysis-induced changes in plasma glucose and insulin concentrations in diabetic patients: Comparison between the hemodialysis and non-hemodialysis days. *Ther. Apher. Dial.* **2007**, *11*, 288–295. [CrossRef]
68. Hayashi, A.; Shimizu, N.; Suzuki, A.; Matoba, K.; Momozono, A.; Masaki, T.; Ogawa, A.; Moriguchi, I.; Takano, K.; Kobayashi, N.; et al. Hemodialysis-Related Glycemic Disarray Proven by Continuous Glucose Monitoring; Glycemic Markers and Hypoglycemia. *Diabetes Care* **2021**, *44*, 1647–1656. [CrossRef] [PubMed]
69. Mori, K.; Emoto, M.; Abe, M.; Inaba, M. Visualization of Blood Glucose Fluctuations Using Continuous Glucose Monitoring in Patients Undergoing Hemodialysis. *J. Diabetes. Sci. Technol.* **2019**, *13*, 413–414. [CrossRef] [PubMed]
70. Abe, M.; Okada, K.; Soma, M. Antidiabetic agents in patients with chronic kidney disease and end-stage renal disease on dialysis: Metabolism and clinical practice. *Curr. Drug Metab.* **2011**, *12*, 57–69. [CrossRef] [PubMed]
71. Kidney Disease Outcomes Quality Initiative (KDOQI). KDOQI Clinical Practice Guidelines and Clinical Practice Recommendations for Diabetes and Chronic Kidney Disease. *Am. J. Kidney Dis.* **2007**, *49*, S62–S73.
72. Guideline Development Group. Clinical Practice Guideline on management of patients with diabetes and chronic kidney disease stage 3b or higher (eGFR < 45 mL/min). *Nephrol. Dial. Transplant.* **2015**, *30* (Suppl. S2), ii1–ii142.
73. Maruyama, N.; Abe, M. Targets and Therapeutics for Glycemic Control in Diabetes Patients on Hemodialysis. *Contrib. Nephrol.* **2018**, *196*, 37–43.
74. Abe, M.; Okada, K. DPP-4 Inhibitors in Diabetic Patients with Chronic Kidney Disease and End-Stage Kidney Disease on Dialysis in Clinical Practice. *Contrib. Nephrol.* **2015**, *185*, 98–115.
75. Park, S.H.; Nam, J.Y.; Han, E.; Lee, Y.H.; Lee, B.W.; Kim, B.S.; Cha, B.S.; Kim, C.S.; Kang, E.S. Efficacy of different dipeptidyl peptidase-4 (DPP-4) inhibitors on metabolic parameters in patients with type 2 diabetes undergoing dialysis. *Medicine* **2016**, *95*, e4543. [CrossRef]
76. Chacra, A.; Gantz, I.; Mendizabal, G.; Durlach, L.; O'Neill, E.A.; Zimmer, Z.; Suryawanshi, S.; Engel, S.S.; Lai, E. A randomised, double-blind, trial of the safety and efficacy of omarigliptin (a once-weekly DPP-4 inhibitor) in subjects with type 2 diabetes and renal impairment. *Int. J. Clin. Pract.* **2017**, *71*, e12955. [CrossRef]
77. Kaku, K.; Ishida, K.; Shimizu, K.; Achira, M.; Umeda, Y. Efficacy and safety of trelagliptin in Japanese patients with type 2 diabetes with severe renal impairment or end-stage renal disease: Results from a randomized, phase 3 study. *J. Diabetes Investig.* **2020**, *11*, 373–381. [CrossRef]

78. Wanner, C.; Inzucchi, S.E.; Lachin, J.M.; Fitchett, D.; von Eynatten, M.; Mattheus, M.; Johansen, O.E.; Woerle, H.J.; Broedl, U.C.; Zinman, B.; et al. Empagliflozin and Progression of Kidney Disease in Type 2 Diabetes. *N. Engl. J. Med.* **2016**, *375*, 323–334. [CrossRef] [PubMed]
79. Packer, M.; Anker, S.D.; Butler, J.; Filippatos, G.; Ferreira, J.P.; Pocock, S.J.; Carson, P.; Anand, I.; Doehner, W.; Haass, M.; et al. Effect of Empagliflozin on the Clinical Stability of Patients With Heart Failure and a Reduced Ejection Fraction: The EMPEROR-Reduced Trial. *Circulation* **2021**, *143*, 326–336. [CrossRef] [PubMed]
80. Neal, B.; Perkovic, V.; Mahaffey, K.W.; de Zeeuw, D.; Fulcher, G.; Erondu, N.; Shaw, W.; Law, G.; Desai, M.; Matthews, D.R.; et al. Canagliflozin and Cardiovascular and Renal Events in Type 2 Diabetes. *N. Engl. J. Med.* **2017**, *377*, 644–657. [CrossRef] [PubMed]
81. Perkovic, V.; Jardine, M.J.; Neal, B.; Bompoint, S.; Heerspink, H.J.L.; Charytan, D.M.; Edwards, R.; Agarwal, R.; Bakris, G.; Bull, S.; et al. Canagliflozin and Renal Outcomes in Type 2 Diabetes and Nephropathy. *N. Engl. J. Med.* **2019**, *380*, 2295–2306. [CrossRef]
82. Heerspink, H.J.L.; Stefánsson, B.V.; Correa-Rotter, R.; Chertow, G.M.; Greene, T.; Hou, F.F.; Mann, J.F.E.; McMurray, J.J.V.; Lindberg, M.; Rossing, P.; et al. Dapagliflozin in Patients with Chronic Kidney Disease. *N. Engl. J. Med.* **2020**, *383*, 1436–1446. [CrossRef]
83. McMurray, J.J.V.; Solomon, S.D.; Inzucchi, S.E.; Køber, L.; Kosiborod, M.N.; Martinez, F.A.; Ponikowski, P.; Sabatine, M.S.; Anand, I.S.; Bělohlávek, J.; et al. Dapagliflozin in Patients with Heart Failure and Reduced Ejection Fraction. *N. Engl. J. Med.* **2019**, *381*, 1995–2008. [CrossRef]
84. Granhall, C.; Søndergaard, F.L.; Thomsen, M.; Anderson, T.W. Pharmacokinetics, Safety and Tolerability of Oral Semaglutide in Subjects with Renal Impairment. *Clin. Pharmacokinet.* **2018**, *57*, 1571–1580. [CrossRef]
85. Yajima, T.; Yajima, K.; Hayashi, M.; Takahashi, H.; Yasuda, K. Improved glycemic control with once-weekly dulaglutide in addition to insulin therapy in type 2 diabetes mellitus patients on hemodialysis evaluated by continuous glucose monitoring. *J. Diabetes Complicat.* **2018**, *32*, 310–315. [CrossRef]
86. Bomholt, T.; Idorn, T.; Knop, F.K.; Jørgensen, M.B.; Ranjan, A.G.; Resuli, M.; Hansen, P.M.; Borg, R.; Persson, F.; Feldt-Rasmussen, B.; et al. The Glycemic Effect of Liraglutide Evaluated by Continuous Glucose Monitoring in Persons with Type 2 Diabetes Receiving Dialysis. *Nephron* **2021**, *145*, 27–34. [CrossRef]
87. Idorn, T.; Knop, F.K.; Jørgensen, M.B.; Jensen, T.; Resuli, M.; Hansen, P.M.; Christensen, K.B.; Holst, J.J.; Hornum, M.; Feldt-Rasmussen, B. Safety and Efficacy of Liraglutide in Patients With Type 2 Diabetes and End-Stage Renal Disease: An Investigator-Initiated, Placebo-Controlled, Double-Blind, Parallel-Group, Randomized Trial. *Diabetes Care* **2016**, *39*, 206–213. [CrossRef]
88. Fonseca, V.A.; Alvarado-Ruiz, R.; Raccah, D.; Boka, G.; Miossec, P.; Gerich, J.E.; EFC6018 GetGoal-Mono Study Investigators. Efficacy and safety of the once-daily GLP-1 receptor agonist lixisenatide in monotherapy: A randomized, double-blind, placebo-controlled trial in patients with type 2 diabetes (GetGoal-Mono). *Diabetes Care* **2012**, *35*, 1225–1231. [CrossRef] [PubMed]
89. Snyder, R.W.; Berns, J.S. Use of insulin and oral hypoglycemic medications in patients with diabetes mellitus and advanced kidney disease. *Semin. Dial.* **2004**, *17*, 365–370. [CrossRef] [PubMed]
90. Charpentier, G.; Riveline, J.P.; Varroud-Vial, M. Management of drugs affecting blood glucose in diabetic patients with renal failure. *Diabetes. Metab.* **2000**, *26*, 73–85. [PubMed]
91. Reilly, J.B.; Berns, J.S. Selection and dosing of medications for management of diabetes in patients with advanced kidney disease. *Semin. Dial.* **2010**, *23*, 163–168. [CrossRef] [PubMed]
92. Shoji, T.; Emoto, M.; Mori, K.; Morioka, T.; Fukumoto, S.; Takahashi, T.; Matsumoto, A.; Nishizawa, Y.; Inaba, M. Thrice-weekly insulin injection with nurse's support for diabetic hemodialysis patients having difficulty with self injection. *Osaka City Med. J.* **2012**, *58*, 35–38.
93. Fouque, D.; Vennegoor, M.; ter Wee, P.; Wanner, C.; Basci, A.; Canaud, B.; Haage, P.; Konner, K.; Kooman, J.; Martin-Malo, A.; et al. European Best Practice Guideline on nutrition. *Nephrol. Dial. Transplant.* **2007**, *22* (Suppl. S2), ii45–ii87. [CrossRef]
94. National Kidney Foundation. Clinical practice guidelines for nutrition in chronic renal failure. *Am. J. Kidney. Dis.* **2000**, *35*, S17–S104.
95. UK Renal Association. Nutrition in Chronic Kidney Disease Clinical Practice Guidelines. 2009–2010. Available online: https://ukkidney.org/sites/renal.org/files/nutrition-in-ckd-5th-edition-1.pdf (accessed on 8 August 2022).
96. Naylor, H.L.; Jackson, H.; Walker, G.H.; Macafee, S.; Magee, K.; Hooper, L.; Stewart, L.; MacLaughlin, H.L.; Renal Nutrition Group of the British Dietetic Association; British Dietetic Association. British Dietetic Association Renal Nutrition Group Evidence Based Dietetic Guidelines Protein Requirements Of Adults On Haemodialysis And Peritoneal Dialysis. *J. Hum. Nutr. Diet.* **2013**, *26*, 315–328. [CrossRef]
97. Leavey, S.F.; McCullough, K.; Hecking, E.; Goodkin, D.; Port, F.K.; Young, E.W. Body mass index and mortality in 'healthier' as compared with 'sicker' haemodialysis patients: Results from the Dialysis Outcomes and Practice Patterns Study (DOPPS). *Nephrol. Dial. Transplant.* **2001**, *16*, 2386–2394. [CrossRef]
98. Fissell, R.B.; Bragg-Gresham, J.L.; Gillespie, B.W.; Goodkin, D.A.; Bommer, J.; Saito, A.; Akiba, T.; Port, F.K.; Young, E.W. International variations in vitamin prescription and association with mortality in the Dialysis Outcomes and Practice Patterns Study (DOPPS). *Am. J. Kidney. Dis.* **2004**, *44*, 293–299. [CrossRef]
99. Kalantar-Zadeh, K.; Block, G.; McAllister, C.J.; Humphreys, M.H.; Kopple, J.D. Appetite and inflammation, nutrition, anemia, and clinical outcome in hemodialysis patients. *Am. J. Clin. Nutr.* **2004**, *80*, 299–307. [CrossRef] [PubMed]
100. Pupim, L.B.; Heimburger, O.; Qureshi, A.R. Accelerated lean body mass loss in incident chronic dialysis patients with diabetes mellitus. *Kidney Int.* **2005**, *68*, 2638–2674. [CrossRef]

101. Cano, N.J.; Roth, H.; Aparicio, M.; Azar, R.; Canaud, B.; Chauveau, P.; Combe, C.; Fouque, D.; Laville, M.; Leverve, X.M.; et al. Malnutrition in haemodialysis diabetic patients:evaluation and prognostic influence. *Kidney Int.* **2002**, *62*, 593–601. [CrossRef]
102. Fouque, D.; Kalantar-Zadeh, K.; Kopple, J.; Cano, N.; Chauveau, P.; Cuppari, L.; Franch, H.; Guarnieri, G.; Ikizler, T.A.; Kaysen, G.; et al. A proposed nomenclature and diagnostic criteria for protein-energy wasting in acute and chronic kidney disease. *Kidney Int.* **2008**, *73*, 391–398. [CrossRef]
103. Pupim, L.B.; Flakoll, P.J.; Majchrzak, K.M.; Aftab Guy, D.L.; Stenvinkel, P.; Ikizler, T.A. Increased muscle protein breakdown in chronic haemodialysis patient with type 2 diabetes mellitus. *Kidney Int.* **2005**, *68*, 1857–1865. [CrossRef] [PubMed]
104. Noori, N.; Kopple, J.D. Effect of diabetes mellitus on protein-energy wasting and protein wasting in end-stage renal disease. *Semin. Dial.* **2010**, *23*, 178–184. [CrossRef]
105. Kopple, J.D. Pathophysiology of protein-energy wasting in chronic renal failure. *J. Nutr.* **1999**, *129*, 2475–2515. [CrossRef] [PubMed]
106. Matsuo, S.; Nakamoto, M.; Nishihara, G.; Yasunaga, C.; Yanagida, T.; Matsuo, K.; Sakemi, T. Impaired taste acuity in patients with diabetes on maintenance haemodialysis. *Nephron Clin. Pract.* **2003**, *94*, 46–50. [CrossRef]
107. Masakane, I.; Taniguchi, M.; Nakai, S.; Tsuchida, K.; Goto, S.; Wada, A.; Ogata, S.; Hasegawa, T.; Hamano, T.; Hanafusa, N.; et al. Annual Dialysis Data Report 2015, JSDT Renal Data Registry. *Ren. Replace. Ther.* **2018**, *4*, 19. [CrossRef]

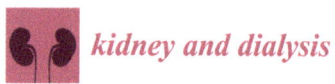 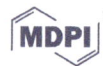

Perspective

Non-Ischemic Myocardial Fibrosis in End-Stage Kidney Disease Patients: A New Perspective

Kenji Nakata and Nobuhiko Joki *

Department of Nephrology, Toho University Ohashi Medical Center, Tokyo 153-8515, Japan
* Correspondence: jokinobuhiko@gmail.com; Tel.: +81-3-3468-1251; Fax: +81-3-5433-3067

Abstract: Cardiovascular medicine, especially for ischemic heart disease, has evolved and advanced over the past two decades, leading to substantially improved outcomes for patients, even those with chronic kidney disease. However, the prognosis for patients with end-stage kidney disease (ESKD) has not improved so greatly. Recent studies have reported that myocardial fibrosis in chronic kidney disease patients is characterized by patchy and interstitial patterns. Areas of fibrosis have been located in the perivascular space, and severe fibrotic lesions appear to spread into myocardial fiber bundles in the form of pericellular fibrosis. These findings are fully consistent with known characteristics of reactive fibrosis. In hemodialysis patients, a greater extent of myocardial fibrosis is closely associated with a poorer prognosis. In this review, we focus on non-ischemic cardiomyopathy, especially reactive myocardial fibrosis, in ESKD patients.

Keywords: reactive fibrosis; type 2 myocardial infarction; biomarker

Citation: Nakata, K.; Joki, N. Non-Ischemic Myocardial Fibrosis in End-Stage Kidney Disease Patients: A New Perspective. *Kidney Dial.* 2023, 3, 311–321. https://doi.org/10.3390/kidneydial3030027

Academic Editors: Ken Tsuchiya, Norio Hanafusa and Vladimir Tesar

Received: 5 April 2023
Revised: 22 July 2023
Accepted: 31 August 2023
Published: 6 September 2023

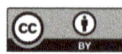

Copyright: © 2023 by the authors. Licensee MDPI, Basel, Switzerland. This article is an open access article distributed under the terms and conditions of the Creative Commons Attribution (CC BY) license (https://creativecommons.org/licenses/by/4.0/).

1. Introduction

About 20 years have passed since chronic kidney disease (CKD) was first recognized as a contributor to atherosclerotic cardiovascular disease [1,2]. This condition is considered to correspond to group 4 in the CRS classification [3]. The pathogenesis of CRS4 has been predominantly explained by narrowing of the artery and tissue ischemia due to atherosclerosis, as typically seen in coronary artery disease. Cardiovascular medicine, especially for atherosclerosis, has evolved and improved over the past two decades, even for patients with CKD, however its effect is limited. The short-term prognosis after myocardial infarction in CKD patients has improved, however long-term prognosis has not yet improved [4].

The pathophysiology may change as CKD progresses. In CKD 1–3, about 60% of myocardial infarctions are ST-segment elevation myocardial infarction, whereas in CKD 5, about 60% are non-ST-segment elevation myocardial infarction [5]. This implies that in advanced CKD, myocardial injury due to non-atherosclerotic conditions may occur. It is well known that lipid-lowering therapies appear much less effective in patients with advanced stages of CKD, including end-stage kidney disease (ESKD) [6–8], compared with early-stage CKD patients. On the other hand, vascular dysfunction such as arterial distensibility and stiffness is present in the early stage of CKD, and plays an important mediator in the chronic impairment of cardiac function [9]. It has been reported that left ventricular remodeling occurs with the progression of CKD and is often complicated by cardiac hypertrophy [10,11]. It has also been reported that fibrosis of the myocardium appears early in the course of CKD [12,13]. To establish a better prognosis for CKD patients, we must first understand the mechanism and pathophysiology of non-ischemic cardiomyopathy in CKD. In this review, we focus on non-ischemic cardiomyopathy, especially cardiac fibrosis, in end-stage kidney disease (ESKD) patients.

2. Myocardial Fibrosis in CKD

Research into non-atherosclerotic pathology has focused on myocardial fibrosis. Aoki et al. performed a coronary angiography on 40 maintenance hemodialysis patients with left ventricular systolic dysfunction (ejection fraction <50%) and dilated cardiomyopathy. They checked for the absence of significant coronary artery narrowing lesions, and then carried out myocardial biopsies for the purpose of histological study [14]. Fifty patients with dilated cardiomyopathy who were not on dialysis were enrolled as controls. The area of fibrosis in cardiomyocyte cells was found to be 22% in both groups. However, severe fibrosis, defined as an area of 45% or more, was often observed in the dialysis patients compared with the controls. Areas of fibrosis of 30% or more were associated with significantly poorer prognoses in the dialysis group, but not in the control group. Histologically, cardiac fibrosis is broadly categorized into two types: replacement fibrosis and reactive fibrosis, also known as diffuse myocardial fibrosis because of its manifestation as a diffuse and excessive deposition of extracellular matrix components in interstitial and perivascular areas (Figure 1).

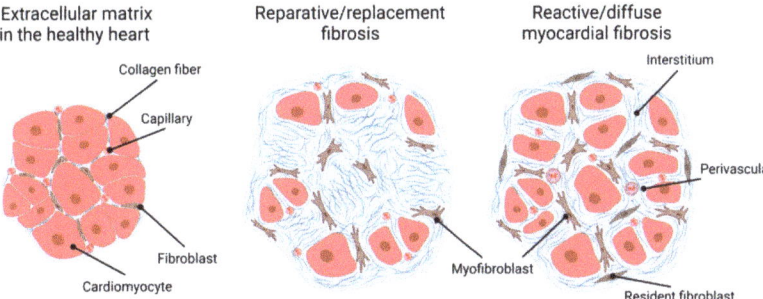

Figure 1. Types of cardiac fibrosis [15]. The extracellular matrix in the healthy heart (**left**) is a three-dimensional network of collagen fibers that embeds cardiac cells such as cardiomyocytes, capillaries, and fibroblasts. "Replacement/reparative fibrosis" (**middle**) is visible as a collagen-based scar that is formed during a healing process and replaces dying cardiomyocytes after ischemic insults. "Reactive/diffuse myocardial fibrosis" (**right**) manifests as diffuse deposition of cross-linked collagens in interstitial and perivascular areas.

Replacement fibrosis is the result of a healing process after acute myocardial infarction, or the result of cardiomyocyte death brought about by other causes. It is visible as a fibrotic scar triggered by ischemic cell death. Reactive fibrosis is caused by the diffuse deposition and cross-linking of collagens in interstitial and perivascular areas that occur in chronic cardiac conditions [15–17]. Researchers have considered non-ischemic myocardial fibrosis as expressing the pathological pattern of reactive fibrosis, and it has been observed in hypertensive cardiomyopathy [18], diabetic cardiomyopathy [19], aortic valve stenosis [20], and hypertrophic cardiomyopathy [21].

Diabetic kidney disease is the greatest cause of dialysis-dependent ESKD [22,23]. In addition, CKD patients often exhibit left ventricular hypertrophy [24], which may be due to compensatory mechanisms of pressure overload [25]. The process of CKD progression is now thought to be part of the progression process of reactive cardiac fibrosis. One review article concerning cardiovascular disease clearly states that the myocardial fibrosis in patients with CKD is characterized by patchy fibrosis [26], which is consistent with known characteristics of reactive fibrosis. Izumaru et al. conducted a histological study of 334 autopsy cases [27] to evaluate the myocardial cell width and areas of myocardial fibrosis according to the GFR. As the GFR decreases, both the myocardial wall thickness and myocyte width increase. This phenomenon persists even after an adjustment for confounding factors such as age, sex, hypertension, and diabetes mellitus. Similarly, the area of myocardial fibrosis increases from 3.22% to 6.14% as the GFR declines from >60 to <30 mL/min/1.73 m^2. The fibrosis itself exhibits patchy and interstitial patterns, and areas of fibrosis are found mainly in the perivascular space. In addition, some severe fibrotic lesions appear to spread into myocardial fiber bundles in the form of pericellular fibrosis (Figure 2). These findings are fully consistent with reactive fibrosis development. Even after adjustment for confounding factors such as hypertension and diabetes, fibrosis exhibits a tendency to increase as eGFR declines. Additionally, a uremic milieu may also be considered an important pathological condition that may contribute to reactive fibrosis development. Renal anemia, iron deficiency [28], and hyperphosphatemia [29] all may play some role in increasing the area of myocardial fibrosis with decreasing levels of eGFR.

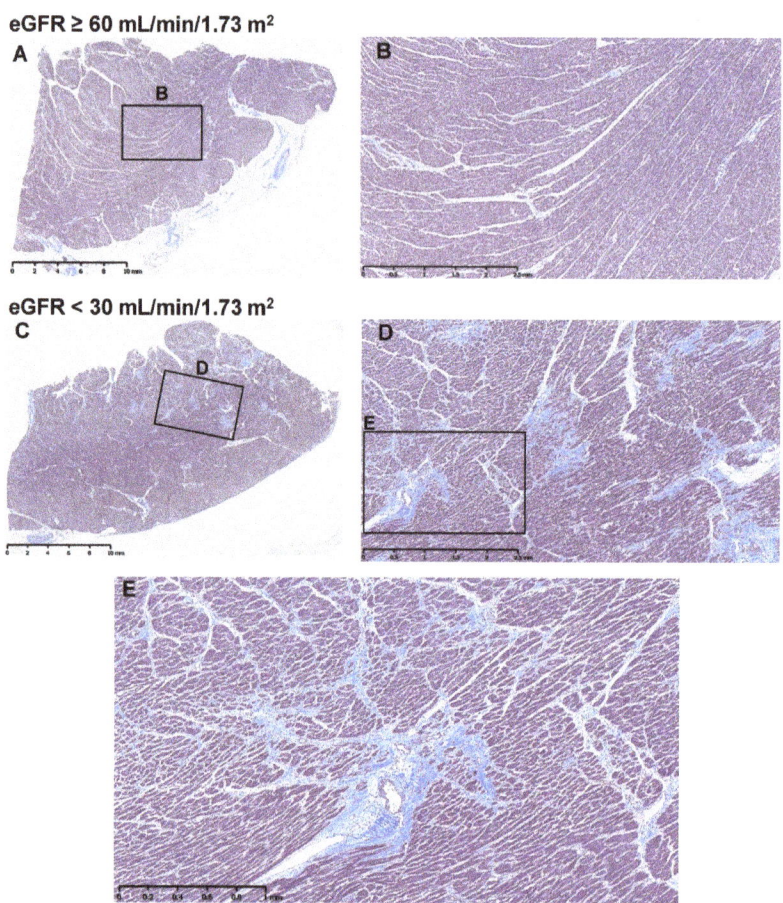

Figure 2. Myocardial tissues in samples with estimated glomerular filtration rates (eGFRs) ≥60 and <30 mL/min/1.73 m² (Masson trichrome staining). Reproduced with permission from Izumaru et al., [27], approved by Elsevier. (**A,C**) Light microscopic views of myocardial tissues in samples with eGFRs (**A**) ≥60 and (**C**) <30 mL/min/1.73 m². (**B,D**) Corresponding lesions from the boxed areas indicated in (**A,C**), respectively. (**E**) Corresponding lesion from the boxed area indicated in (**D**), which shows the pattern of patchy and interstitial fibrosis. The area of fibrosis was found mainly in the perivascular space.

3. Mechanism of Reactive Myocardial Interstitial Fibrosis

Fibrosis is an essential process in the repair of damaged tissue and wounds. In general, fibrosis occurs when there is an imbalance between collagen synthesis and degradation irrespective of tissue repair. Some pathological factors promote synthesis more than degradation of collagen, resulting in an accumulation of collagenous tissue and leading to organ dysfunction. In pathologically, fibrosis is the excessive deposition of extracellular matrix (ECM), such as collagens and fibronectin [30]. For this process, myofibroblast-mediated fibrosis in the myocardium is the hallmark of pathophysiological cardiac fibrosis and remodeling [31]. A common feature of cardiac fibrotic diseases is the activation of fibroblasts and their differentiation into myofibroblasts, which express and secrete much higher levels of ECM proteins. Myofibroblasts are not usually present in healthy cardiac tissue, with the exception of heart valve leaflets. However, the transition from fibroblasts to myofibroblasts can be induced by changes in the physical environmental condition of the body. Among them, three factors, mechanical stress, inflammation, cytokines, and growth factors are particularly closely related to the pathogenesis of chronic kidney disease [31].

Pressure loading of the heart, as in aortic valve stenosis and systemic hypertension, is known to increase wall stress and promote reactive fibrosis in the left ventricle chamber. A gradient of fibrosis extends from the endocardial to the epicardial surface. This reflects the gradient in chamber wall stress that results from the increased pressure load. Fibroblasts can also become activated by mechanical stress. This phenomenon can be explained by the fact that fibroblasts sense mechanical forces through mechanosensitive receptors, such as integrins, ion channels, G-protein coupled receptors, and growth factor receptors [15], and activate downstream pathways that promote matrix transcription. As we are well aware, the frequency of hypertension in patients with chronic kidney disease increases with advanced stages and is more frequent in patients with end-stage kidney disease. Another mechanical force for the left ventricle is volume overload, and it is often seen in ESKD patients. In patients with severe aortic regurgitation, a model of left ventricular volume overload, fibrotic remodeling has been extensively documented [32]. However, in contrast to pressure loading, the network of molecular cascades activated by volume overload-induced mechanical stress for cardiac fibrosis has not been characterized [31].

It is well known that the activity of the renin–angiotensin–aldosterone system and sympathetic nervous system activity are increased in patients with chronic kidney disease. These two neurohormonal factors are representative factors that activate fibroblasts and induce differentiation into myofibroblasts [33,34]. Furthermore, diseases or conditions that trigger inflammatory responses, either systemically or locally, can also cause reactive fibrosis to develop. These include obesity, diabetes, metabolic syndrome, infections of the heart, drugs, and radiation. Depending on the stimulus, reactive fibrosis can develop in a relatively homogeneous pattern throughout the myocardium (interstitial fibrosis), or it may be more prominent in the tissue surrounding intracardiac blood vessels (perivascular fibrosis) [35].

4. Detection of Myocardial Fibrosis in a Clinical Setting

The best means for properly evaluating myocardial fibrosis is a histological approach. Myocardial biopsy is a highly invasive method that requires hospitalization. Recently, Holmstrom et al. carried out a unique histological study that evaluated the severity of non-ischemic myocardial fibrosis by using heart samples of 1100 autopsies [36]. To achieve noninvasive detection of moderate or severe fibrosis, they sought an association between the severity of non-ischemic cardiac fibrosis and the findings from resting 12-lead electrocardiograms. They considered that QRS widths greater than 100 ms were associated with advanced myocardial fibrosis. Also, negative T waves on aVR becoming shallower and closer to flat were potential candidates for more volume of myocardial fibrosis. They found that T wave depressions of -0.1 mV or less in aVR were associated with advanced myocardial fibrosis. There is no further evidence of a link between aVR-T wave changes and myocardial fibrosis, which may limit its use in clinical practice. However, it is of interest that two Japanese cohort studies previously confirmed that the flat or elevation of a T wave on aVR is closely associated with prognosis in dialysis patients [37,38]. In particular, Sato et al. classified patients into four groups according to the T wave of aVR, as shown in Figure 3, and verified the association with prognosis. It can be confirmed that the prognosis is worse in the group with shallower negative T waves [38].

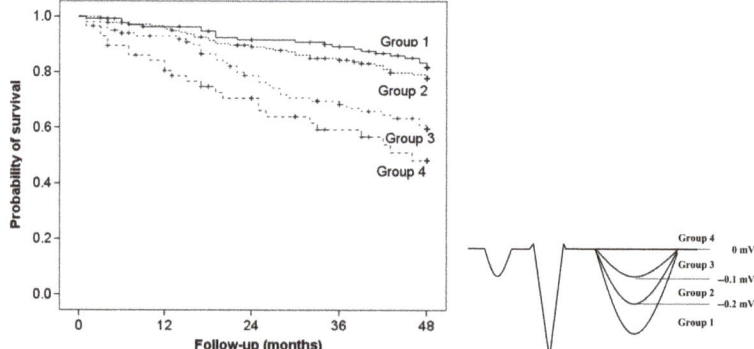

Figure 3. Schematic presentation of T-wave amplitude of lead aVR (aVRT)-based groupings. Patients were divided into four groups according to aVRT amplitude as follows: Group 1, aVRT < −0.2 mV; Group 2, −0.2 ≤ aVRT < −0.1 mV; Group 3, −0.1 ≤ aVRT < 0 mV; and Group 4, aVRT ≥ 0 mV. Composite cardiovascular disease (CVD) events-free survival curves according to T-wave amplitude of lead aVR (aVRT) based grouping. (p < 0.001, by log-rank test). Ref. [38], approved by Wiley.

Two representative cardiac biomarkers, BNP and troponin T, already used in routine practice have been suggested to be indicators of myocardial fibrosis in CKD patients. Marker of increased LV wall stress, NT-pro BNP, and of myocardial injury, hs-cTnT, were independently associated with native T1, which is evaluated by cardiovascular magnetic resonance and marker for myocardial fibrosis [39]. With regard to possible biomarkers for myocardial fibrosis, two collagen precursors, carboxy-terminal propeptide of procollagen type I and amino-terminal pro-peptide of pro-collagen type III (PIIINP), have been found to correlate with the levels of collagen deposition in dilated cardiomyopathy and in ischemic or hypertensive heart disease [40,41]. Nishimura et al. proposed a cut-off value for PIIINP for cardiovascular events in hemodialysis patients [42]. The cardiovascular-event-free survival rates at five years were lower in patients with serum PIIINP ≥1.75 U/mL, compared with those with that <1.75 U/mL (31.9% vs. 88.2%) (Figure 4). Although it is still unclear whether PIIINP levels are histologically associated with the prevalence of myocardial fibrosis in hemodialysis patients, serum PIIINP might yet be a new biomarker for predicting cardiovascular events in patients undergoing hemodialysis.

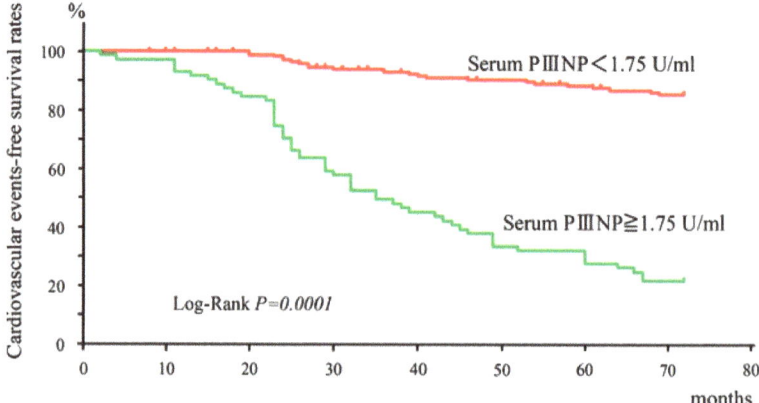

Figure 4. Kaplan–Meier analysis of cardiovascular-event-free survival rates for two levels of serum PIIINP concentration (1.75 U/mL) [42]. The cardiovascular-event-free survival rates at 5 years were lower in patients with serum PIIINP ≥1.75 U/mL than in those with <1.75 U/mL (31.9% vs. 88.2%).

The gold standard for the recognition and quantification of cardiac fibrosis is cardiac magnetic resonance using gadolinium-based contrast agents [43]. Gadolinium does not cross the membranes of intact cardiomyocyte cells but is distributed in the extracellular space [44]. A higher distribution volume and slower washout in cases of myocardial scarring or edema results in a hyperintense area in late post-contrast phases when compared to the iso-hypointense normal myocardium [45,46]. By means of such an observation, late gadolinium enhancement can enable the detection of myocardial fibrosis. The association between myocardial fibrosis as measured by LGE and the findings of histological assessments is well-established, showing high sensitivity and specificity [47,48]. However, the use of gadolinium is contraindicated in renal dysfunction patients with GFR levels below 15, including patients on maintenance dialysis, due to concerns about nephrogenic systemic fibrosis. Therefore, a method that does not use gadolinium is required. To this end, the T1 mapping method represents a promising candidate [49,50]. T1 measures the longitudinal relaxation time, which is a specific time constant depending on the tissue composition. Myocardial T1 mapping is a purely parametric technique that physically measures the absolute values of T1 rather than relative differences in signal intensity. Measurements may be taken before (native T1) or after gadolinium administration. Native T1 mapping has been reported as useful in detecting myocardial fibrosis in dialysis patients [51,52].

5. Potential Means of Preventing Cardiac Fibrosis

One potential method for retarding the progression of cardiac fibrosis involves interfering with the renin–angiotensin–aldosterone axis. Patients with hypertensive heart disease who were treated using the angiotensin-converting enzyme inhibitor lisinopril [53] exhibited a reduction in the extent of fibrotic deposits, as evaluated by endomyocardial biopsy, as well as an improvement in LV diastolic dysfunction and reduction in LV stiffness. Similar treatment with the angiotensin receptor blocker losartan led to almost identical results [54]. These findings imply that blocking the renin–angiotensin–aldosterone system, along with appropriate control of blood pressure, may be important for the prevention of reactive cardiac fibrosis in cases of hypertensive cardiomyopathy. Myocardial biopsy assessments of heart failure patients have also revealed that the mineralocorticoid receptor antagonist spironolactone reduces areas of myocardial fibrosis [55]. The effect of inhibiting the renin–angiotensin–aldosterone system on prognosis in end-stage renal disease patients is still controversial, with some studies reporting clinical benefit [56], while others report no such benefit [57]. However, a meta-analysis does suggest that aldosterone antagonists reduce the risk of death and morbidity due to cardiovascular and cerebrovascular disease in CKD patients requiring dialysis [58].

In a recent large phase 3 clinical study for patients with heart failure reduced ejection fraction (HFrEF), the risk of hospitalization for heart failure or death from cardiovascular causes was lower among those who received the sodium-glucose cotransporter 2 (SGLT2) inhibitor than among those who received the placebo, regardless of the presence or absence of diabetes [59,60]. It is very interesting that the sub-analysis confirms a significant reduction in the primary endpoint in the SGLT2 inhibitor group, regardless of whether the cardiomyopathy is ischemic or non-ischemic. Furthermore, similar effects have been observed in large clinical trials in heart failure preserved ejection fraction (HFpEF) [61,62]. This suggests that SGLT2 inhibitors may have an inhibitory effect on myocardial fibrosis. It has been shown that the SGLT2 inhibitor empagliflozin reduces myocardial interstitial fibrosis and is linked to improved diastolic dysfunction in diabetic mice [63].

Another possible means to reduce myocardial fibrosis is the loop diuretic torasemide. A study of patients with chronic heart failure suggest that torasemide might inhibit the progression of myocardial fibrosis as an additional benefit to patients receiving standard therapy with RAS-system inhibitors for heart failure [64]. This positive finding has not been reported for furosemide, the most popular loop diuretic in clinical settings. This may be a direct effect of torasemide itself rather than any effect of reduced volume overload in the left ventricle. Lopez et al. found that the activation of the enzyme procollagen type

I carboxy-terminal proteinase (PCP), which catalyzes the extracellular conversion of the precursor procollagen type I into the fibril-forming molecule collagen type I, abnormally increased in the myocardium of heart failure patients [65]. Such activation decreased in torasemide-treated patients and remained unchanged in furosemide-treated patients [65]. Studies of the myocardium in rats found that torasemide, but not furosemide, reduced the expression of aldosterone synthase and transforming growth factor-beta1, both of which can activate PCP in fibrogenic cells [66,67]. A recently published study compared the effects of torasemide and furosemide in patients with diabetes-mellitus-associated heart failure with preserved ejection fraction using changes in the serum levels of C-terminal propeptide of procollagen type I as a biomarker of myocardial fibrosis. No differences in biomarker changes were found between the two treatment groups [68]. The potential use of diuretics in maintenance dialysis patients may be limited; however, torasemide might be a potential treatment option for ESKD patients not on dialysis with volume overload [69]. Further study is needed to confirm the effect of torasemide on cardiac fibrosis in ESKD patients. Experimental studies indicate that several additional antifibrotic therapeutic interventions, including inhibition of fibrosis-promoting inflammatory cytokines such as IL-1 [70], anti-TGF-β approaches [71], and ECM cross-linking enzyme inhibition strategies [72]. Unfortunately, it is undeniable that it will take a long time for these treatments to become available for use in clinical practice.

6. Future Directions

To improve the cardiac prognosis of ESKD patients, it is essential to act to prevent myocardial fibrosis or clinically termed HFpEF. However, there are two reasons why their management is very difficult in a clinical setting. One is that there are no laboratory tests, such as blood tests or imaging tests, that can accurately determine the degree of myocardial fibrosis precisely. This means that even if preventive strategies are taken, there is no way to determine their efficacy.

Second, there is still no effective therapy that can retard already advanced myocardial fibrosis. It has been reported that patients with ESKD already have suffered from advanced myocardial fibrosis. This means that it is not possible to regress myocardial fibrosis in patients with ESKD, nor is it expected to improve their prognosis. What can be done today is to first identify the clinical risk factors for myocardial fibrosis. Then, it is suggested that the only preventive approach is to reduce the progression of myocardial fibrosis by strictly correcting these factors. It is important to take these preventive approaches early in the course of CKD.

7. Summary

During the course of CKD development, accelerated progression of myocardial fibrosis is caused by well-known factors such as hypertension, diabetes, dyslipidemia, and fluid overload, as well as lesser-known factors associated with the uremic milieu. Diagnostic and therapeutic strategies for reactive myocardial fibrosis are still not established. Because gadolinium is not appropriate for patients with end-stage renal disease, novel diagnostic methods, including biomarkers, are needed. Renin–angiotensin-system inhibitors, SGLT2 inhibitors, and torasemide are candidates for the treatment of myocardial fibrosis, however there is not enough evidence to show that each treatment is effective for myocardial fibrosis in patients with ESKD. To ensure a comprehensive approach to the prevention and management of nonatherosclerotic cardiovascular disease in ESKD patients, multidisciplinary care and collaboration among nephrologists, cardiologists, and other health care providers is necessary.

Author Contributions: Original draft preparation, K.N. and N.J.; writing, N.J. All authors have read and agreed to the published version of the manuscript.

Funding: This research received no external funding.

Institutional Review Board Statement: Not applicable.

Informed Consent Statement: Not applicable.

Data Availability Statement: No new data were created or analyzed in this study. Data sharing is not applicable to this article.

Conflicts of Interest: The authors declare no conflict of interest.

References

1. Sarnak, M.J.; Levey, A.S.; Schoolwerth, A.C.; Coresh, J.; Culleton, B.; Hamm, L.L.; McCullough, P.A.; Kasiske, B.L.; Kelepouris, E.; Klag, M.J.; et al. Kidney disease as a risk factor for development of cardiovascular disease: A statement from the American Heart Association Councils on Kidney in Cardiovascular Disease, High Blood Pressure Research, Clinical Cardiology, and Epidemiology and Prevention. *Circulation* **2003**, *108*, 2154–2169. [CrossRef]
2. Ronco, C.; McCullough, P.; Anker, S.D.; Anand, I.; Aspromonte, N.; Bagshaw, S.M.; Bellomo, R.; Berl, T.; Bobek, I.; Cruz, D.N.; et al. Cardio-renal syndromes: Report from the consensus conference of the acute dialysis quality initiative. *Eur. Heart J.* **2010**, *31*, 703–711. [CrossRef]
3. Rangaswami, J.; Bhalla, V.; Blair, J.E.A.; Chang, T.I.; Costa, S.; Lentine, K.L.; Lerma, E.V.; Mezue, K.; Molitch, M.; Mullens, W.; et al. Cardiorenal Syndrome: Classification, Pathophysiology, Diagnosis, and Treatment Strategies: A Scientific Statement from the American Heart Association. *Circulation* **2019**, *139*, e840–e878. [CrossRef]
4. Nauta, S.T.; van Domburg, R.T.; Nuis, R.J.; Akkerhuis, M.; Deckers, J.W. Decline in 20-year mortality after myocardial infarction in patients with chronic kidney disease: Evolution from the prethrombolysis to the percutaneous coronary intervention era. *Kidney Int.* **2013**, *84*, 353–358. [CrossRef]
5. Bae, E.H.; Lim, S.Y.; Cho, K.H.; Choi, J.S.; Kim, C.S.; Park, J.W.; Ma, S.K.; Jeong, M.H.; Kim, S.W. GFR and cardiovascular outcomes after acute myocardial infarction: Results from the Korea Acute Myocardial Infarction Registry. *Am. J. Kidney Dis.* **2012**, *59*, 795–802. [CrossRef]
6. Massy, Z.A.; de Zeeuw, D. LDL cholesterol in CKD—To treat or not to treat? *Kidney Int.* **2013**, *84*, 451–456. [CrossRef]
7. Wanner, C.; Krane, V.; Marz, W.; Olschewski, M.; Mann, J.F.; Ruf, G.; Ritz, E. Atorvastatin in patients with type 2 diabetes mellitus undergoing hemodialysis. *N. Engl. J. Med.* **2005**, *353*, 238–248. [CrossRef]
8. Fellstrom, B.C.; Jardine, A.G.; Schmieder, R.E.; Holdaas, H.; Bannister, K.; Beutler, J.; Chae, D.W.; Chevaile, A.; Cobbe, S.M.; Gronhagen-Riska, C.; et al. Rosuvastatin and cardiovascular events in patients undergoing hemodialysis. *N. Engl. J. Med.* **2009**, *360*, 1395–1407. [CrossRef]
9. Zanoli, L.; Lentini, P.; Briet, M.; Castellino, P.; House, A.A.; London, G.M.; Malatino, L.; McCullough, P.A.; Mikhailidis, D.P.; Boutouyrie, P. Arterial Stiffness in the Heart Disease of CKD. *J. Am. Soc. Nephrol.* **2019**, *30*, 918–928. [CrossRef]
10. London, G.M. Cardiovascular disease in chronic renal failure: Pathophysiologic aspects. *Semin. Dial.* **2003**, *16*, 85–94. [CrossRef]
11. London, G.M. Left ventricular alterations and end-stage renal disease. *Nephrol. Dial. Transpl.* **2002**, *17* (Suppl. S1), 29–36. [CrossRef] [PubMed]
12. Hayer, M.K.; Price, A.M.; Liu, B.; Baig, S.; Ferro, C.J.; Townend, J.N.; Steeds, R.P.; Edwards, N.C. Diffuse Myocardial Interstitial Fibrosis and Dysfunction in Early Chronic Kidney Disease. *Am. J. Cardiol.* **2018**, *121*, 656–660. [CrossRef]
13. Edwards, N.C.; Moody, W.E.; Yuan, M.; Hayer, M.K.; Ferro, C.J.; Townend, J.N.; Steeds, R.P. Diffuse interstitial fibrosis and myocardial dysfunction in early chronic kidney disease. *Am. J. Cardiol.* **2015**, *115*, 1311–1317. [CrossRef] [PubMed]
14. Aoki, J.; Ikari, Y.; Nakajima, H.; Mori, M.; Sugimoto, T.; Hatori, M.; Tanimoto, S.; Amiya, E.; Hara, K. Clinical and pathologic characteristics of dilated cardiomyopathy in hemodialysis patients. *Kidney Int.* **2005**, *67*, 333–340. [CrossRef] [PubMed]
15. Schimmel, K.; Ichimura, K.; Reddy, S.; Haddad, F.; Spiekerkoetter, E. Cardiac Fibrosis in the Pressure Overloaded Left and Right Ventricle as a Therapeutic Target. *Front. Cardiovasc. Med.* **2022**, *9*, 886553. [CrossRef]
16. Frangogiannis, N.G.; Kovacic, J.C. Extracellular Matrix in Ischemic Heart Disease, Part 4/4: JACC Focus Seminar. *J. Am. Coll. Cardiol.* **2020**, *75*, 2219–2235. [CrossRef] [PubMed]
17. Diez, J.; Gonzalez, A.; Kovacic, J.C. Myocardial Interstitial Fibrosis in Nonischemic Heart Disease, Part 3/4: JACC Focus Seminar. *J. Am. Coll. Cardiol.* **2020**, *75*, 2204–2218. [CrossRef] [PubMed]
18. van Hoeven, K.H.; Factor, S.M. A comparison of the pathological spectrum of hypertensive, diabetic, and hypertensive-diabetic heart disease. *Circulation* **1990**, *82*, 848–855. [CrossRef] [PubMed]
19. Shimizu, M.; Umeda, K.; Sugihara, N.; Yoshio, H.; Ino, H.; Takeda, R.; Okada, Y.; Nakanishi, I. Collagen remodelling in myocardia of patients with diabetes. *J. Clin. Pathol.* **1993**, *46*, 32–36. [CrossRef]
20. Treibel, T.A.; Lopez, B.; Gonzalez, A.; Menacho, K.; Schofield, R.S.; Ravassa, S.; Fontana, M.; White, S.K.; DiSalvo, C.; Roberts, N.; et al. Reappraising myocardial fibrosis in severe aortic stenosis: An invasive and non-invasive study in 133 patients. *Eur. Heart J.* **2018**, *39*, 699–709. [CrossRef]
21. Shirani, J.; Pick, R.; Roberts, W.C.; Maron, B.J. Morphology and significance of the left ventricular collagen network in young patients with hypertrophic cardiomyopathy and sudden cardiac death. *J. Am. Coll. Cardiol.* **2000**, *35*, 36–44. [CrossRef] [PubMed]
22. Nitta, K.; Goto, S.; Masakane, I.; Hanafusa, N.; Taniguchi, M.; Hasegawa, T.; Nakai, S.; Wada, A.; Hamano, T.; Hoshino, J.; et al. Annual dialysis data report for 2018, JSDT Renal Data Registry: Survey methods, facility data, incidence, prevalence, and mortality. *Ren. Replace. Ther.* **2020**, *6*, 41. [CrossRef]

23. Boenink, R.; Astley, M.E.; Huijben, J.A.; Stel, V.S.; Kerschbaum, J.; Ots-Rosenberg, M.; Asberg, A.A.; Lopot, F.; Golan, E.; Castro de la Nuez, P.; et al. The ERA Registry Annual Report 2019: Summary and age comparisons. *Clin. Kidney J.* **2022**, *15*, 452–472. [CrossRef] [PubMed]
24. Di Lullo, L.; Gorini, A.; Russo, D.; Santoboni, A.; Ronco, C. Left Ventricular Hypertrophy in Chronic Kidney Disease Patients: From Pathophysiology to Treatment. *Cardiorenal Med.* **2015**, *5*, 254–266. [CrossRef]
25. Paoletti, E.; De Nicola, L.; Gabbai, F.B.; Chiodini, P.; Ravera, M.; Pieracci, L.; Marre, S.; Cassottana, P.; Luca, S.; Vettoretti, S.; et al. Associations of Left Ventricular Hypertrophy and Geometry with Adverse Outcomes in Patients with CKD and Hypertension. *Clin. J. Am. Soc. Nephrol.* **2016**, *11*, 271–279. [CrossRef]
26. Tonelli, M.; Karumanchi, S.A.; Thadhani, R. Epidemiology and Mechanisms of Uremia-Related Cardiovascular Disease. *Circulation* **2016**, *133*, 518–536. [CrossRef]
27. Izumaru, K.; Hata, J.; Nakano, T.; Nakashima, Y.; Nagata, M.; Fukuhara, M.; Oda, Y.; Kitazono, T.; Ninomiya, T. Reduced Estimated GFR and Cardiac Remodeling: A Population-Based Autopsy Study. *Am. J. Kidney Dis.* **2019**, *74*, 373–381. [CrossRef]
28. Toblli, J.E.; Cao, G.; Rivas, C.; Giani, J.F.; Dominici, F.P. Intravenous iron sucrose reverses anemia-induced cardiac remodeling, prevents myocardial fibrosis, and improves cardiac function by attenuating oxidative/nitrosative stress and inflammation. *Int. J. Cardiol.* **2016**, *212*, 84–91. [CrossRef] [PubMed]
29. Amann, K.; Breitbach, M.; Ritz, E.; Mall, G. Myocyte/capillary mismatch in the heart of uremic patients. *J. Am. Soc. Nephrol.* **1998**, *9*, 1018–1022. [CrossRef]
30. Bonnans, C.; Chou, J.; Werb, Z. Remodelling the extracellular matrix in development and disease. *Nat. Rev. Mol. Cell Biol.* **2014**, *15*, 786–801. [CrossRef]
31. Frangogiannis, N.G. Cardiac fibrosis. *Cardiovasc. Res.* **2021**, *117*, 1450–1488. [CrossRef]
32. Lee, J.K.T.; Franzone, A.; Lanz, J.; Siontis, G.C.M.; Stortecky, S.; Grani, C.; Roost, E.; Windecker, S.; Pilgrim, T. Early Detection of Subclinical Myocardial Damage in Chronic Aortic Regurgitation and Strategies for Timely Treatment of Asymptomatic Patients. *Circulation* **2018**, *137*, 184–196. [CrossRef] [PubMed]
33. Schnee, J.M.; Hsueh, W.A. Angiotensin II, adhesion, and cardiac fibrosis. *Cardiovasc. Res.* **2000**, *46*, 264–268. [CrossRef]
34. Leask, A. Getting to the heart of the matter: New insights into cardiac fibrosis. *Circ. Res.* **2015**, *116*, 1269–1276. [CrossRef]
35. Cowling, R.T.; Kupsky, D.; Kahn, A.M.; Daniels, L.B.; Greenberg, B.H. Mechanisms of cardiac collagen deposition in experimental models and human disease. *Transl. Res.* **2019**, *209*, 138–155. [CrossRef] [PubMed]
36. Holmstrom, L.; Haukilahti, A.; Vahatalo, J.; Kentta, T.; Appel, H.; Kiviniemi, A.; Pakanen, L.; Huikuri, H.V.; Myerburg, R.J.; Junttila, J. Electrocardiographic associations with myocardial fibrosis among sudden cardiac death victims. *Heart (Br. Card. Soc.)* **2020**, *106*, 1001–1006. [CrossRef] [PubMed]
37. Matsukane, A.; Hayashi, T.; Tanaka, Y.; Iwasaki, M.; Kubo, S.; Asakawa, T.; Takahashi, Y.; Imamura, Y.; Hirahata, K.; Joki, N.; et al. Usefulness of an Upright T-Wave in Lead aVR for Predicting the Short-Term Prognosis of Incident Hemodialysis Patients: A Potential Tool for Screening High-Risk Hemodialysis Patients. *Cardiorenal Med.* **2015**, *5*, 267–277. [CrossRef]
38. Sato, Y.; Hayashi, T.; Joki, N.; Fujimoto, S. Association of Lead aVR T-wave Amplitude With Cardiovascular Events or Mortality Among Prevalent Dialysis Patients. *Ther. Apher. Dial.* **2017**, *21*, 287–294. [CrossRef]
39. Arcari, L.; Engel, J.; Freiwald, T.; Zhou, H.; Zainal, H.; Gawor, M.; Buettner, S.; Geiger, H.; Hauser, I.; Nagel, E.; et al. Cardiac biomarkers in chronic kidney disease are independently associated with myocardial edema and diffuse fibrosis by cardiovascular magnetic resonance. *J. Cardiovasc. Magn. Reson.* **2021**, *23*, 71. [CrossRef] [PubMed]
40. Querejeta, R.; Varo, N.; Lopez, B.; Larman, M.; Artinano, E.; Etayo, J.C.; Martinez Ubago, J.L.; Gutierrez-Stampa, M.; Emparanza, J.I.; Gil, M.J.; et al. Serum carboxy-terminal propeptide of procollagen type I is a marker of myocardial fibrosis in hypertensive heart disease. *Circulation* **2000**, *101*, 1729–1735. [CrossRef] [PubMed]
41. Klappacher, G.; Franzen, P.; Haab, D.; Mehrabi, M.; Binder, M.; Plesch, K.; Pacher, R.; Grimm, M.; Pribill, I.; Eichler, H.G.; et al. Measuring extracellular matrix turnover in the serum of patients with idiopathic or ischemic dilated cardiomyopathy and impact on diagnosis and prognosis. *Am. J. Cardiol.* **1995**, *75*, 913–918. [CrossRef]
42. Nishimura, M.; Tokoro, T.; Takatani, T.; Sato, N.; Hashimoto, T.; Kobayashi, H.; Ono, T. Circulating Aminoterminal Propeptide of Type III Procollagen as a Biomarker of Cardiovascular Events in Patients Undergoing Hemodialysis. *J. Atheroscler. Thromb.* **2019**, *26*, 340–350. [CrossRef] [PubMed]
43. Gupta, S.; Ge, Y.; Singh, A.; Grani, C.; Kwong, R.Y. Multimodality Imaging Assessment of Myocardial Fibrosis. *JACC Cardiovasc. Imaging* **2021**, *14*, 2457–2469. [CrossRef] [PubMed]
44. Scully, P.R.; Bastarrika, G.; Moon, J.C.; Treibel, T.A. Myocardial Extracellular Volume Quantification by Cardiovascular Magnetic Resonance and Computed Tomography. *Curr. Cardiol. Rep.* **2018**, *20*, 15. [CrossRef] [PubMed]
45. Schelbert, E.B.; Hsu, L.Y.; Anderson, S.A.; Mohanty, B.D.; Karim, S.M.; Kellman, P.; Aletras, A.H.; Arai, A.E. Late gadolinium-enhancement cardiac magnetic resonance identifies postinfarction myocardial fibrosis and the border zone at the near cellular level in ex vivo rat heart. *Circ. Cardiovasc. Imaging* **2010**, *3*, 743–752. [CrossRef]
46. Kim, R.J.; Fieno, D.S.; Parrish, T.B.; Harris, K.; Chen, E.L.; Simonetti, O.; Bundy, J.; Finn, J.P.; Klocke, F.J.; Judd, R.M. Relationship of MRI delayed contrast enhancement to irreversible injury, infarct age, and contractile function. *Circulation* **1999**, *100*, 1992–2002. [CrossRef]

47. Azevedo, C.F.; Nigri, M.; Higuchi, M.L.; Pomerantzeff, P.M.; Spina, G.S.; Sampaio, R.O.; Tarasoutchi, F.; Grinberg, M.; Rochitte, C.E. Prognostic significance of myocardial fibrosis quantification by histopathology and magnetic resonance imaging in patients with severe aortic valve disease. *J. Am. Coll. Cardiol.* **2010**, *56*, 278–287. [CrossRef] [PubMed]
48. Moon, J.C.; Reed, E.; Sheppard, M.N.; Elkington, A.G.; Ho, S.Y.; Burke, M.; Petrou, M.; Pennell, D.J. The histologic basis of late gadolinium enhancement cardiovascular magnetic resonance in hypertrophic cardiomyopathy. *J. Am. Coll. Cardiol.* **2004**, *43*, 2260–2264. [CrossRef]
49. Puntmann, V.O.; Voigt, T.; Chen, Z.; Mayr, M.; Karim, R.; Rhode, K.; Pastor, A.; Carr-White, G.; Razavi, R.; Schaeffter, T.; et al. Native T1 mapping in differentiation of normal myocardium from diffuse disease in hypertrophic and dilated cardiomyopathy. *JACC Cardiovasc. Imaging* **2013**, *6*, 475–484. [CrossRef] [PubMed]
50. Iles, L.M.; Ellims, A.H.; Llewellyn, H.; Hare, J.L.; Kaye, D.M.; McLean, C.A.; Taylor, A.J. Histological validation of cardiac magnetic resonance analysis of regional and diffuse interstitial myocardial fibrosis. *Eur. Heart J. Cardiovasc. Imaging* **2015**, *16*, 14–22. [CrossRef]
51. Hayer, M.K.; Radhakrishnan, A.; Price, A.M.; Liu, B.; Baig, S.; Weston, C.J.; Biasiolli, L.; Ferro, C.J.; Townend, J.N.; Steeds, R.P.; et al. Defining Myocardial Abnormalities Across the Stages of Chronic Kidney Disease: A Cardiac Magnetic Resonance Imaging Study. *JACC Cardiovasc. Imaging* **2020**, *13*, 2357–2367. [CrossRef] [PubMed]
52. Rutherford, E.; Talle, M.A.; Mangion, K.; Bell, E.; Rauhalammi, S.M.; Roditi, G.; McComb, C.; Radjenovic, A.; Welsh, P.; Woodward, R.; et al. Defining myocardial tissue abnormalities in end-stage renal failure with cardiac magnetic resonance imaging using native T1 mapping. *Kidney Int.* **2016**, *90*, 845–852. [CrossRef] [PubMed]
53. Brilla, C.G.; Funck, R.C.; Rupp, H. Lisinopril-mediated regression of myocardial fibrosis in patients with hypertensive heart disease. *Circulation* **2000**, *102*, 1388–1393. [CrossRef] [PubMed]
54. Diez, J.; Querejeta, R.; Lopez, B.; Gonzalez, A.; Larman, M.; Martinez Ubago, J.L. Losartan-dependent regression of myocardial fibrosis is associated with reduction of left ventricular chamber stiffness in hypertensive patients. *Circulation* **2002**, *105*, 2512–2517. [CrossRef]
55. Izawa, H.; Murohara, T.; Nagata, K.; Isobe, S.; Asano, H.; Amano, T.; Ichihara, S.; Kato, T.; Ohshima, S.; Murase, Y.; et al. Mineralocorticoid receptor antagonism ameliorates left ventricular diastolic dysfunction and myocardial fibrosis in mildly symptomatic patients with idiopathic dilated cardiomyopathy: A pilot study. *Circulation* **2005**, *112*, 2940–2945. [CrossRef]
56. Suzuki, H.; Kanno, Y.; Sugahara, S.; Ikeda, N.; Shoda, J.; Takenaka, T.; Inoue, T.; Araki, R. Effect of angiotensin receptor blockers on cardiovascular events in patients undergoing hemodialysis: An open-label randomized controlled trial. *Am. J. Kidney Dis.* **2008**, *52*, 501–506. [CrossRef]
57. Iseki, K.; Arima, H.; Kohagura, K.; Komiya, I.; Ueda, S.; Tokuyama, K.; Shiohira, Y.; Uehara, H.; Toma, S.; Olmesartan Clinical Trial in Okinawan Patients Under OKIDS (OCTOPUS) Group. Effects of angiotensin receptor blockade (ARB) on mortality and cardiovascular outcomes in patients with long-term haemodialysis: A randomized controlled trial. *Nephrol. Dial. Transpl.* **2013**, *28*, 1579–1589. [CrossRef]
58. Hasegawa, T.; Nishiwaki, H.; Ota, E.; Levack, W.M.; Noma, H. Aldosterone antagonists for people with chronic kidney disease requiring dialysis. *Cochrane Database Syst. Rev.* **2021**, *2*, CD013109. [CrossRef]
59. McMurray, J.J.V.; Solomon, S.D.; Inzucchi, S.E.; Kober, L.; Kosiborod, M.N.; Martinez, F.A.; Ponikowski, P.; Sabatine, M.S.; Anand, I.S.; Belohlavek, J.; et al. Dapagliflozin in Patients with Heart Failure and Reduced Ejection Fraction. *N. Engl. J. Med.* **2019**, *381*, 1995–2008. [CrossRef]
60. Packer, M.; Anker, S.D.; Butler, J.; Filippatos, G.; Pocock, S.J.; Carson, P.; Januzzi, J.; Verma, S.; Tsutsui, H.; Brueckmann, M.; et al. Cardiovascular and Renal Outcomes with Empagliflozin in Heart Failure. *N. Engl. J. Med.* **2020**, *383*, 1413–1424. [CrossRef]
61. Solomon, S.D.; McMurray, J.J.V.; Claggett, B.; de Boer, R.A.; DeMets, D.; Hernandez, A.F.; Inzucchi, S.E.; Kosiborod, M.N.; Lam, C.S.P.; Martinez, F.; et al. Dapagliflozin in Heart Failure with Mildly Reduced or Preserved Ejection Fraction. *N. Engl. J. Med.* **2022**, *387*, 1089–1098. [CrossRef]
62. Anker, S.D.; Butler, J.; Filippatos, G.; Ferreira, J.P.; Bocchi, E.; Bohm, M.; Brunner-La Rocca, H.P.; Choi, D.J.; Chopra, V.; Chuquiure-Valenzuela, E.; et al. Empagliflozin in Heart Failure with a Preserved Ejection Fraction. *N. Engl. J. Med.* **2021**, *385*, 1451–1461. [CrossRef]
63. Habibi, J.; Aroor, A.R.; Sowers, J.R.; Jia, G.; Hayden, M.R.; Garro, M.; Barron, B.; Mayoux, E.; Rector, R.S.; Whaley-Connell, A.; et al. Sodium glucose transporter 2 (SGLT2) inhibition with empagliflozin improves cardiac diastolic function in a female rodent model of diabetes. *Cardiovasc. Diabetol.* **2017**, *16*, 9. [CrossRef] [PubMed]
64. Lopez, B.; Querejeta, R.; Gonzalez, A.; Sanchez, E.; Larman, M.; Diez, J. Effects of loop diuretics on myocardial fibrosis and collagen type I turnover in chronic heart failure. *J. Am. Coll. Cardiol.* **2004**, *43*, 2028–2035. [CrossRef]
65. Lopez, B.; Gonzalez, A.; Beaumont, J.; Querejeta, R.; Larman, M.; Diez, J. Identification of a potential cardiac antifibrotic mechanism of torasemide in patients with chronic heart failure. *J. Am. Coll. Cardiol.* **2007**, *50*, 859–867. [CrossRef]
66. Veeraveedu, P.T.; Watanabe, K.; Ma, M.; Thandavarayan, R.A.; Palaniyandi, S.S.; Yamaguchi, K.; Suzuki, K.; Kodama, M.; Aizawa, Y. Comparative effects of torasemide and furosemide in rats with heart failure. *Biochem. Pharmacol.* **2008**, *75*, 649–659. [CrossRef]
67. Veeraveedu, P.T.; Watanabe, K.; Ma, M.; Palaniyandi, S.S.; Yamaguchi, K.; Suzuki, K.; Kodama, M.; Aizawa, Y. Torasemide, a long-acting loop diuretic, reduces the progression of myocarditis to dilated cardiomyopathy. *Eur. J. Pharmacol.* **2008**, *581*, 121–131. [CrossRef] [PubMed]

68. Trippel, T.D.; Van Linthout, S.; Westermann, D.; Lindhorst, R.; Sandek, A.; Ernst, S.; Bobenko, A.; Kasner, M.; Spillmann, F.; Gonzalez, A.; et al. Investigating a biomarker-driven approach to target collagen turnover in diabetic heart failure with preserved ejection fraction patients. Effect of torasemide versus furosemide on serum C-terminal propeptide of procollagen type I (DROP-PIP trial). *Eur. J. Heart Fail.* **2018**, *20*, 460–470. [CrossRef]
69. Lopez, B.; Gonzalez, A.; Hermida, N.; Laviades, C.; Diez, J. Myocardial fibrosis in chronic kidney disease: Potential benefits of torasemide. *Kidney Int. Suppl.* **2008**, *74*, S19–S23. [CrossRef] [PubMed]
70. Kraft, L.; Erdenesukh, T.; Sauter, M.; Tschope, C.; Klingel, K. Blocking the IL-1beta signalling pathway prevents chronic viral myocarditis and cardiac remodeling. *Basic Res. Cardiol.* **2019**, *114*, 11. [CrossRef]
71. Edgley, A.J.; Krum, H.; Kelly, D.J. Targeting fibrosis for the treatment of heart failure: A role for transforming growth factor-beta. *Cardiovasc. Ther.* **2012**, *30*, e30–e40. [CrossRef] [PubMed]
72. Shinde, A.V.; Su, Y.; Palanski, B.A.; Fujikura, K.; Garcia, M.J.; Frangogiannis, N.G. Pharmacologic inhibition of the enzymatic effects of tissue transglutaminase reduces cardiac fibrosis and attenuates cardiomyocyte hypertrophy following pressure overload. *J. Mol. Cell. Cardiol.* **2018**, *117*, 36–48. [CrossRef] [PubMed]

Disclaimer/Publisher's Note: The statements, opinions and data contained in all publications are solely those of the individual author(s) and contributor(s) and not of MDPI and/or the editor(s). MDPI and/or the editor(s) disclaim responsibility for any injury to people or property resulting from any ideas, methods, instructions or products referred to in the content.

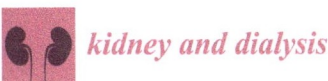

Perspective

How Can We Improve the Appetite of Older Patients on Dialysis in Japan?

Yukie Kitajima

Department of Medical Nutrition, Faculty of Healthcare, Tokyo Healthcare University, Tokyo 154-8568, Japan; y-kitajima@thcu.ac.jp

Abstract: It is necessary to ensure adequate energy and protein intake in dialysis patients. However, in addition to the decline in dietary intake in older dialysis patients due to aging, the rate of anorexia is high in dialysis patients, which increases the risk of protein–energy wasting (PEW), sarcopenia, and frailty. There are many causes of anorexia in dialysis patients, including older dialysis patients, and approaches to improve the appetite of such patients have been reported; however, there has been no established approach to improve appetite adequately. Therefore, a key practical goal is to identify anorexia early and implement timely interventions before weight loss occurs. Appetite assessment tools and weight loss assessments are helpful for the screening and early identification of anorectic signs. Nutritional interventions include reducing dietary restrictions, using oral nutritional supplements, and intradialytic parenteral nutrition, as well as replenishing energy, protein, and zinc to prevent the development of nutritional disorders among older dialysis patients. Appetite assessments, early intervention, and dietary and nutritional counseling are key to improving appetite in these patients. The aging rate of dialysis patients in Japan is unprecedented globally, and I believe that this is a situation that will eventually occur in other countries as well. I discuss the factors that contribute to anorexia, especially in older dialysis patients, and Japan's efforts to address this problem, such as the relaxation of dietary restrictions and the use of oral nutritional supplements.

Keywords: aged; anorexia; appetite; dialysis; diet

1. Introduction

The goal of nutritional therapy for dialysis patients is to maintain good nutritional and physical status, prevent the onset and severity of complications such as heart failure, infectious disease, cerebrovascular disease, etc. while maintaining the quality of life and activities of daily living. Although it is necessary to ensure adequate energy and protein intake, in addition to the decline in dietary intake in older dialysis patients due to aging, the rate of anorexia is high in dialysis patients, which increases the risk of protein–energy wasting (PEW), sarcopenia, and frailty. There are many causes of anorexia in dialysis patients, including older dialysis patients, and approaches to improving appetite have been reported, including early appetite assessment, consideration of dialysis conditions, and prescription of medications. However, there has been no established approach to adequately improve appetite. Therefore, the practical goal is to identify anorexia early and implement timely interventions before weight loss occurs. The number of chronic dialysis patients in Japan is 344,640 [1], and the prevalence of dialysis patients is the second highest in the world (after Taiwan) [2]. In Japan, the aging dialysis population is remarkable, with an average age of 69.67 years, and the average age is increasing every year [1]. While the age group with the highest percentage is 70–74 years old for both men and women, the number of patients younger than 70 years has been decreasing since 2017; the increase in the number of dialysis patients in Japan is primarily due to the increase in the number of patients older than 70 years. I believe that this unprecedented aging of dialysis patients is a situation that will eventually occur in other countries. In this study, I discuss the factors that contribute to anorexia, especially in older dialysis patients, as well as the steps that are being taken to address this issue in Japan.

2. Loss of Appetite in Dialysis Patients

Appetite is regulated by various factors, such as hormones and peptides, that stimulate the appetite when hungry and suppress it when full. However, the aging process reduces the ability to control these factors, making older adults more likely to have a decreased appetite [3,4]. Appetite loss has been observed in approximately 40% of patients undergoing dialysis [5,6].

In addition to factors specific to renal failure (e.g., uremic substances and inflammation), gastrointestinal disorders, taste abnormalities, poor oral hygiene, depression, and social and economic poverty, the effects of comorbidities have been implicated as causes of decreased appetite in patients undergoing dialysis [6,7]. End-stage renal failure has been associated with the retention of uremic substances and the short-term dysregulation of appetite-regulating substances in the gastrointestinal tract, resulting in early satiety and delayed gastric emptying [8]. Thus, the conditions of older patients on dialysis are further complicated by aging, their psychological and social backgrounds, and other factors that can lead to appetite loss.

Loss of appetite on dialysis days in hemodialysis patients affects energy and protein intake on both dialysis and non-dialysis days. In particular, many patients have decreased appetite on dialysis days [9], with average intakes on dialysis days reported to be 77.5 kcal/day lower in energy and 4.79 g/day lower in protein than on non-dialysis days [8]. One report compared appetite and hunger between dialysis and non-dialysis days and found that appetite decreased the most at lunch and dinner on dialysis days [10,11].

Following the spread of the coronavirus disease (COVID-19) in 2020, some facilities in Japan stopped serving food and beverages during dialysis, and patients stopped eating food when they underwent dialysis. Notomi et al. [12] investigated the relationship between the discontinuation of cafeteria services at a dialysis facility (as part of the measures taken against the spread of COVID-19) and dry weight. They reported no changes in dry weight in the group that did not patronize cafeteria services before COVID-19 (non-users). However, a reduction in dry weight was observed in the group of patients who patronized cafeteria services until discontinuation due to COVID-19 (0.8% at 7 months and 1.2% at 10 months), which was significantly different from that observed in non-users (7 months, $p = 0.007$; 10 months, $p < 0.001$). Thus, it was concluded that dialysis patients need to take action to compensate for the lack of energy and nutrients in response to their altered eating rhythms associated with dialysis and the discontinuation of food provision due to COVID-19 infection control.

Moreover, action must be taken to detect and intervene early in appetite loss, especially in older patients on dialysis. As anorexia in dialysis patients becomes more severe, the complication rates of hypoalbuminemia and underweight increase, which are associated with a higher risk of hospitalization [4] and prolonged recovery time after the completion of dialysis [13]. Decreased appetite progresses from increased protein catabolism to the development and severity of PEW, sarcopenia, and frailty, with a consequent impact on life expectancy [14].

3. Appetite Assessment and Appetite-Related Factors

Including older patients, the causes of anorexia in patients undergoing dialysis are diverse, making definitive treatment difficult. A systematic review of the treatment of age-related anorexia revealed a lack of evidence and an overlap between nutritional interventions for anorexia and nutritional disorders. Megestrol acetate is a drug that improves appetite [15]; however, relevant evidence is lacking, and its cautious use has been called for [16]. Based on the action points for treating anorexia, the implementation of a nutritional assessment and plan should be considered [17] (Figure 1). Early detection of anorexia may enable timely intervention before weight loss occurs. Action points related to appetite assessment and appetite loss are as follows.

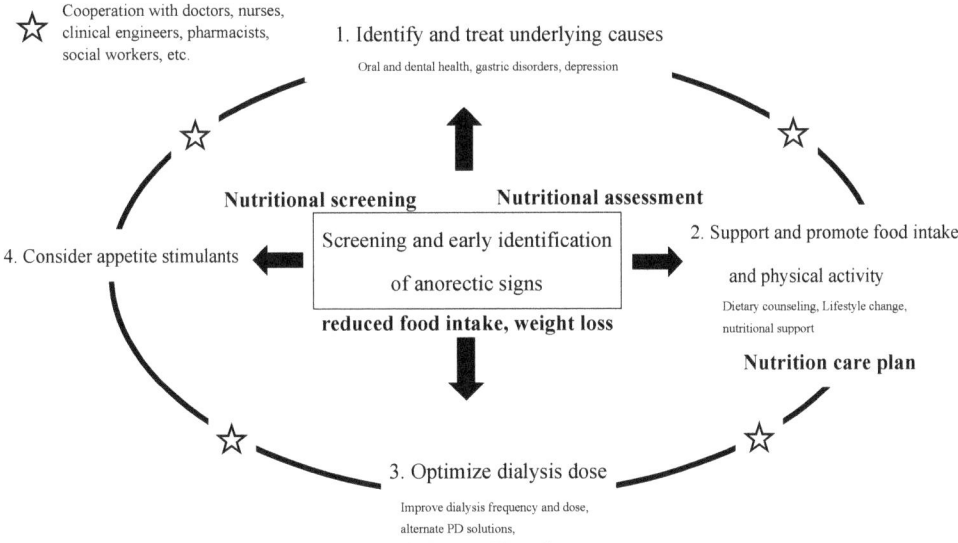

Figure 1. Proposed action points including nutritional intervention to treat anorexia in patients with CKD. Reproduced with permission from Carrero JJ et al., Nutrition Management of Renal Disease; published by Elsevier, 2021.

3.1. Appetite Assessment

Common items in various nutritional screening and assessment tools include weight loss and decreased or altered dietary intake. This indicates that weight loss and decreased food intake are important factors in nutritional status, not only in hemodialysis patients.

Simple methods for assessing anorexia include the numerical rating scale (NRS) [18], the Council on Nutrition appetite questionnaire (CNAQ) [19], the Simplified Nutrition Assessment Questionnaire (SNAQ) [19], Appetite and Diet Assessment Tool (ADAT) [20], self-assessment of appetite changes [21], subjective assessment of appetite [6,10], Visual analogue scale (VAS) [22], Functional Assessment of Anorexia/Cachexia Therapy (FAACT) score [23], and Anorexia Questionnaire (AQ) [21] (Table 1). The VAS and FAACT are significantly associated with decreased food intake in patients on dialysis. These methods can also be used for monitoring anorexia. In contrast, a method that does not use an assessment chart and only asks the dialysis patient whether they have an appetite during dialysis is simpler and can become a routine part of daily practice.

Table 1. Characteristics of selected appetite assessment tools.

Appetite Assessment Tool	Time Frame of Assessment	Description
numerical rating scale (NRS) [18]	Dietary habits for a week	Simple and easy to quantify. Determines present appetite indicated with a line on a scale (each end of the scale: 'Appetite' or 'No appetite').
Council on Nutrition appetite questionnaire (CNAQ) [19]	Dietary habits for a month	Contains 8 questions related to appetite, food intake, satiety, and number of meals consumed per day derived from the Appetite, Hunger and Sensory Perception Questionnaire (AHSPQ).

Table 1. *Cont.*

Appetite Assessment Tool	Time Frame of Assessment	Description
Simplified Nutrition Assessment Questionnaire (SNAQ) [19]	Dietary habits for a month	Contains four questions related to appetite, food intake, satiety, and number of meals consumed per day.
Appetite and Diet Assessment Tool (ADAT) [20]	everyday	44-Item self-administered questionnaire divided into three sections about appetite and eating habits in general, on dialysis, and on non-dialysis days, respectively.
self-assessment of appetite changes [21]	Last month (30 days)	Compares present appetite vs. appetite over the last month (increased, decreased, or unchanged).
subjective assessment of appetite [6,10]	Last week (7 days)	Compares present appetite vs. appetite last week (increased, decreased, or unchanged).
Visual analogue scale (VAS) [22]	At that point	Simple and easy to quantify. Determines present appetite indicated with a line on a scale (scale extremities: 0 mm, 'no hunger'; 100 mm, 'hunger').
Functional Assessment of Anorexia/Cachexia Therapy (FAACT) score [23]	At that point	12 questions related to appetite and food intake. Each question allows for 5 answers (i.e., not at all, a little bit, somewhat, quite a bit, very much.)
Anorexia questionnaire (AQ) [21]	At that point	4 questions on the presence of early satiety, taste/smell alterations, meat aversion, and nausea/vomiting.

3.2. Consideration of Dialysis Conditions

Increased appetite and the frequency of dialysis with hemodiafiltration have been suggested to improve nutritional status, appetite, and food intake [24]. Information should be shared with the clinical staff to discuss dialysis requirements (e.g., method, membrane, volume, and duration).

However, it should be noted that increased dialysis efficiency, while potentially improving appetite [24], can lead to a loss of amino acids [25,26] and the removal of micronutrients. Thus, the dialysis conditions should be determined based on the nutritional status of the patient.

Metabolic acidosis is also known to cause loss of appetite and easy fatigability. In their analysis of the DOPPS (dialysis outcomes and practice patterns study) of approximately 17,000 hemodialysis patients, Tentori et al. reported that the lower the pre-dialysis bicarbonate concentration, the higher the risk of all-cause mortality [27]. In addition, Vashistha et al. reported that a low pre-dialysis bicarbonate concentration was associated with a higher risk of all-cause mortality, cardiovascular death, and infection-related death based on data from approximately 110,000 hemodialysis patients in the Da Vita group [28]. Therefore, the adequate correction of metabolic acidosis is considered important, and the K/DOQI (National Kidney Foundation Kidney Disease Outcomes Quality Initiative) guidelines recommend a pre-dialysis bicarbonate concentration of at least 22 mEq/L [29,30]. Blood bicarbonate is negatively correlated with serum albumin and phosphorus levels and normalized protein nitrogen appearance; furthermore, in cases of high blood bicarbonate, poor protein intake may be the cause [31]. Therefore, ensuring adequate dietary intake—including protein intake—is necessary to improve metabolic acidosis. If a dietary approach is difficult to implement for dialysis patients with decreased appetite, one approach is to consider dialysate solutions. Acetic-acid-free dialysate with a high bicarbonate concentration of 35 mEq/L is excellent for improving metabolic acidosis, and there have been reports of increased protein intake after switching to acetic acid-free dialysate [32].

3.3. Review of Drug Prescription

In a study examining the association between anorexia and polypharmacy, the total number of medications prescribed did not significantly differ between the two groups; however, the anorexia group received significantly more sleeping pills [33].

Taste abnormalities are present in approximately 30% of patients on dialysis, which are associated with poor nutritional status and life expectancy [34]. One of the main causes of dysgeusia in dialysis patients is inadequate zinc intake, which is associated with dietary restriction, anorexia, intestinal malabsorption [35], and chronic kidney disease. Zinc administration has been reported to increase protein intake [36]. Antihypertensive medications also decrease zinc levels, such as angiotensin-converting enzyme inhibitors, angiotensin II receptor blockers, and calcium channel blockers. Appropriate and periodic prescription reviews are necessary in the treatment of anorexia. The cause of dysgeusia should be identified, and appropriate actions should be taken to address it.

3.4. Oral Care

Poor oral health affects appetite. As the number of natural teeth and appetite are independently associated with changes in body weight, tooth loss may increase the risk of dysphagia, leading to changes in food preference, food avoidance, and decreased energy intake [37].

3.5. Post-Dialysis Fatigue (PDF)

Dialysis patients often experience symptoms of fatigue and discomfort after dialysis [38]. More than 80% of dialysis patients experience symptoms of fatigue [39] and have been reported to rest or nap within 5 h of dialysis [40]. PDF [41] has been assessed on the basis of 'time', 'frequency', and 'intensity' by asking about 'time to recover from haemodialysis' (recovery time) [38–42], and various measures have been studied, but no international guidelines have been established for optimal measurement methods; if PDF is severe, it may indicate reduced food intake or missed meals after dialysis. A study of the new PDF scale reported that patients with normalized protein catabolic rate (nPCR) less than 0.8 had lower nPCR and serum albumin as the new PDF scale increased [43]. As reduced food intake and habitual skipping of meals can lead to decreased appetite, assessing symptoms of fatigue and malaise after dialysis can be effective in preventing decreased appetite. Standard dialysis is a type of dialysis in which patients go to a dialysis center three times a week. The rule that the medical staff ask a simple question before starting dialysis—"How long did it take you to feel better after your last dialysis session?"—is a simple assessment, but we believe it is a means of early detection of appetite loss.

3.6. Physical Activity

In a cross-sectional observational study of elderly hospitalized patients, good appetite during hospitalization was associated with higher habitual physical activity in the week before admission [44]. In this study, habitual physical activity was assessed using the Physical Activity Scale for the Elderly (PASE), which included leisure-time activities as well as home and work-related activities. A study of elderly maintenance hemodialysis patients reported that the frequency of exercise per week was independently associated with anorexia, and in addition to low muscle mass, slow walking speed was strongly associated with anorexia [45]. Although specific types of exercise and exercise duration were not specified, maintaining physical activity in daily life may be closely related to appetite. Therefore, exercise and rehabilitation interventions to maintain physical function and physical activity may improve appetite loss in dialysis patients.

4. Nutritional Intervention during Anorexia and Decreased Food Intake

If an older patient undergoing dialysis complains of anorexia, the risk of nutritional problems is increased. Anorexia and decreased or absent food intake should be suspected when there is little or no weight gain. When anorexia or decreased food intake occurs, the following interventions should be considered.

4.1. Relaxation or Removal of Diet Restriction or Diet Therapy

Dietary energy deficiency (<35 kcal/kg body weight (BW)/day) and protein deficiency (<0.8 g/kg body weight (BW)/day) are found in 52–92% and 32.3–81% of dialysis patients, respectively [46]. Consuming enough energy and protein is a major challenge for dialysis patients. It is clear that patients with reduced appetite have even lower energy and nutrient intakes. Therefore, there is little need to continue their dialysis diet.

The patient's interest in and satisfaction with food may be restored through the relaxation or removal of dietary restrictions.

4.2. Supplement Energy and Protein with Snacks and Frequent Meals

Ways to increase energy intake include adding fried foods that absorb a lot of oil or fatty meats in dishes or using butter or honey. Older adults may have difficulty eating enough fatty foods, but they can supplement energy and protein by eating small amounts of doughnuts, sandwiches, croissants, etc., outside of mealtimes. In addition, medium-chain triglycerides (MCTs) oil is tasteless, odorless, and can be easily used like a dressing. MCTs are useful as an energy source because they do not form micelles, enter the general circulation quickly through the portal vein. And MCTs consumption may trigger acylation (activation) of ghrelin, leading to increased appetite [47]. In addition to their use in the diet, they can be added to ice cream or yogurt during supplementary meals to increase energy levels in addition to protein intake; elderly dialysis patients treated with 12 g/day of amino acids for 6 months had improved appetite [48]. While a balanced diet of amino acid-rich meats, fish, eggs, beans, and dairy products is important, patients with decreased appetite may also benefit from the use of amino acid-rich oral nutritional supplements (ONS).

4.3. Use of ONS

ONS with limited protein should not be used; those that are high in energy and protein should be used instead. Some reports have suggested that ONS ingestion before meals promotes satisfaction and influences food intake [49]. To address the reduced food intake due to decreased appetite, the use of ONS as part of a meal or during or after dialysis has been considered, and significantly reduced mortality and readmission rates in dialysis patients who received ONS have been reported [49–51]. The recommended amount of nutritional intake from ONS in dialysis patients is 7–10 kcal/kg BW of energy and 0.3–0.4 g/kg BW of protein. Once the amount of supplemental nutrition from ONS has been determined, it is recommended that it be divided into two to three portions per day and continued for a minimum of 3 months [29].

Compared to hemodialysis, hemodiafiltration dialysis—which has recently been implemented in many facilities in Japan—is more efficient in removing medium molecular weight proteins and other substances, while albumin leakage is high [25,26]. Hemodialysis accelerates the breakdown of systemic and muscle proteins, and muscle protein breakdown is accelerated in the 2 h after the end of treatment [52]. Although muscle protein breakdown decreases 2 h after the end of treatment, systemic protein breakdown continues to increase. This suggests the importance of nutritional intake during or immediately after dialysis. Therefore, the use of food or ONS during or immediately after dialysis should be actively sought.

4.4. Intradialytic Parenteral Nutrition (IDPN) Study

In the ESPEN study, nutritional intervention in dialysis patients with nutritional disorders was the first attempt to improve their nutritional status through nutritional guidance. If this was inadequate, ONS were attempted. The next step was to consider an IDPN [26]. In this case, the use of IDPN is conducted for nutritional supplementation. As IDPN alone cannot meet the nutritional requirements of patients, adjustments should be made while considering the concomitant use of diet, enteral nutrition, and ONS.

5. Specific Nutritional Counseling

Nutrient requirements are set based on guidelines [26,29], but no standard diet exists. Specific individualized suggestions are required for a patient to consume the necessary energy and protein in the form of foods and dishes, and how to practice the management of minerals such as salt and potassium must be considered as well. The patient's dietary status and intentions should be ascertained—such as the extent to which the patient can or cannot cook, whether the patient mainly consumes home-cooked meals, what kinds of foods are often purchased, who the key persons are, and so on—and suggestions should be made regarding food choices and how to adjust the amount of food used. The patient's dietary situation can also be assessed, following which suggestions can be made regarding food selection and usage [53]. Dietary suggestions that do not compromise food satisfaction and happiness may influence the food intake of patients [34].

During nutritional guidance, the dietitian may tell the patient something along the lines of "The recommended daily protein intake is 45 g". However, the patient may not understand correctly that the guideline is "up to 45 g of meat (protein food) per day". Therefore, those who provide dietary guidance must give patients specific amounts (guideline amounts), rather than numerical values (g). Next, suggestions for food use and cooking methods should be made, according to the individual's life background [54]. Improving the eating environment may be a more effective strategy for improving the appetite of patients [55].

In addition, attention should be paid to nutritional counseling techniques. Incremental behavior-change techniques can increase confidence in behavior-change self-effectiveness by gradually and incrementally raising the goal toward achieving the behavior [56]. According to social cognitive theory, two factors determine whether an individual can perform a behavior: outcome expectations, which are expectations or images associated with the outcome of performing a certain behavior, and self-efficacy, which is the confidence in one's ability to perform the behavior required to achieve that outcome successfully [56]. The likelihood of performing a behavior is high if both of these factors are high. When providing nutritional counseling to patients, they should be aware of the goals to focus on. Dieticians should set goals that the patient will follow and aim to achieve [53]. Patients need to be able to follow their daily diet without difficulty.

6. Support from Conservative Phase to Dialysis Phase (Dialysis Transition Phase)

Before and after the induction of dialysis, patients are often physically and emotionally unstable. During the transition to dialysis, the patient's diet changes according to the renal replacement therapy (e.g., outpatient hemodialysis, home hemodialysis, or peritoneal dialysis) chosen by the patient, and the treatment methods and diet change significantly. In particular, the diet from the conservative phase to the dialysis phase includes increased protein intake as well as fluid, potassium, and phosphorus management [26,29]. As the patient's physical condition and appetite improve with dialysis therapy, it is important to educate the patient about diet, not only at the time of dialysis induction, but also after one month when the patient has settled into dialysis, or at the time of transfer to a maintenance dialysis facility. In this case, the incremental behavior-change technique described above should be utilized [56].

7. Conclusions

There are many causes of anorexia in dialysis patients, including older patients. To improve appetite in older patients on dialysis, we must identify anorexic conditions early, identify the associated cause(s), and intervene to resolve the problem. Nutritional interventions include reducing dietary restrictions, using ONS and IDPN, and supplementing with energy, protein, and micronutrients to prevent the development of nutritional disorders. Specific recommendations and educational techniques are key to nutritional counseling (Figure 2). This paper described the practicalities of improving the appetite of elderly dialysis patients in Japan at this time from a dietitian's perspective. It is difficult to provide a clear answer on how to improve appetite in older patients on dialysis. However, the proportion of elderly dialysis patients in Japan will not decrease. Therefore, appropriate interventions to increase appetite become even more necessary. Food and food culture are unique to each country. I suggest that research should focus on traditional Japanese dietary patterns in order to suggest dietary patterns for Japanese dialysis patients to prevent appetite loss and dietary guidance to improve appetite. And dialysis treatment is a multi-professional collaborative treatment. Dietitians alone cannot intervene to solve problems. Therefore, in countries with an ageing population of dialysis patients, it is important to combine the assessments of different professions and consider methods to improve the appetite of individual elderly dialysis patients.

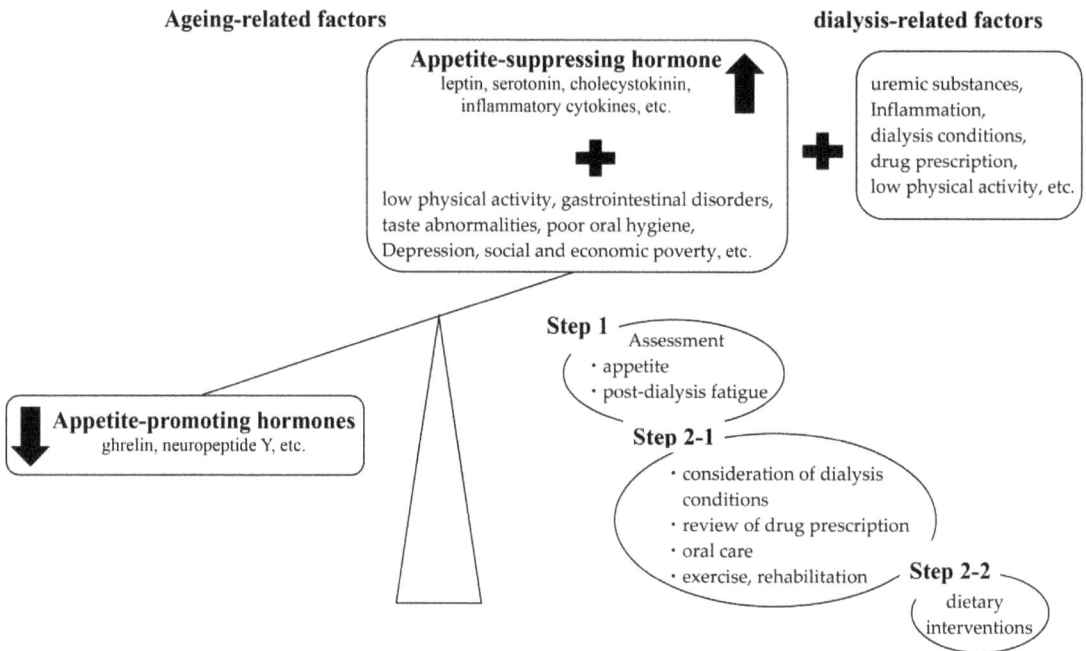

Figure 2. The causes of anorexia with the countermeasures against loss of appetite.

Funding: This research received no external funding.

Institutional Review Board Statement: Not applicable.

Informed Consent Statement: Not applicable.

Data Availability Statement: No new data was created or analyzed in this study. Data sharing is not applicable to this article.

Conflicts of Interest: The author declares no conflict of interest.

References

1. Hanafusa, N.; Abe, M.; Joki, N.; Ogawa, T.; Kanda, E.; Kikuchi, K.; Goto, S.; Taniguchi, M.; Nakai, S.; Naganuma, T.; et al. Annual Dialysis Data Report 2019, JSDT Renal Data Registry. *Ren. Replace. Ther.* **2023**, *9*, 47. [CrossRef]
2. United States Renal Data System. *2020 USRDS Annual Data Report: Epidemiology of Kidney Disease in the United States*; National Institutes of Health, National Institute of Diabetes and Digestive and Kidney Diseases: Bethesda, MD, USA, 2020.
3. Wysokiński, A.; Sobów, T.; Kłoszewska, I.; Kostka, T. Mechanisms of the anorexia of aging—A review. *Age* **2015**, *37*, 9821. [CrossRef]
4. Merchant, R.A.; Vathsala, A. Healthy aging and chronic kidney disease. *Kidney Res. Clin. Pract.* **2022**, *41*, 644–656. [CrossRef]

5. Bossola, M.; Muscaritoli, M.; Tazza, L.; Panocchia, N.; Liberatori, M.; Giungi, S.; Tortorelli, A.; Rossi Fanelli, F.; Luciani, G. Variables associated with reduced dietary intake in HD patients. *J. Renal Nutr.* **2005**, *15*, 244–252. [CrossRef]
6. Kalantar-Zadeh, K.; Block, G.; McAllister, C.J.; Humphreys, M.H.; Kopple, J.D. Appetite and inflammation, nutrition, anemia, and clinical outcome in hemodialysis patients. *Am. J. Clin. Nutr.* **2004**, *80*, 299–307. [CrossRef]
7. Bossola, M.; Muscaritoli, M.; Tazza, L.; Giungi, S.; Tortorelli, A.; Rossi Fanelli, F.; Luciani, G. Malnutrition in HD patients: What therapy. *Am. J. Kidney Dis.* **2005**, *46*, 371–386. [CrossRef]
8. Wright, M.; Woodrow, G.; O'Brien, S.; King, N.; Dye, L.; Blundell, J.; Brownjohn, A.; Turney, J. Disturbed appetite patterns and nutrient intake in peritoneal dialysis patients. *Perit. Dial. Int.* **2003**, *23*, 550–556. [CrossRef]
9. Carrero, J.J. Identification of patients with eating disorders: Clinical and biochemical signs of appetite loss in dialysis patients. *J. Ren. Nutr.* **2009**, *19*, 10–15. [CrossRef]
10. Burrowes, J.D.; Larive, B.; Chertow, G.M.; Cockram, D.B.; Dwyer, J.T.; Greene, T.; Kusek, J.W.; Leung, J.; Rocco, M.V.; Hemodialysis (HEMO) Study Group. Self-reported appetite, hospitalization and death in HD patients: Findings from the HD (HEMO) Study. *Nephrol. Dial. Transplant.* **2005**, *20*, 2765–2774. [CrossRef] [PubMed]
11. Wright, M.J.; Woodrow, G.; O'Brien, S.; King, N.A.; Dye, L.; Blundell, J.E.; Brownjohn, A.M.; Turney, J.H. A novel technique to demonstrate disturbed appetite profiles in haemodialysis patients. *Nephrol. Dial. Transplant.* **2001**, *16*, 1424–1429. [CrossRef]
12. Notomi, S.; Kitamura, M.; Yamaguchi, K.; Harada, T.; Nishino, T.; Funakoshi, S.; Kuno, K. Impact of Cafeteria Service Discontinuation at a Dialysis Facility on Medium-Term Nutritional Status of Elderly Patients Undergoing Hemodialysis. *Nutrients* **2022**, *14*, 1628. [CrossRef]
13. Bossola, M.; Tazza, L. Appetite is associated with the time of recovery after the dialytic session in patients on chronic hemodialysis. *Nephron Clin. Pract.* **2013**, *123*, 129–133. [CrossRef]
14. Kim, J.C.; Kalantar-Zadeh, K.; Kopple, J.D. Frailty and protein-energy wasting in elderly patients with end stage kidney disease. *J. Am. Soc. Nephrol.* **2013**, *24*, 337–351. [CrossRef]
15. Cox, N.J.; Ibrahim, K.; Sayer, A.A.; Robinson, S.M.; Roberts, H.C. Assessment and treatment of the anorexia of aging: A systematic review. *Nutrients* **2019**, *11*, 144. [CrossRef]
16. Wazny, L.D.; Nadurak, S.; Orsulak, C.; Giles-Smith, L.; Tangri, N. The Efficacy and Safety of Megestrol Acetate in Protein-Energy Wasting due to Chronic Kidney Disease: A Systematic Review. *J. Ren. Nutr.* **2016**, *26*, 168–176. [CrossRef]
17. Carrero, J.J.; Qureshi, A.R.; Axelsson, J. Anorexia and appetite stimulants in chronic kidney disease. In *Nutrition Management of Renal Disease*, 4th ed.; Kopple, J., Massry, S., Kalantar-Zadeh, K., Fouque, D., Eds.; Elsevier: Amsterdam, The Netherlands, 2021; pp. 893–906.
18. Carrero, J.J.; Qureshi, A.R.; Axelsson, J.; Avesani, C.M.; Suliman, M.E.; Kato, S.; Bárány, P.; Snaedal-Jonsdottir, S.; Alvestrand, A.; Heimbürger, O.; et al. Comparison of nutritional and inflammatory markers in dialysis patients with reduced appetite. *Am. J. Clin. Nutr.* **2007**, *85*, 695–701. [CrossRef]
19. Wilson, M.M.; Thomas, D.R.; Rubenstein, L.Z.; Chibnall, J.T.; Anderson, S.; Baxi, A.; Diebold, M.R.; Morley, J.E. Appetite assessment: Simple appetite questionnaire predicts weight loss in community-dwelling adults and nursing home residents. *Am. J. Clin. Nutr.* **2005**, *82*, 1074–1081. [CrossRef] [PubMed]
20. Burrowes, J.D.; Powers, S.N.; Cockram, D.B.; Cunniff, P.J.; Paranandi, L.; Kusek, J.W. Use of an appetite and diet assessment tool in the pilot phase of a hemodialysis clinical trial: Mortality and morbidity in hemodialysis study. *J. Ren. Nutr.* **1996**, *6*, 229–232. [CrossRef]
21. Molfino, A.; Kaysen, G.A.; Chertow, G.M.; Doyle, J.; Delgado, C.; Dwyer, T.; Laviano, A.; Rossi Fanelli, F.; Johansen, K.L. Validating appetite assessment tools among patients receiving hemodialysis. *J. Ren. Nutr.* **2016**, *26*, 103–110. [CrossRef] [PubMed]
22. Zabel, R.; Ash, S.; Bauer, J.; King, N. Assessment of subjective appetite sensations in hemodialysis patients. Agreement and feasibility between traditional paper and pen and a novel electronic appetite rating system. *Appetite* **2009**, *52*, 525–527. [CrossRef] [PubMed]
23. Ribaudo, J.M.; Cella, D.; Hahn, E.A.; Lloyd, S.R.; Tchekmedyian, N.S.; Von Roenn, J.; Leslie, W.T. Re-validation and shortening of the Functional Assessment of Anorexia/Cachexia Therapy (FAACT) questionnaire. *Qual. Life Res.* **2000**, *9*, 1137–1146. [CrossRef]
24. Molina, P.; Vizcaíno, B.; Molina, M.D.; Beltrán, S.; González-Moya, M.; Mora, A.; Castro-Alonso, C.; Kanter, J.; Ávila, A.I.; Górriz, J.L.; et al. The effect of high-volume online haemodiafiltration on nutritional status and body composition: The ProtEin Stores prEservaTion (PESET) study. *Nephrol. Dial. Transplant.* **2018**, *33*, 1223–1235. [CrossRef]
25. Sakurai, K. Biomarkers for evaluation of clinical outcomes of hemodiafiltration. *Blood Purif.* **2013**, *35*, 64–68. [CrossRef] [PubMed]
26. Cano, N.J.; Aparicio, M.; Brunori, G.; Carrero, J.J.; Cianciaruso, B.; Fiaccadori, E.; Lindholm, B.; Teplan, V.; Fouque, D.; Guarnieri, G. ESPEN Guidelines on Parenteral Nutrition: Adult renal failure. *Clin. Nutr.* **2009**, *28*, 401–414. [CrossRef] [PubMed]
27. Tentori, F.; Karaboyas, A.; Robinson, B.M.; Morgenstern, H.; Zhang, J.; Sen, A.; Ikizler, T.A.; Rayner, H.; Fissell, R.B.; Vanholder, R.; et al. Association of dialysate bicarbonate concentration with mortality in the dialysis outcomes and practice patterns study (DOPPS). *Am. J. Kidney Dis.* **2013**, *62*, 738–746. [CrossRef] [PubMed]
28. Vashistha, T.; Kalantar–Zadeh, K.; Molnar, M.Z.; Torlén, K.; Mehrotra, R. Dialysis modality and correction of uremic metabolic acidosis: Relationship with all– cause and cause–specific mortality. *Clin. J. Am. Nephrol.* **2013**, *8*, 254–264. [CrossRef]
29. Ikizler, T.A.; Burrowes, J.D.; Byham-Gray, L.D.; Campbell, K.L.; Carrero, J.J.; Chan, W.; Fouque, D.; Friedman, A.N.; Ghaddar, S.; Goldstein-Fuchs, D.J.; et al. KDOQI Clinical Practice Guideline for Nutrition in CKD: 2020 Update. *Am. J. Kidney Dis.* **2020**, *76*, S1–S107. [CrossRef] [PubMed]

30. National Kidney Foundation. K/DOQI clinical practice guideline for bone metabolism and disease in chronic kidney disease. *Am. J. Kidney Dis.* **2003**, *42*, S1–S201. [CrossRef]
31. Bommer, J.; Locatelli, F.; Satayathum, S.; Keen, M.L.; Goodkin, D.A.; Saito, A.; Akiba, T.; Port, F.K.; Young, E.W. Association of predialysis serum bicarbonate levels with risk of mortality and hospitalization in the Dialysis Outcomes and Practice Patterns Study (DOPPS). *Am. J. Kidney Dis.* **2004**, *44*, 661–671. [CrossRef]
32. Movilli, E.; Camerini, C.; Zein, H.; D'Avolio, G.; Sandrini, M.; Strada, A.; Maiorca, R. A prospective comparison of bicarbonate dialysis, hemodiafiltration, and acetate-free biofiltration in the elderly. *Am. J. Kidney Dis.* **1996**, *27*, 541–547. [CrossRef]
33. Notomi, S.; Kitamura, M.; Yamaguchi, K.; Komine, M.; Sawase, K.; Nishino, T.; Funakoshi, S. Anorexia Assessed by Simplified Nutritional Appetite Questionnaire and Association with Medication in Older Patients Undergoing Hemodialysis. *Biol. Pharm. Bull.* **2003**, *46*, 286–291. [CrossRef] [PubMed]
34. Lynch, K.E.; Lynch, R.; Curhan, G.C.; Brunelli, S.M. Altered taste perception and nutritional status among hemodialysis patients. *J. Ren. Nutr.* **2013**, *23*, 288–295.e1. [CrossRef] [PubMed]
35. Mahajan, S.K.; Bowersox, E.M.; Rye, D.L.; Abu-Hamdan, D.K.; Prasad, A.S.; McDonald, F.D.; Biersack, K.L. Factors underlying abnormal zinc metabolism in uremia. *Kidney Int. Suppl.* **1989**, *27*, S269–S273. [PubMed]
36. Wang, L.J.; Wang, M.Q.; Hu, R.; Hu, R.; Yang, Y.; Huang, Y.S.; Xian, S.X.; Lu, L. Effect of Zinc Supplementation on Maintenance Hemodialysis Patients: A Systematic Review and Meta-Analysis of 15 Randomized Controlled Trials. *Biomed. Res. Int.* **2017**, *2017*, 1024769. [CrossRef] [PubMed]
37. Takehara, S.; Hirani, V.; Wright, F.A.C.; Naganathan, V.; Blyth, F.M.; Le Couteur, D.G.; Waite, L.M.; Seibel, M.J.; Handelsman, D.J.; Cumming, R.G. Appetite, oral health and weight loss in community-dwelling older men: An observational study from the Concord Health and Ageing in Men Project (CHAMP). *BMC Geriatr.* **2021**, *16*, 255. [CrossRef] [PubMed]
38. Bossola, M.; Tazza, L. Postdialysis fatigue: A frequent and debilitating symptom. *Semin. Dial.* **2016**, *29*, 222–227. [CrossRef] [PubMed]
39. Gordon, P.L.; Doyle, J.W.; Johansen, K.L. Postdialysis fatigue is associated with sedentary behavior. *Clin. Nephrol.* **2011**, *75*, 426–433. [PubMed]
40. Artom, M.; Moss-Morris, R.; Caskey, F.; Chilcot, J. Fatigue in advanced kidney disease. *Kidney Int.* **2014**, *86*, 497–505. [CrossRef] [PubMed]
41. Jhamb, M.; Weisbord, S.D.; Steel, J.L.; Unruh, M. Fatigue in patients receiving maintenance dialysis: A review of definitions, measures, and contributing factors. *Am. J. Kidney Dis.* **2008**, *52*, 353–365. [CrossRef] [PubMed]
42. Lindsay, R.M.; Heidenheim, P.A.; Nesrallah, G.; Garg, A.X.; Suri, R. Minutes to recovery after a hemodialysis session: A simple health-related quality of life question that is reliable, valid, and sensitive to change. *Clin. J. Am. Soc. Nephrol.* **2006**, *1*, 952–959. [CrossRef]
43. Kodama, H.; Togari, T.; Konno, Y.; Tsuji, A.; Fujinoki, A.; Kuwabara, S.; Inoue, T. A new assessment scale for post-dialysis fatigue in hemodialysis patients. *Renal Replacement Therapy* **2020**, *6*, 1. [CrossRef]
44. Cox, N.J.; Howson, F.; Ibrahim, K.; Morrison, L.; Sayer, A.A.; Roberts, H.C.; Robinson, S.M. Mood and physical activity are associated with appetite in hospitalised older men and women. *Age Ageing* **2022**, *51*, afac297. [CrossRef] [PubMed]
45. Li, C.; Chen, L.; He, L.; Zhang, Y.; Chen, H.; Liu, Y.; Tang, S.; Zheng, H. Study on the relationship between sarcopenia and its components and anorexia in elderly maintenance haemodialysis patients. *Nurs. Open* **2022**, *9*, 1096–1104. [CrossRef] [PubMed]
46. Sahathevan, S.; Khor, B.H.; Ng, H.M.; Gafor, A.H.A.; Mat Daud, Z.A.; Mafra, D.; Karupaiah, T. Understanding development of malnutrition in hemodialysis patients: A narrative review. *Nutrients* **2020**, *12*, 3147. [CrossRef] [PubMed]
47. Yoshimura, Y.; Shimazu, S.; Shiraishi, A.; Nagano, F.; Tominaga, S.; Hamada, T.; Kudo, M.; Yamasaki, Y.; Noda, S.; Bise, T. Ghrelin activetion by ingestion of medium-chain triglycerides in healthy adults: A pilot trial. *J. Aging Res. Clin. Pract.* **2018**, *7*, 42–46.
48. Hiroshige, K.; Sonta, T.; Suda, T.; Kanegae, K.; Ohtani, A. Oral supplementation of branched-chain amino acid improves nutritional status in elderly patients on chronic haemodialysis. *Nephrol. Dial. Transplant.* **2001**, *16*, 1856–1862. [CrossRef] [PubMed]
49. Boudville, N.; Rangan, A.; Moody, H. Oral nutritional supplementation increases caloric and protein intake in peritoneal dialysis patients. *Am. J. Kidney Dis.* **2003**, *41*, 658–663. [CrossRef] [PubMed]
50. Weiner, D.E.; Tighiouart, H.; Ladik, V.; Meyer, K.B.; Zager, P.G.; Johnson, D.S. Oral intradialytic nutritional supplement use and mortality in hemodialysis patients. *Am. J. Kidney Dis.* **2014**, *63*, 276–285. [CrossRef] [PubMed]
51. Leonberg-Yoo, A.K.; Wang, W.; Weiner, D.E.; Lacson, E., Jr. Oral nutritional supplements and 30-day readmission rate in hypoalbuminemic maintenance hemodialysis patients. *Hemodial. Int.* **2019**, *23*, 93–100. [CrossRef]
52. Ikizler, T.A.; Pupim, L.B.; Brouillette, J.R.; Levenhagen, D.K.; Farmer, K.; Hakim, R.M.; Flakoll, P.J. Hemodialysis stimulates muscle and whole body protein loss and alters substrate oxidation. *Am. J. Physiol. Endocrinol. Metab.* **2002**, *282*, E107–E116. [CrossRef]
53. Pace, R.C.; Kirk, J. Academy of Nutrition and Dietetics and National Kidney Foundation: Revised 2020 Standards of Practice and Standards of Professional Performance for Registered Dietitian Nutritionists (Competent, Proficient, and Expert) in Nephrology Nutrition. *J. Ren. Nutr.* **2021**, *31*, 100–115.e41. [CrossRef]
54. Nakanishi, T.; Kogirima, M.; Hayashi, F.; Kitajima, Y. Standards of professional practice and the qualities or abilities required for registered dietitians: Findings from a surgery of practicing registered dietitians. *Jpn. J. Nutr. Diet.* **2019**, *77*, 44–56. [CrossRef]

55. Tentori, F.; Elder, S.J.; Thumma, J.; Pisoni, R.L.; Bommer, J.; Fissell, R.B.; Fukuhara, S.; Jadoul, M.; Keen, M.L.; Saran, R.; et al. Physical exercise among participants in the Dialysis Outcomes and Practice Patterns Study (DOPPS): Correlates and associated outcomes. *Nephrol. Dial. Transplant.* **2010**, *25*, 3050–3062. [CrossRef]
56. Krebs, P.; Norcross, J.C.; Nicholson, J.M.; Prochaska, J.O. Stages of change and psychotherapy outcomes: A review and meta-analysis. *J. Clin. Psychol.* **2018**, *74*, 1964–1979. [CrossRef]

Disclaimer/Publisher's Note: The statements, opinions and data contained in all publications are solely those of the individual author(s) and contributor(s) and not of MDPI and/or the editor(s). MDPI and/or the editor(s) disclaim responsibility for any injury to people or property resulting from any ideas, methods, instructions or products referred to in the content.

MDPI
St. Alban-Anlage 66
4052 Basel
Switzerland
www.mdpi.com

Kidney and Dialysis Editorial Office
E-mail: kidneydial@mdpi.com
www.mdpi.com/journal/kidneydial

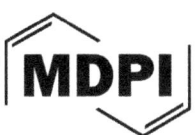

Disclaimer/Publisher's Note: The statements, opinions and data contained in all publications are solely those of the individual author(s) and contributor(s) and not of MDPI and/or the editor(s). MDPI and/or the editor(s) disclaim responsibility for any injury to people or property resulting from any ideas, methods, instructions or products referred to in the content.

www.ingramcontent.com/pod-product-compliance
Lightning Source LLC
LaVergne TN
LVHW070605100526
838202LV00012B/570